Pediatric Robotic Surgery

Girolamo Mattioli • Paolo Petralia
Editors

Pediatric Robotic Surgery

Technical and Management Aspects

Springer

Editors
Girolamo Mattioli
School of Pediatric Surgery, DINOGMI
Istituto Giannina Gaslini
Genova
Italy

Paolo Petralia
Istituto Giannina Gaslini
Genova
Italy

ISBN 978-3-319-41862-9 ISBN 978-3-319-41863-6 (eBook)
DOI 10.1007/978-3-319-41863-6

Library of Congress Control Number: 2017951241

Printed on acid-free paper

This Springer imprint is published by Springer Nature
The registered company is Springer International Publishing AG
The registered company address is: Gewerbestrasse 11, 6330 Cham, Switzerland

Foreword

Pediatric robotic surgery is developed over the years especially in pediatric urology, but recently this technology is applied for other pediatric diseases. For the first time a book on pediatric robotic surgery is presented, covering all the fields of pediatric surgical pathology (thoracic, abdominal, oncology, gynecological, and urinary). All the principal international pioneers of pediatric robotic surgery are involved, providing current indications to robotic surgery; technical notes are illustrated to show patient position, robotic assessment, and the optimal use of robotic instruments. Managerial aspects are provided to give suggestions to start robotic surgical approach in each pediatric department. This book is addressed to the hospital general managers, medical directors, pediatric surgeons, and pediatric urologist.

Genoa, Italy Luca Pio

Preface

The field of pediatric minimally invasive surgery has undergone remarkable changes in the last few years.

The growing technology offered more and more miniaturized and precise instruments up to the creation of a robotic system able to support the surgeon in more and more complex surgical procedures.

Despite this the current robotic systems are still not able to replace the surgeon who maintains a key role in the performance of surgical procedure and that above all has to decide the surgical indications, the operative setting, and know how to manage surgical complications.

This book is intended to provide all the instruments to start a pediatric robotic surgical program in a pediatric surgical unit. Managerial insights were provided in order to face up to the high purchase and maintenance cost of a robotic system.

All the fields of pediatric general surgery and urology are covered including the most recently reported techniques.

The authors were selected from Europe and the United States and each chapter was written by an authority in that field.

The overall objective of this book is to improve the offer of the minimally invasive approach to those children that actually received open surgical procedures due to the limitations of the traditional laparoscopy/thoracoscopy.

Genoa, Italy — Girolamo Mattioli and Paolo Petralia

Acknowledgments

The editors gratefully acknowledge the contributing authors for their work and for sharing their wisdom for the preparation of their individual chapters.

We thank Dr. Luca Pio for his work on book conception and authors coordination.

We express our thanks to Madona Samuel, project coordinator at Springer Nature, the executive editor Donatella Rizza, and the editor Elisa Geranio who provided professional support, without whom this book would never have reached print.

Contents

Part 1

Strategy Planning, Training and Preoperative Setup

From Laparoscopy to Robotic Surgery: Sense and Nonsense

1

Girolamo Mattioli and Paolo Petralia

The very first study relating to the use of robotic surgery in pediatrics was released in 2001 by Meininger with a case report about the execution of a Nissen fundoplication on a 10-year-old female, in which they analyzed the standard intraoperative monitoring parameters and some other more specific parameters such as the invasive pressure monitoring throughout the entire procedure; the results showed that the robotic procedure didn't cause instability nor difficulties in the anesthesiological management [1].

Starting from these earliest promising results several other publications about robotic surgery in pediatrics were released: in 2002 Hollands published a case report on the comparison among four different procedures (entero-enteric ostomy, hepaticojejunostomy, portal-enteric ostomy, esophagus-esophageal ostomy) performed both with laparoscopic and robotic approach, using the Zeus system (Zeus Robotic Surgical System—Computer Motion, Inc., Goleta, CA, USA), on animal models; despite the initial difficulties (mostly technical difficulties due to the robotic tool management) the results highlighted the potentialities of the robot and the possibility of expanding minimally invasive surgery through different fields [2].

In a 2002 retrospective study by Gutt, a series of personal 14 robot-assisted (using DaVinci robot) procedures (11 fundoplications, 2 cholecystectomies, and 1 salpingo-oophorectomy) were analyzed, focusing on the positive aspects such as the absence of intra- and postoperative complications, 3D vision of the operative field, larger degrees of the instruments, better ergonomics felt by the surgeon, as well as negative ones, such as high costs and long-lasting docking time [3].

In 2007 Najmaldin analyzed through a prospective study the data related to 50 different robot-assisted procedures performed on 40 patients, with 3 conversions to open surgery (one of them related to instrumental problems), and with 2 postoperative complications not directly correlated to the robotic technique. Also this study highlights the great potentiality of the use of robotic surgery in pediatrics and the need of deeper studies to define its limits [4].

Meehan retrospectively analyzed a wide series of 100 robot-assisted procedures performed by 2 surgeons and including 24 different procedures (89 abdominal and 11 thoracic) and they defined a rate of conversion to open surgery of 12% and a rate of conversion to minimally invasive surgery of 1% (diaphragmatic hernia repair converted to thoracoscopy). Their study proves that the learning curve for robotic surgery is shorter

G. Mattioli (✉)
Pediatric Surgery Unit, Istituto Giannina Gaslini, Genoa, Italy

DINOGMI, University of Genoa, Genoa, Italy
e-mail: girolamomattioli@gaslini.org

P. Petralia
General Director, Istituto Giannina Gaslini, Genoa, Italy

G. Mattioli, P. Petralia (eds.), *Pediatric Robotic Surgery*, DOI 10.1007/978-3-319-41863-6_1

(an average of 15 cases vs. 25–50), and underlines the importance of a specialized nursing team, of an accurate selection of the cases (minimum patient weight 2.5 kg) in relation to the available tools, and of the space organization inside the operating room [5].

Another wide retrospective study counting 144 different procedures, and mostly fundoplications (39), cholecystectomies (34), gastric bandings (15), and splenectomies (13), was published by Alqahtani et al. [6], who pointed out the advantages robotics has in pediatrics as well as in adult patients, and especially when the tightness of the operative field makes it hard to proceed through the dissection and reconstruction phases; they also highlighted the importance and need to make randomized studies in order to validate the benefits and the potential development of even more specific tools for the pediatric use (which point of view limits the use of the robot on younger patients here and now) [6].

There are also two further retrospective studies, respectively, published by Camps and de Lambert, which proved that robotic surgery can be applied in pediatrics, guaranteeing a safety level as high as in laparoscopy, and even extended its use in some procedures which turn out to be technically difficult when using a laparoscopic approach. This last point of view is an important cause for reflection especially in relation to the high costs of robotic surgery compared to laparoscopy [7, 8].

The comparison between laparoscopic, robotic, and open surgery was widely analyzed by Sinha, who conducted a literature review and took into consideration 31 studies (4 case-control, 1 perspective, and other case series and case report) for a total of 566 patients: what emerges from their analysis is that the most performed procedures in pediatrics are pyeloplasty (141 cases) and fundoplication (122 cases) and that robot-assisted surgery faces a lower complications ratio and the same number of conversions when compared to laparoscopic surgery. They also debate the economic matter as a cause for reflection for the spread of this technology on a large scale, and the limitation of its use in younger patients, such as newborns, due to the unsuitableness of the instrumentation which exists so far [9].

Another review by Van Haasteren evaluated 13 studies (8 case series and 5 comparative studies concerning robotic vs. open or robotic vs. laparoscopic surgery). This review stated that robotic surgery doesn't guarantee a better outcome compared to open surgery or conventional minimally invasive surgery, but it does have advantages in situations in which the accessibility to the operative field using an open or a laparoscopic approach would be very hard and it permits to perform dissections, resections, and reconstructions in complex anatomic structures in a certainly easier way comparing to the other two surgical techniques [10].

Another wide review published in 2013 by Cundy analyzed data from 137 studies including gastrointestinal, genitourinary, and thoracic robot-assisted surgical procedures for a total of 1840 patients and 2393 procedures [11]. They noticed that the most performed procedures in pediatrics are, again, pyeloplasty (672) and fundoplication (424) and that in the last few years there was a progressive growth of the number of urological cases compared to the earlier years, thus reflecting the high potential of this technology.

One of the most important application fields of robotic surgery in pediatrics is without a doubt urology, relating to both number of scientific studies and number of procedures. One of the most significant studies in this area of interest is the recent publication by Chung, who wrote a meta-analysis on robotic and open surgery of the obstruction of the pyelo-ureteral junction, analyzing data from seven different comparative studies (robotic vs. open) and three other studies based on national databases, for a total of 20,691 patients (robotic:open = 1956:18,735). The authors examined different aspects such as operative time, which turned out to be longer by 64.26 min (95% CI 37.58–90.93; $p < 0.00001$) with the robotic approach, blood losses which turned out to be smaller with the robotic approach, and a minor postoperative analgesic need in patients who had robotic surgery [12]. For what concerns conversions no robotic procedure had to be converted to open surgery and only one of the studies reported three cases of conversion (two of them finished with a laparoscopic approach and one of them finished with the robot after solving the mechanical problem). For what concerns the hospital stay length, it was shorter for patients within the robotic group by 0.95 days (95% CI 0.38–1.52; $p = 0.001$); relating to the economic comparison the robotic group turned out to be more expensive compared to the open group by 3.26 thousand USD (95% CI 1.79–4.73 thousand USD; $p < 0.00001$). By analyzing the success rate there are no statistically significant differences between the two groups (RR: 0.99, 95 CI 0.94–1.05), and for what concerns complications the robotic group has a higher ratio with a significant statistic (RR = 1.29, 95 CI 1.05–1.58, $p = 0.001$).

In conclusion, in the light of the analyzed data, the authors affirm that the robotic approach to the obstruction of the pyelo-ureteral junction isn't advantageous compared to the traditional open approach, although they don't exclude the possibility that the robotic approach will be reevaluated and become advantageous in the future, thanks to a wider availability of a purely pediatric instrumentation and a reduction of the instrument management costs [12].

Besides the treatment of obstruction of the pyelo-ureteral junction, pediatric robotic surgery could gain a great application field in bladder reconstruction surgery (appendicovesicostomy, bladder augmentation, and ureteral reimplantations).

Among other publications, Casale analyzed the employment of robot-assisted surgery in ureteral reimplant with a transtrigonal approach on a total of 41 patients with a mean age of 38 months (16–81), and they proved that it's possible to preserve the pelvic plexus and thus preserve the patient's continence, even if spending a significant amount of operative time. In the light of this aspect and taking into consideration the high percentage of success (97.6% in 40 patients out of 41) in terms of vescicoureteral reflux resolution, the authors agree that the operation is useful [13].

In a further retrospective case-control study Marchini compared robotic assisted ureteral reimplant (39 patients for a total of 19 intravescical and 20 extravescical approaches) and open ureteral reimplant (39 patients for a total of 22 intravescical and 17 extravescical approaches) and obtained a similar success rate between the two open and robotic surgery groups but a shorter hospital stay length and a lower need of postoperative analgesia in the robotic intravescical group compared to the equivalent open surgery group. The authors stressed the need of new studies, and especially long-term studies, in order to define costs and benefits of robot-assisted surgery, as expressed concerning the other robotic procedures [14].

Kasturi analyzed in a prospective way long-term outcomes (2-year follow-up) of robot-assisted nerve sparing for bilateral ureteral reimplantation. They took into consideration 150 patients, all of them suffering from higher than third-grade vescicoureteral reflux, and they observed a resolution of VUR in 97.3% of cases at third postoperative month CUM and a mean residual urine volume corresponding to 3.2% of mean bladder capacity (range 0–11%). All patients had urodynamic test before CUM, and the results were a mean flux of 14.6 mL/s (range 8.9–28.6) and a mean residual urine volume of 3.8% (range 0–13%) (same results as preoperative ones). Those data aren't significantly different from those obtained with robotic surgery, but it's proved again that with a robotic approach a more detailed view of the pelvic plexus and the involved anatomic structures is possible, thus guaranteeing a better preservation of them [15].

Gargollo published a retrospective study about 38 robotic assisted Leadbetter/Mitchell procedures with vesical neck sling and Mitrofanoff appendicovesicostomy, in which he gained good results and a percentage of 82% (31 out of 38) of "dry" patients through CIC every 3 h. Four of the seven "not-dry" patients weren't compliant to CIC; one of them wasn't dry from uretra and Monti channel; two patients developed a reduction of bladder compliance which wasn't responsive to medical therapy or Botox injection, thus heading for ileocystoplasty. Mean operative time was 5.6 hours (3.6–12.25) with longer time in the earlier 10 operations compared to the last 28 with evidence of statistically significant difference

(p = 0.0001). In the light of these results the author recommends this technique even if stressing that its usefulness is strictly linked to a wide surgery experience in robot-assisted pyeloplasty and ureteral reimplantation [16].

Another major application field for robotic surgery is fundoplication. Among many important studies we want to mention Cundy meta-analysis, in which the authors compared the robotic approach to laparoscopy in the making of fundoplications. They involved six studies (four cohort and two case-control studies, one of them a prospective study and the others retrospective observational studies) for a total of 135 robot-assisted and 162 laparoscopic procedures and they found out that conversion rate is 3.0% (4/135) for the robotic group and 6.2% (10/162) for the laparoscopic group, which means a 51% lower rate for the robotic group comparing to the laparoscopic one, but not statistically significant (OR = 0.49; 95%; CI 0.14–1.72; $p = 0.27$). By analyzing operative time, there is no significant difference in length of robotic group. For what concerns hospital stay length there are no significant differences between the groups. Complication rate is 12/135 (8.9%) for the robotic group and 13/162 (8.0%) for the laparoscopy group and it isn't significant either. A cost analysis highlights the fact that even eliminating robotic instrumentation maintenance costs the robotic group appears to be still more expensive (€9584 vs. €8982). Within the population of the meta-analysis they noticed only three relapses (two in those who had laparoscopy and one in those who had robotic surgery) and a similar success rate in follow-up. The authors who collected these data define the two different procedures as similar, so we can't say that robotic surgery has great advantages here, but they highlight that other long-term follow-up studies are needed in order to better define the efficacy of a robotic approach, which can be used today only for specifically selected cases such as redo surgery or tough anatomic situations that couldn't be approached via laparoscopy. Moreover they stress that cost-effectiveness analysis must be periodically reassessed since robotic surgery costs are destined to change when other competitors enter the market, thus lowering the indirect fixed costs which now strongly weight on the economic analysis of robotic surgery [17].

In 2007 Meehan published a retrospective study about the first 50 robot-assisted fundoplications. Seventy percentage of the 50 patients suffered from some neurological disease. The data analysis doesn't stress the results as much in terms of operative time (docking, total operative time) nor hospital stay length or complications and relapses, but rather in terms of fast learning curve, such as they saw a decreasing of docking time and operative time already at fifth case, which proves a great improvement of all the robotic team (doctors and nurses); moreover, they assert that from that fifth operation on the one operating at the console was the resident, who was proved to have rapidly improved his abilities when comparing operative times at the end of the series. This confirms the thesis that, compared to laparoscopy, the learning curve is significantly faster.

The authors specify that all the robotic involved team improved with a fast learning curve [18].

Another work was published by Cundy about robotic learning curve, through the analysis of the different phases of a robot-assisted operation (docking, console, and total) in a progressive way and highlighting the faster peak compared to laparoscopy, the following plateau phase and the final new peak, which is however decreasing compared to the shortening of operative time. This kind of evolution traces a Gaussian function, which parts represent learning phases: the rapid ascending part corresponds with the learning phase, the plateau corresponds with the learning strengthening, and the descending part corresponds with the sharpening and perfectioning of the abilities. The authors stress that the improvement and learning of the whole involved robotic team determine the rapidity of the ascending part of the curve, and especially the subanalysis of docking phase showed that the plateau is reached at 12th operation [19].

In a prospective study Granéli decided to take GERD evaluation indices and the need for antiacid secretory agents and antiasthmatics as outcome parameters of fundoplications. They analyzed 40 patients and saw that there was a widely reduced need for antiacid secretory agents and antiasthmatics comparing to preoperative need, respectively, from 100% to 20% ($p < 0.001$) and from 55% to 30% ($p < 0.04$), and also a reduction of the acid exposition in 24 h from a mean 11% to 1% ($p < 0.001$) and a DeMeester score from 40 to 5 ($p < 0.001$) [20].

Other procedures have been done with robotic surgery such as the treatment of choledochal cyst, which was described by Kim in his retrospective study about a comparison between robot-assisted and open surgery: he took into consideration a series of 79 cases, and 39 of them had a robotic approach, and he affirmed that this kind of approach doesn't lead to significant outcome differences comparing to traditional open surgery (in terms of hospital stay length, complications, analgesic need, alimentation time, operative time) and it can be an efficient surgical option which needs to be supported by further studies and by the development of a more and more specific instrumentation devoted to this certain type of population [21].

Pediatric robot-assisted surgery found an application field in thoracic surgery but there are few studies with a wide series of cases.

Ballouhey analyzed their first experience (2018–2013) with robot-assisted thoracic surgery. It included 11 cases (3 esophageal third-type atresias, 4 mediastinal cysts, 2 diaphragmatic hernias, 1 gastric tubulization with transposition, 1 Heller myotomy); three of the patients were newborn. Three procedures were converted into open thoracic surgery because of a reduction of the internal space (two esophageal atresias and one diaphragmatic hernia); there were no periprocedural complications. Mean hospital stay length was 13.5 days and 6.2 days if newborn excluded. Mean operative time was 190 min (120–310). There were two postoperative complications, one conservatively treated T-E fistula recurrence and the other after bronchogenic cyst removal dysphagia which spontaneously resolved within a month. Authors confirm that thoracic robot-assisted surgery can bring benefits especially on children weighing more than 20 kg, based on their analysis. This is due to instrumental unsuitability for smaller patients, especially in mediastinal cyst treatment. This is what Meehan affirms in his 2008 clinical records on mediastinal cyst treatment [22], in which there were no complications nor conversions and he emphasized the usefulness of robot approach in dissecting solid masses inside thoracic cage [23].

In conclusion the sense of introduction of robotic surgery in children is the extension of minimally invasive surgery to some procedures that were widely performed in traditional open surgery and to perform redo procedure that will be extremely difficult with conventional lapar\ thoracoscopic surgery.

References

1. Meininger DD, Byhahn C, Heller K, Gutt CN, Westphal K. Totally endoscopic Nissen fundoplication with a robotic system in a child. Surg Endosc. 2001;15(11):1360.
2. Hollands CM, Dixey LN. Applications of robotic surgery in pediatric patients. Surg Laparosc Endosc Percutan Tech. 2002;12(1):71–6.
3. Gutt CN, Markus B, Kim ZG, Meininger D, Brinkmann L, Heller K. Early experiences of robotic surgery in children. Surg Endosc. 2002;16(7):1083–6.
4. Najmaldin A, Antao B. Early experience of tele-robotic surgery in children. Int J Med Robot. 2007;3(3): 199–202.
5. Meehan JJ, Sandler A. Pediatric robotic surgery: a single-institutional review of the first 100 consecutive cases. Surg Endosc. 2008;22(1):177–82.
6. Alqahtani A, Albassam A, Zamakhshary M, Shoukri M, Altokhais T, Aljazairi A, Alzahim A, Mallik M, Alshehri A. Robot-assisted pediatric surgery: how far can we go? World J Surg. 2010;34(5):975–8. doi:10.1007/s00268-010-0431-6.
7. Camps JI. The use of robotics in pediatric surgery: my initial experience. Pediatr Surg Int. 2011;27(9):991–6. doi:10.1007/s00383-011-2901-9.
8. de Lambert G, Fourcade L, Centi J, Fredon F, Braik K, Szwarc C, Longis B, Lardy H. How to successfully implement a robotic pediatric surgery program: lessons learned after 96 procedures. Surg Endosc. 2013;27(6):2137–44.
9. Sinha CK, Haddad M. Robot-assisted surgery in children: current status. J Robot Surg. 2008;1(4):243–6.
10. van Haasteren G, Levine S, Hayes W. Pediatric robotic surgery: early assessment. Pediatrics. 2009;124(6): 1642–9.
11. Cundy TP, Shetty K, Clark J, Chang TP, Sriskandarajah K, Gattas NE, Najmaldin A, Yang GZ, Darzi A. The first decade of robotic surgery in children. J Pediatr Surg. 2013;48(4):858–65.

12. Chang SJ, Hsu CK, Hsieh CH, Yang SS. Comparing the efficacy and safety between robotic-assisted versus open pyeloplasty in children: a systemic review and meta-analysis. World J Urol. 2015;33(11): 1855–65.
13. Casale P, Patel RP, Kolon TF. Nerve sparing robotic extravesical ureteral reimplantation. J Urol. 2008; 179(5):1987–9. discussion 1990
14. Marchini GS, Hong YK, Minnillo BJ, Diamond DA, Houck CS, Meier PM, Passerotti CC, Kaplan JR, Retik AB, Nguyen HT. Robotic assisted laparoscopic ureteral reimplantation in children: case matched comparative study with open surgical approach. J Urol. 2011;185(5):1870–5.
15. Kasturi S, Sehgal SS, Christman MS, Lambert SM, Casale P. Prospective long-term analysis of nerve-sparing extravesical robotic-assisted laparoscopic ureteral reimplantation. Urology. 2012;79(3): 680–3.
16. Gargollo PC. Robotic-assisted bladder neck repair: feasibility and outcomes. Urol Clin North Am. 2015; 42(1):111–20.
17. Cundy TP, Harling L, Marcus HJ, Athanasiou T, Darzi AW. Meta analysis of robot-assisted versus conventional laparoscopic fundoplication in children. J Pediatr Surg. 2014;49(4):646–52.
18. Meehan JJ, Meehan TD, Sandler A. Robotic fundoplication in children: resident teaching and a single institutional review of our first 50 patients. J Pediatr Surg. 2007;42(12):2022–5.
19. Cundy TP, Rowland SP, Gattas NE, White AD, Najmaldin AS. The learning curve of robot-assisted laparoscopic fundoplication in children: a prospective evaluation and CUSUM analysis. Int J Med Robot. 2015;11(2):141–9.
20. Granéli C, Kockum CC, Arnbjornsson E, Anderberg M. Outcome after computer-assisted (robotic) Nissen fundoplication in children measured as pre- and postoperative acid reducing and asthma medications use. Eur J Pediatr Surg. 2014;25(6):532–6.
21. Kim NY, Chang EY, Hong YJ, Park S, Kim HY, Bai SJ, Han SJ. Retrospective assessment of the validity of robotic surgery in comparison to open surgery for pediatric choledochal cyst. Yonsei Med J. 2015;56(3):737–43.
22. Ballouhey Q, Villemagne T, Cros J, Vacquerie V, Bérenguer D, Braik K, Szwarc C, Longis B, Lardy H, Fourcade L. Assessment of paediatric thoracic robotic surgery. Interact Cardiovasc Thorac Surg. 2015;20(3):300–3.
23. Meehan JJ, Sandler AD. Robotic resection of mediastinal masses in children. J Laparoendosc Adv Surg Tech A. 2008;18(1):114–9.

2 Management Aspects, Cost Analysis and Training

Paolo Petralia, Nicolò Maria Buffi, Pasquale Cardone, Ubaldo Rosati, Paola Barabino, Luca Pio, and Girolamo Mattioli

The DaVinci robot is a technological system which allows the surgeon to "easily" perform advanced surgery with a minimally invasive approach [1]. However, there aren't strong evidences but only expert opinions and feasibility studies as far as paediatrics is concerned [2–7].

Besides confirming the advantages brought by robotic surgery in the execution of some procedures, this review introduces the theme of the four stages, defined by Balliol Collaboration [8, 9] which follow one another in the evolution of a technological innovation, thus presenting the concept of IDEAL [10, 11]:

- Innovation
- Development
- Early dispersion and exploration
- Assessment
- Long-term implementation and monitoring

Today the studies about robotic paediatric surgery are at stage 2b, and the aim to go over this phase and enter stage 3 (assessment) reflects the need to promote controlled perspective trials, to analyse the aspect of the patient benefits and the cost-effectiveness of this new surgical technique [12].

Therefore, a cost-effectiveness study still has to be done, particularly in paediatrics, and that makes it impossible to realise an HTA standards study.

The tools for the economic analysis are well known:

- Cost-effectiveness [13] cost utility [14]—CEA/CUA—individual profit
- Budget impact analysis [15]—BIA—sustainability for the national health service, equity
- Break-even point—BEP [16]—activity volumes, organisational business aspects

Based on the international literature and the current clinical research state, there is a clear evidence of feasibility and studies prove the relevance of this kind of approach; however this awareness isn't expressible because of the high cost of the technology.

P. Petralia, M.D. (✉)
General Direction, Istituto Giannina Gaslini, Genoa, Italy
e-mail: paolopetralia@gaslini.org

N.M. Buffi • P. Cardone
Department of Urology, Humanitas Clinical and Research Centre, Milan, Rozzano, Italy

U. Rosati
Quality Control Unit, Istituto Giannina Gaslini, Genoa, Italy

P. Barabino
Pharmacy Unit, Istituto Giannina Gaslini, Genoa, Italy

L. Pio • G. Mattioli
Pediatric Surgery Unit, Istituto Giannina Gaslini, Genoa, Italy

DINOGMI, University of Genoa, Genoa, Italy

G. Mattioli, P. Petralia (eds.), *Pediatric Robotic Surgery*, DOI 10.1007/978-3-319-41863-6_2

Nevertheless, it's not easy to build the economic bases on scientific evidences when talking about paediatrics, which isn't statistically significant yet, since the only experience concerns adults and should be shifted to significantly lower numbers.

The ethical point of view is just as relevant: if robotic surgery guarantees a better functional outcome compared to open surgery, and if robotic surgery makes advanced minimally invasive surgery easy, then it's morally mandatory to treat paediatric patients according to their health-care "specificity" and with the best available technologies, just like adult patients.

Another perspective is represented by centralisation. A first working model can be represented by paediatrics chronic inflammatory bowel diseases monitored by SIGENP [17]. Pelvic surgery (prostate) must be performed in robotic surgery because it guarantees the best functional result. And rectal surgery has the same benefits. Therefore the hypothesis is that every child with ulcerative colitis heading to surgery should have surgery in a robotic centre. And moreover, they have to be guaranteed a paediatric specificity. The problem is that there isn't a sufficient number of cases to offer an economically sustainable result. This leads to the necessity to centralise in order to increase the expertise and thus reduce the adverse events. There are lots of examples also concerning neonatal malformations, but feasibility studies still have to be done in this field.

Feasibility of robotic surgery is undeniable. In adult males, for example, there is evidence of a better post-prostatectomy erectile function compared to open surgery [18–20].

Today there is no evidence in paediatrics, but only expert opinions. However this experience leads us to pursue the same clinical results for children, too.

Also surgical team takes advantage of robotic support: learning curve, technical perfection, physical exertion and its potential damage support robotic surgery compared to laparoscopic and open surgery.

Further research is needed in order to evaluate strength and weakness of the economic sustainability. Many issues are positive and, whatever the final result is, we must purse this project to clarify its potentiality and find scientific evidences. This is the specific (and social) task of IRCCS to guarantee a paediatric specificity.

It seems like there are good starting points: teams of experts and a centre giving great importance to paediatric care quality, ethics and paediatric specificity (children must be treated by experts in a specific paediatric hospital).

Hence, paediatric surgery should use the DaVinci robot in routine minimally invasive surgery as well as in discovering new techniques where to adopt advanced minimally invasive surgery.

2.1 Cost Analysis

There are many studies about economical aspects in robotic surgery applied to adults but there is a lack of them in paediatrics. Among many studies, the one published by Mahida JB is relevant. He made a complete economical analysis of paediatric robotic surgery compared to laparoscopic and open approaches collecting data from 47 national third-level health centres (USA) [21].

His detailed analysis (including a health technology assessment) demonstrated that robotic approach is more expensive than laparoscopic and open surgery, both in general surgery and in urology, even if he observed a shortening of hospital stay length in urology. Especially hospitalisation costs are higher in robotics [21].

All recent studies are in agreement that this innovative technology is at very high costs but further evaluations are needed [21–26]. Scenario will change when new instrumentations are available, and new companies and products enter the market lowering the prices, making that technology more available and increasing the application fields and user constituency, thus making economic return easier.

Economic sustainability is the main aspect to take into consideration when evaluating health technology assessment (HTA). HTA is a multidimensional and multidisciplinary approach to analyse medical-clinic, social, management, economic, ethic and legal implications of a new technology, through the evaluation of efficacy, safety, costs, social and organisational effect [27–29]. HTA analyses real and potential effects of the technology, both before the beginning and during its entire life cycle, along with the consequences that introducing or excluding it will bring to the health system, economy and society.

The evaluation of health-care, economic, social and ethic consequences determined by new technologies' introduction must be based on strict method: pertinence and sustainability of treatments. In other words it is mandatory to consider the effects of a new technology on health, and availability and allocation of sources and other aspects describing the health system performance, such as equity and capability to respond properly to population needs.

This kind of study isn't proper of medical approach, since it's not sufficient to demonstrate a new technology efficacy. The amount of applied sources must be considered as well. Since sources are limited, using them for a new technology necessarily means to renounce other alternative uses.

Parameters to evaluate are technological characteristics, safety, efficacy in clinical practice, ethical impact, social impact and economical aspects. Therefore before investing we must consider how much value this technology makes and in advantage of whom.

Break-even point (BEP) [16] calculated for paediatric robotic surgery needs more than 500 cases/year.

The purpose of budget impact analysis [30] is to calculate financial consequences of adopting a new health-care intervention in a specific context with source restrictions. To know the value for money of a new treatment it's not enough but we need to now its impact in absolute terms on budget, and there are no complete studies on robotic surgery.

There are situations where a technology is cost effective but BIA results say that it isn't sustainable or it can be granted only to few (equity).

Concerning cost evaluation discussion:

- Health direct costs: treatment and health-care sources
- Non-health direct costs: non-health sources used by enti assistenziali non sanitari, patients and families
- Indirect costs: sources not produced because of disease both by patients and relatives
- Intangible costs: psychological and physical pain consequences

Literature agrees and recognises that the only real difference in terms of costs is between laparoscopic and open surgery: hospital stay length is short and so is operative time.

There are no further savings between laparoscopy and robot-assisted surgery but there is a wide difference in costs. Fixed costs are critically higher which means that in order to respect the break-even point several operations are needed.

The key question is how to increase clinical records:

1. Network among different paetiatric hospitals—centralisation in specific paediatric hospitals for rare diseases in order to improve the outcome
2. Increasing out-of-region attraction (higher perceived quality)
3. Switch of 70–80% of open surgery approaches to minimally invasive robotic surgery (way less tiring for surgeons than laparoscopy)

This step would lead very close to the BEP and remarkably decrease costs (hospital stay and operative time), thus partially offsetting fixed robot cost.

Benefits are hardly valuable in terms of money. This aspect should consider different stakeholders [31]:

a. Child and his family
b. Hospital
c. Training system
d. Research system

Benefits for children and his family can be summarised as follows:

- Paediatric environment and paediatric staff (specificity)
- Pain decrease (painless hospital)
- Other savings (movements, drugs, etc.)
- Ethical issues

Moreover there would be potential benefits for the hospital in terms of attractivity increase and out-of-region operations, growth of clinical reports, decrease of open surgery in favour of minimally invasive surgery, higher satisfaction of surgeons and possibility of extending the use of robots to other fields (gynaecology, head and neck surgery).

Benefits involve research and training too: shorter learning curves, training simulators, set-up of prospective trials, ad hoc clinical trial funding and increase of research outcomes. Moreover it's possible to start partnerships aimed at academic research and training (paediatric nurse school and paediatric surgery residency) and interdisciplinary among all surgery branches.

2.2 Training in Paediatric Robotic Surgery

Robotic surgery has emerged as a new technology over the last decade and has brought with it new challenges, particularly in terms of teaching and training. One of the greatest benefits of robot-assisted laparoscopic surgery (RALS) has been the ability to spread the applications of minimally invasive surgery to paediatric surgical patients [32]. While adult surgical procedures are, for the most part, extirpative in nature, children often require reconstructive procedures. In this context, the adoption of laparoscopic paediatric surgery lagged significantly behind the adult population. Moreover despite refinements in laparoscopic instrumentation, including the development of needlescopic 3-mm instruments, paediatric laparoscopic reconstructive surgery is extremely tedious and challenging. The limited working space commonly forces the surgeon to perform surgical procedures using very difficult angles and non-ergonomic positions. The chance of port-site conflicts and instrument collision is significantly greater in children.

RALS provides the surgeon with better three-dimensional vision, seven degrees of freedom truly mimicking the movements made during standard open surgery and motion scaling with tremor cancellation and it is far better ergonomically than standard laparoscopy. Indeed, these advantages make this technology ideal for children with congenital anomalies who often require reconstructive procedures. Moreover, the system can generate extremely delicate movements in a confined working space, such as that found in the paediatric population.

As with the introduction of any new surgical technology, a structured training program has to be developed to ensure better surgical outcomes and patient safety, which must not be compromised during the learning process [33, 34]. A well-organised educational curriculum [35] as well as proficiency-based credentialing processes are required to ensure the safe and efficacious clinical application of new technologies. To my knowledge, due to the heterogeneous indications to paediatric surgery there are no validated training programs for this reason it may benefit from the experience developed in adult robotic surgery [33].

The trainees must understand robotic technology. It is essential to become familiar with the tool, the Da Vinci surgical system, which is currently the only commercially available robotic surgery platform. The trainee has to be educated about the device parameters and functions and, more important, instructed on basic troubleshooting and limitations of the system. The right educational curriculum should begin with practical skill training. To increase the knowledge of robotic technology, highly intensive dry and wet laboratory training should be undertaken. Several simulators are now available to increase robotic skills. The dry lab guarantees good coordination development and allows trainees to start getting in touch with the instruments. In such a context, bimanuality, dissection, and suturing techniques are easily developed. The main disadvantages of this training strategy relate to the lack of bleeding and the fact that surgical procedures often are not reproducible, as they are in the laboratory. The best way to simulate technical procedures is in the wet lab. Few dedicated training centres are available around Europe, but new technology can be developed with animal models. The wet lab provides a good simulator of procedures, allowing surgical skills to be developed and scientific models to be studied. The main disadvantages relate to the high cost of such teaching models, large numbers of animals that need to be sacrificed, and requirements of ethics committees. Moreover, surgical procedures are reproducible but with different anatomic characteristics. Before starting with real-life case observation, high-volume robotic training centres should be identified to guarantee real-life case observation in qualified centres. The tips and tricks of each procedure must be shown during live surgery, and different techniques should be discussed with mentors. Bedside assistance must be considered as the first step to get in touch with real-life procedures. The tips and tricks developed during bedside assisting are very important to gain complete knowledge of the procedure. Moreover, the console surgeon will rely on the future assistants to help solve problems at the bedside. Modular training is the best way to learn how to perform a procedure, reducing performance time and complications. The procedure must be divided into steps, and the trainee should gain experience with each step, according to its predefined difficulty. More recently, the use of a dual console has been successfully introduced in training. The dual console has enabled two surgeons to operate at the same time. It is a perfect tool for interaction in real time and for better control of the procedure. Having an experienced surgeon and a trainee each at an individual console makes this tool the perfect choice for training.

Moreover, we have to consider the nontechnical skill issue. Robotic surgery more than other procedure requires a team work that involves scrub nurses, bedside assistant and console surgeon. Scrub nurse must have a good knowledge of robot system including cable connection, basic troubleshooting and sterilisation of the instruments. The bedside assistant requires a dexterity to recognise conflicts between instruments and malfunction of the system and to communicate with the first operator. The console surgeon represents the leader of a group that must coordinate the team.

We can conclude that the success of an educational curriculum depends on the well-done training made by experts and the developing of a good team work to reach a safety surgery.

References

1. Pugin FL, Bucher PAR, Morel P. History of robotic surgery: from AESOP® and ZEUS® to da vinci®. J Visc Surg. 2011;148(5 Suppl):e3–8.
2. Hollands CM, Dixey LN. Applications of robotic surgery in pediatric patients. Surg Laparosc Endosc Percutan Tech. 2002;12(1):71–6.
3. Gutt CN, Markus B, Kim ZG, et al. Early experiences of robotic surgery in children. Surg Endosc. 2002;16(7):1083–6.
4. Najmaldin A, Antao B. Early experience of tele-robotic surgery in children. Int J Med Robot. 2007;3(3):199–202.
5. Meehan JJ, Sandler A. Pediatric robotic surgery: a single-institutional review of the first 100 consecutive cases. Surg Endosc. 2008;22(1):177–82.
6. Alqahtani A, Albassam A, Zamakhshary M, et al. Robot-assisted pediatric surgery: how far can we go? World J Surg. 2010;34(5):975–8. doi:10.1007/s00268-010-0431-6.
7. Camps JI. The use of robotics in pediatric surgery: my initial experience. Pediatr Surg Int. 2011;27(9):991–6. doi:10.1007/s00383-011-2901-9.
8. Barkun JS, Aronson JK, Feldman LS, et al. Evaluation and stages of surgical innovations. Lancet. 2009;374(9695):1089–96.
9. Ergina PL, Cook JA, Blazeby JM, et al. Challenges in evaluating surgical innovation. Lancet. 2009;374(9695):1097–104.
10. McCulloch P, Altman DG, Campbell WB, et al. No surgical innovation without evaluation: the IDEAL recommendations. Lancet. 2009;374(9695):1105–12.
11. Menon M, Abaza R, Sood A, et al. Robotic kidney transplantation with regional hypothermia: evolution of a novel procedure utilizing the IDEAL guidelines (IDEAL phase 0 and 1). Eur Urol. 2014;65(5):1001–9.
12. Cundy TP, Shetty K, Clark J, et al. The first decade of robotic surgery in children. J Pediatr Surg. 2013;48(4):858–65.
13. Smith WF. Cost-effectiveness and cost-benefit analyses for public health programs. Public Health Rep. 1968;83(11):899–906.
14. Berkson J. Cost-utility as a measure of the efficiency of a test. J Am Stat Assoc. 1947;42(238):246–55.
15. Faleiros DR, Álvares J, Almeida AM, et al. Budget impact analysis of medicines: updated systematic review and implications. Expert Rev Pharmacoecon Outcomes Res. 2016;16(2):257–66.
16. Laskaris J, Regan K. The new break-even analysis. Healthc Financ Manage. 2013;67(12):88–95.
17. Aloi M, Lionetti P, Barabino A, et al. Phenotype and disease course of early-onset pediatric inflammatory bowel disease. Inflamm Bowel Dis. 2014;20(4):597–605.
18. Student V Jr, Vidlar A, Grepl M, et al. Advanced reconstruction of Vesicourethral support (ARVUS) during robot-assisted radical prostatectomy: one-year

functional outcomes in a two-group randomised controlled trial. Eur Urol. 2016;71(5):822–30. pii: S0302-2838(16)30201-9
19. Allan C, Ilic D. Laparoscopic versus robotic-assisted radical prostatectomy for the treatment of localised prostate cancer: a systematic review. Urol Int. 2016;96(4):373–8.
20. JC H, Gandaglia G, Karakiewicz PI, et al. Comparative effectiveness of robot-assisted versus open radical prostatectomy cancer control. Eur Urol. 2014;66(4):666–72.
21. Mahida JB, Cooper JN, Herz D, Diefenbach KA, Deans KJ, Minneci PC, McLeod DJ. Utilization and costs associated with robotic surgery in children. J Surg Res. 2015;199(1):169–76.
22. Chang SJ, Hsu CK, Hsieh CH, Yang SS. Comparing the efficacy and safety between robotic-assisted versus open pyeloplasty in children: a systemic review and meta-analysis. World J Urol. 2015;33(11):1855–65.
23. Kim NY, Chang EY, Hong YJ, Park S, Kim HY, Bai SJ, Han SJ. Retrospective assessment of the validity of robotic surgery in comparison to open surgery for pediatric choledochal cyst. Yonsei Med J. 2015;56(3):737–43.
24. Ballouhey Q, Villemagne T, Cros J, Vacquerie V, Bérenguer D, Braik K, Szwarc C, Longis B, Lardy H, Fourcade L. Assessment of paediatric thoracic robotic surgery. Interact Cardiovasc Thorac Surg. 2015;20(3):300–3.
25. Gargollo PC. Robotic-assisted bladder neck repair: feasibility and outcomes. Urol Clin North Am. 2015;42(1):111–20.
26. Cundy TP, Harling L, Marcus HJ, Athanasiou T, Darzi AW. Meta analysis of robot-assisted versus conventional laparoscopic fundoplication in children. J Pediatr Surg. 2014;49(4):646–52.
27. Menon D, Marshall D. The internationalization of health technology assessment. Int J Technol Assess Health Care. 1996;12(1):45–51.
28. Luce BR, Drummond M, Jönsson B, et al. EBM, HTA, and CER: clearing the confusion. Milbank Q. 2010;88(2):256–76.
29. Turchetti G, Pierotti F, Palla I. Comparative health technology assessment of robotic-assisted, direct manual laparoscopic and open surgery: a prospective study. Surg Endosc. 2016;31(2):543–51.
30. Ghabri S, Autin E, Hamers FF, et al. Use of budget impact analysis (Bia) in economic evaluations of drugs and medical devices submitted to the French National Authority for Health (has). Value Health. 2015;18(7):A530.
31. Lee L, Sheikh A. Understanding stakeholder interests and perspectives in evaluations of health IT. Stud Health Technol Inform. 2016;222:53–62.
32. Orvieto MA, Large M, Gundeti MS. Robotic paediatric urology. BJU Int. 2012;110(1):2–13.
33. Gundeti MS. Comment on "education and training in pediatric robotic surgery: lessons learned from an inaugural multinational workshop". J Robot Surg. 2015;9(1):65–6.
34. Buffi N, Van Der Poel H, Guazzoni G, Mottrie A. Methods and priorities of robotic surgery training program. Junior European Association of Urology (EAU) robotic urology section with the collaboration of the EAU young academic urologists robotic section. Eur Urol. 2014;65(1):1–2.
35. Volpe A, Ahmed K, Dasgupta P, Ficarra V, Novara G, van der Poel H, Mottrie A. Pilot validation study of the European Association of Urology robotic training curriculum. Eur Urol. 2015;68(2):292–9.

3 Operating Room Setting and Robotic Instrumentation

Gloria Pelizzo

3.1 Introduction

Robotic surgical systems improve visualization, offer superior dexterity and precision, reduce fatigue on the part of the surgeon, and eliminate operator tremor [1–6]. These systems for minimally invasive surgery are the dominant surgical newcomers and have been proposed in all surgical fields in adult patients.

In recent years many pediatric surgical centers have reported their experience with this technology and most authors agree that robotic surgical procedures in children do require a dedicated skill [7–9]. The lack of specialized instruments for infants and children requires an adapted platform to maximize the efficiency of standard instruments. An understanding of robotic instrumentation is necessary to define the best way to maximize the patient's safety during robotic surgical procedures and minimize the potential for errors.

Proper operating room setup will facilitate surgical training, speed up the learning process, and promote interest in this mini invasive approach in the pediatric setting [10, 11].

G. Pelizzo
Pediatric Surgery Unit, Children's Hospital, Istituto Mediterraneo di Eccellenza Pediatrica, Palermo, Italy
e-mail: gloriapelizzo@gmail.com

3.2 The da Vinci® Surgical System

The da Vinci Surgical System® is available in four different models: standard, streamlined (S), S-high definition (HD), and S integrated (i)-HD.

Each system has three components: the surgeon console, patient cart, and vision cart [12, 13]. The da Vinci Robotic System, the most common "master-slave system," can be equipped with various instruments and camera-endoscope units that attach to the arms of the robot.

The robot arms are capable of holding and manipulating the surgical-laparoscopic camera, fine surgical instruments, and various sources of energy during the operation.

3.2.1 Surgeon Console

The surgeon console is the driver's seat for controlling the da Vinci® system. The system offers the surgeon a three-dimensional view of the surgical field through the stereoviewer; the system is adjusted with the pod controls, while the instrument arms are controlled by using the master controllers and foot pedals. The three-dimensional images of the surgical field are displayed in real-time high resolution under the stereoviewer [12, 14, 15].

The system status icons and messages appear in specific locations within the stereoviewer and alert the surgeon to any changes or errors with the

G. Mattioli, P. Petralia (eds.), *Pediatric Robotic Surgery*, DOI 10.1007/978-3-319-41863-6_3

system. The infrared sensors, which are directly adjacent to the stereoviewer, activate all the instruments when the surgeon's head is placed between them. Robotic instruments are immediately deactivated when the surgeon looks away from the stereoviewer or removes his head from between the infrared sensors [12]. This serves as a security system which prevents unintentional movement of robotic instruments inside the patient's body.

The Si system is also available with two surgeon consoles to improve fellow education and resident training.

3.2.2 Patient Cart

The patient-side cart has three robotic arms and an optional fourth arm (Fig. 3.1). One arm holds the endoscope, while the other arms hold interchangeable surgical instruments. Each arm has several clutch buttons that assist with the gross movements of the arm and to insert or withdraw instruments. The da Vinci system uses EndoWrist® (Intuitive Surgical, Inc., Sunnyvale, CA) surgical instruments, which mimic the movements of the human hand and wrist (Fig. 3.2). The instruments have seven degrees of freedom with 180° of articulation and 540° of rotation simulating a surgeon's hand and wrist movements [2]. Each instrument has a fixed number of uses before becoming deactivated. The system automatically tracks the number of uses remaining on each instrument and communicates this in the stereoviewer. An instrument arm will not function if an outdated instrument is loaded [12, 15].

3.2.3 Vision Cart

The vision system includes the endoscope, cameras, and other equipment to produce a 3D image of the operating field.

There are currently two endoscope sizes on the market, 8.5 mm and 12 mm. The endoscope, available with a 0° and 30° lens (Figs. 3.2 and 3.3), is connected to either a high-magnification (15× magnification with 45° view) or a wide-angle (10× magnification with 60° view) camera. The camera head is also connected to an automatic focus control that is linked to the surgeon console. The optical camera channels are connected to chip camera control units (CCU).

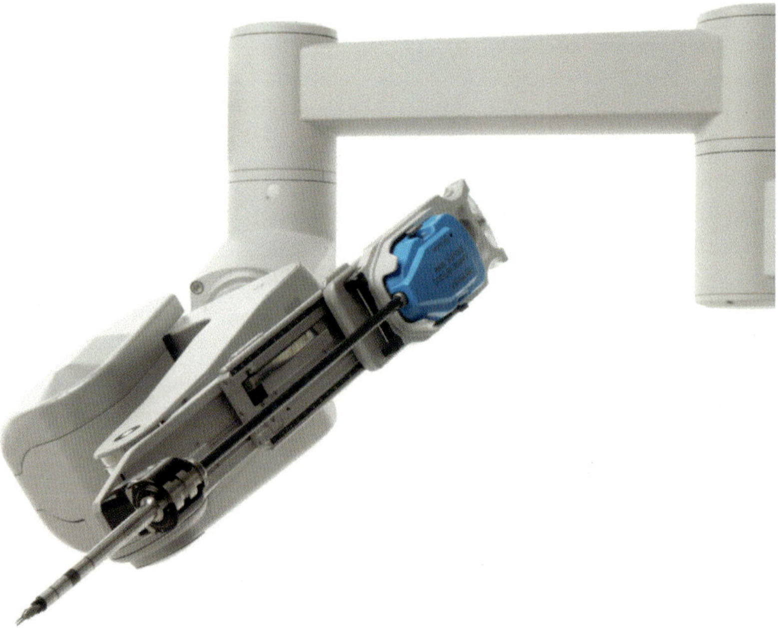

Fig. 3.1 Photograph of the angled instrument arm (courtesy of Intuitive Surgical, Inc.)

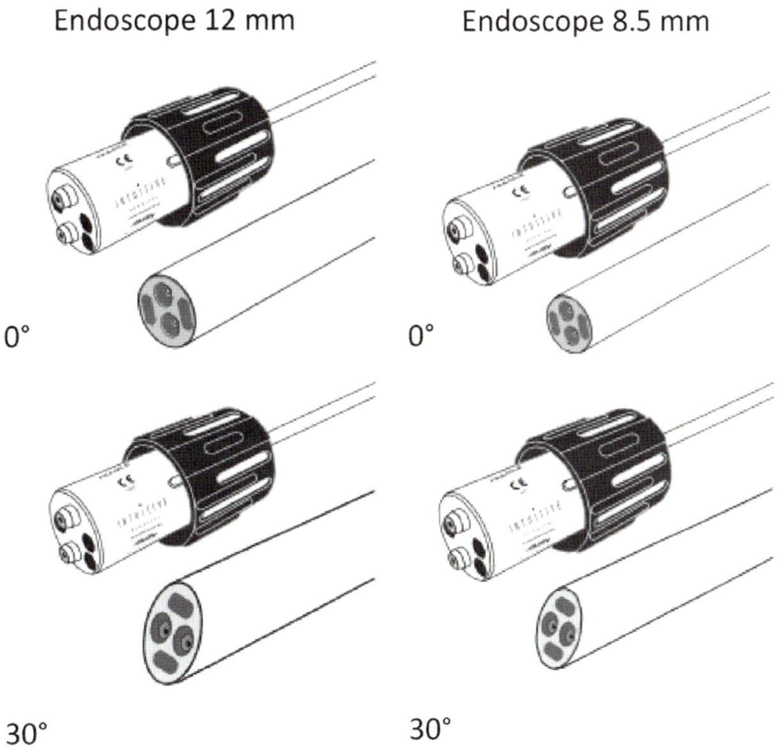

Fig. 3.2 Picture of 12 and 8.5 mm endoscope with 0° and 30° lens

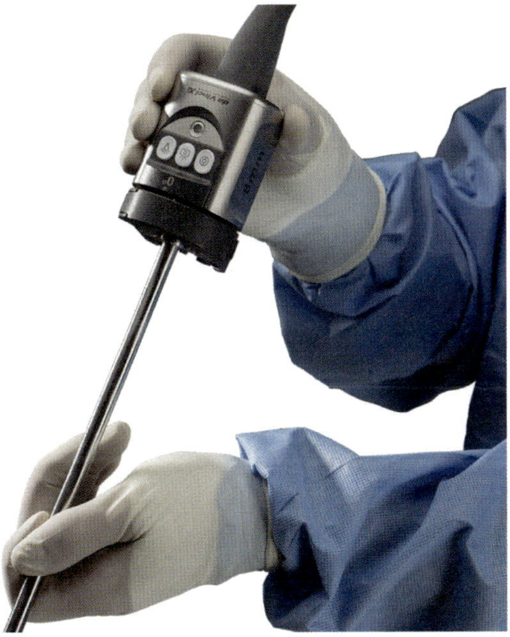

Fig. 3.3 Photograph of the high-resolution endoscope (courtesy of Intuitive Surgical, Inc.)

Definition and resolution of the camera and CCU are defined according to the generation system. The system also has a digital zoom that allows the surgeon to magnify the view of the tissue without moving the endoscope.

3.3 Ports and Instruments

The EndoWrist® instruments simulate a surgeon's hand and wrist movements. All motions originate from the master controllers. The da Vinci® S, the most common system in use, includes a 57 cm blue housing instrument with release levers, instrument shaft, wrist, and a variety of instrument tips (Table 3.1). Also here, each instrument has a fixed number of uses before becoming deactivated. The number of uses is automatically reported on the stereoviewer and when the instrument becomes outdated it does not allow the arm to function. The instruments are not interchangeable between systems.

Table 3.1 Instruments and assistant ports available for pediatric robotic surgery da Vinci® (Intuitive Surgical, Inc., Sunnyvale, CA)

Robotic EndoWrist® instruments (Intuitive Surgical, Inc., Sunnyvale, CA)	Assistant port
• 5 mm Instruments (8.5 mm camera) *EndoWrist* Monopolar Cautery Instruments Ultrasonic energy instrument Needle drivers Scissors *EndoWrist* Graspers • 8 mm Instruments (12 mm camera) *EndoWrist* Needle Drivers *EndoWrist* Graspers *EndoWrist* Scissors *EndoWrist* Scalpels Specialty instruments 8 mm Cautery instruments Monopolar cautery instruments *EndoWrist* Bipolar Cautery Instruments *EndoWrist®* OneTM Instruments Ultrasonic energy instrument *EndoWrist* Clip Appliers • Single-site camera and instruments®	• Laparoscopic trocars 3 or 5 mm: • Needle driver • Endoscopic clip applier • Suction irrigator • Pigtail
Accessories	
• 5 mm Robotic trocars (2–3 depending on the number of instrument arms) • 8 mm Robotic trocars (2–3 depending on the number of instrument arms) • Sterile drapes for camera and instrument arms, camera and telemonitor • Sterile camera mount and camera trocar mount (depending on the type of system) • Sterile trocar mount (depending on the type of system) • Sterile instrument adapter (comes attached to the drape for the S) • Sterile camera adapter	

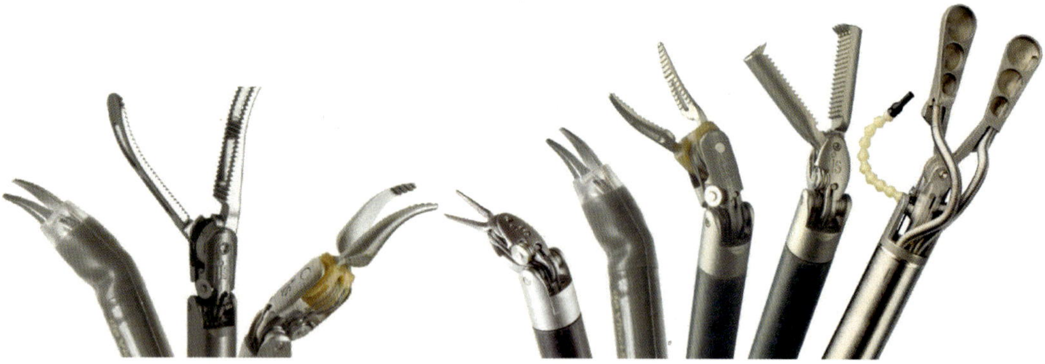

Fig. 3.4 Photograph of EndoWrist® (Intuitive Surgical, Inc., Sunnyvale, CA) 8 mm instruments for the da Vinci Si System (courtesy of Intuitive Surgical, Inc.)

Currently, for pediatric surgery the EndoWrist® instruments available are available only in 8 or 5 mm shaft diameters (Figs. 3.4 and 3.5).

The 8 mm instruments operate on an "angled joint" compared to the 5 mm which move on a "snake joint." The tip of the angled joint instruments rotates with a short radius and the "snake joint" has a larger range of rotation at the tip (3 cm).

The 8 mm set instruments include a 12 mm camera and reusable cannulas (blunt and/or bladeless obturator) with disposable seals. For the 12 mm camera, the blunt-tip trocar is indicated. This consists of a blunt obturator with a balloon and a valve body/cannula assembly. The advantages of using this port include its short intra-abdominal length and superior anchoring to

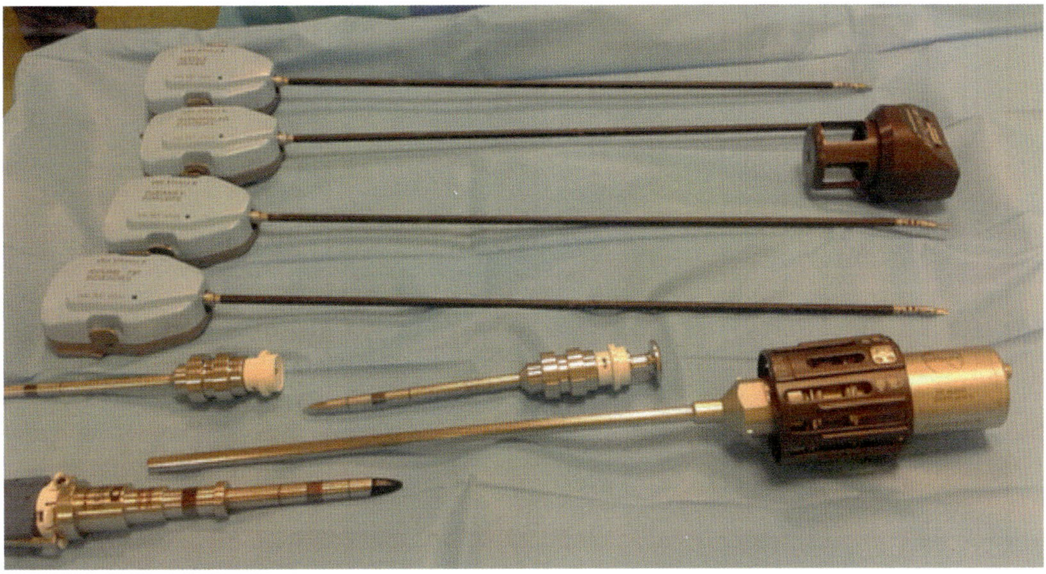

Fig. 3.5 Photograph of EndoWrist® (Intuitive Surgical, Inc., Sunnyvale, CA) 5 mm instruments for the da Vinci Si System

the abdominal wall without the need for suture fixation.

The latest da Vinci surgical system version (Intuitive Surgical, Sunnyvale, CA, USA) includes an 8.5 mm three-dimensional camera and 5 mm working instruments.

This system is also useful in the pediatric age, in the limited working space typical in small children [9]. In these patients, port placement is crucial to accommodate the instruments and represents the most challenging aspect to maximize movement and prevent collisions of the external robotic arms.

The slightest variation in port-site insertion even millimetric can produce limited mobility of the instruments, thus producing robot arm conflicts, and may jeopardize the safety of the procedure. The insertion site requires a wider angulation in comparison with mini access surgery. The smaller the patient, the wider the trocar angulation must be, especially when using 5 mm instruments with less dexterity than the 8 mm instruments. The maximum distance between trocars will benefit the dexterity of the surgeon as ergonomics are quite different with respect to laparoscopy. Working ports should also be placed at a sufficient distance (at least 3 cm) from the superior iliac spine and costal margin in the lower and upper abdomen, respectively [16, 17].

The placement of all the working ports and docking procedure in small patients must be performed under direct vision in the following order: working instruments and lastly the camera port.

The use of the assistant ports is very common in pediatric surgery. The trocars currently in use are reusable 3 mm trocars and laparoscopic instruments for providing retraction, suctioning, or passing pig tails utilized in urologic procedures, and 5 mm laparoscopic trocars and instruments for the passage of scissors, suction, and suture needle holder.

3.3.1 The Single-Site Port

Single-site port is a device nicknamed the “chopstick” surgery technique that enables the use of the robotic arms through a single incision without instrument collision [18–20]. All instruments and optics are placed via this single site (Fig. 3.6). However, the single-site dissecting and cautery instruments do not have wristed action. This system is available for an 8.5 mm camera, as well as for two curved cannulas for robotically controlled instruments, 5 mm instruments for dissection and cautery, and one 5 mm standard laparoscopic grasper for retraction (Fig. 3.7).

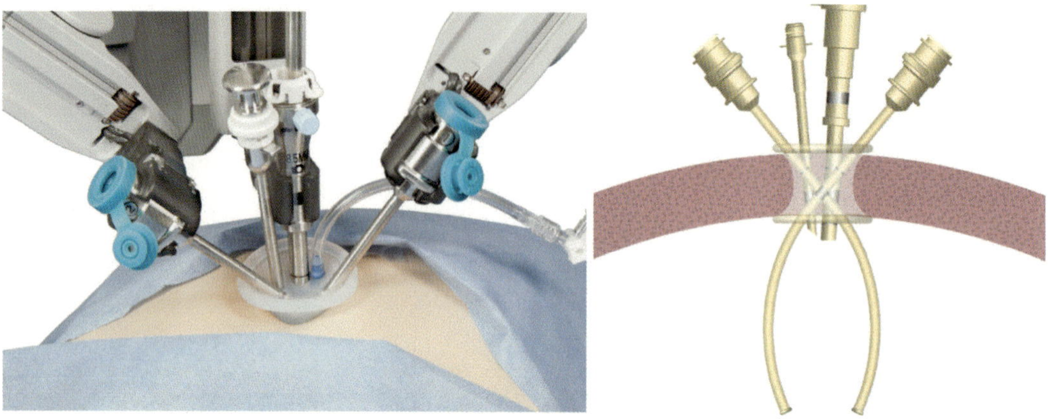

Fig. 3.6 Illustration of the single-site camera and associated instruments (courtesy of Intuitive Surgical, Inc.)

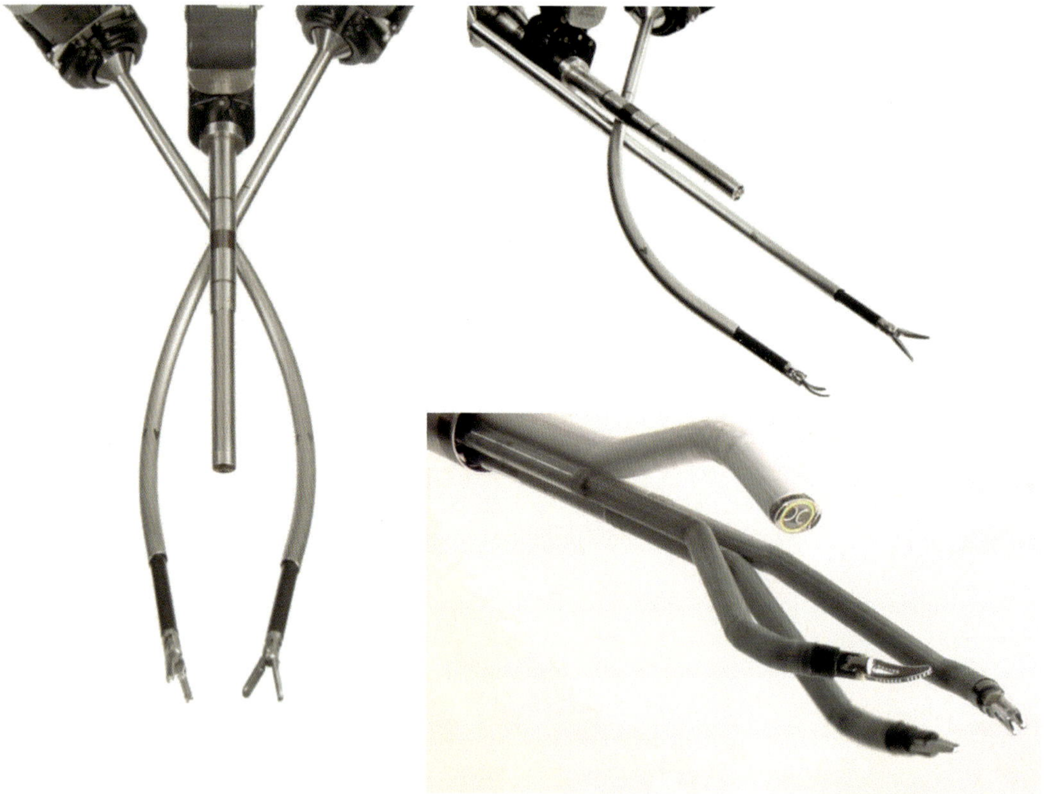

Fig. 3.7 Photograph of the single-site instruments (courtesy of Intuitive Surgical, Inc.)

The da Vinci computer software allows the surgeon to control the dissection in a natural intuitive fashion. Each hand controls the instrument on its own side and triangulation is achieved by crossing the curved cannulas midway through the access port without the need for crossing over.

3.4 Operating Room Set-up

Preparing the operating room for robotic assisted procedures begins before the patient enters the room [12]. An efficient setup and well-organized operating room for pediatric robotic surgery should

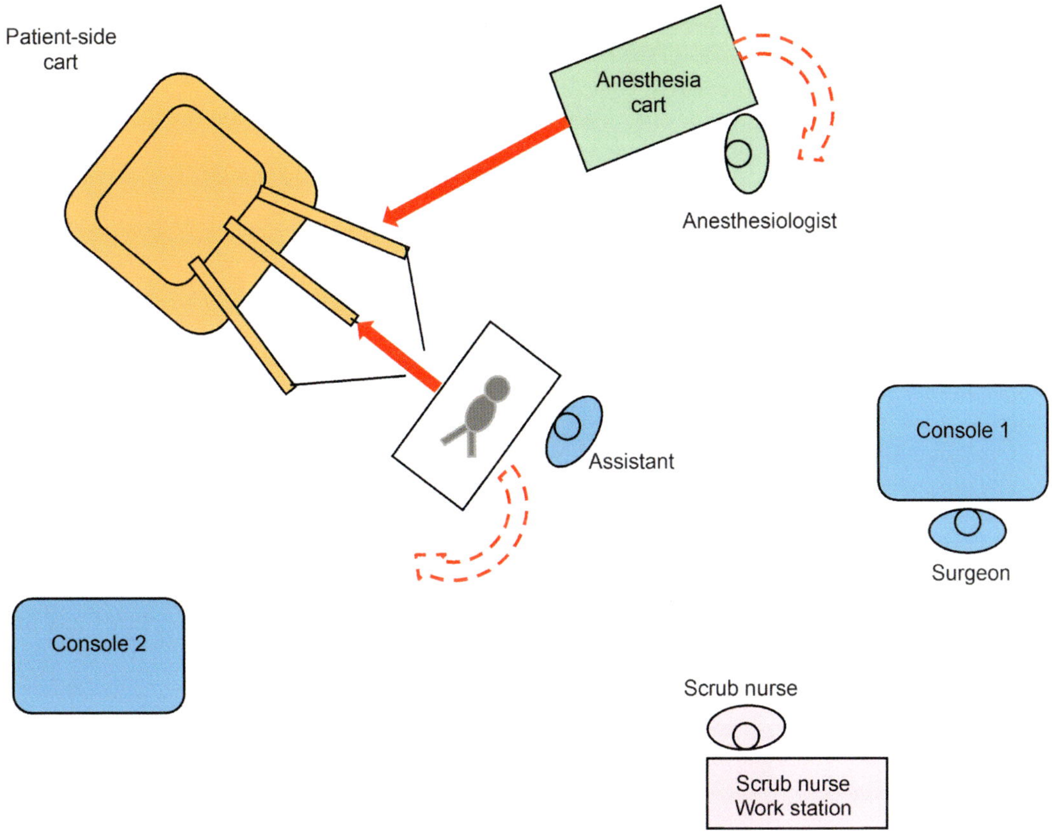

Fig. 3.8 Pediatric robotic room setting. The operating room table may have the choice to move around the robot and the anesthesiologist to move their equipment toward the robot position

provide adequate space for surgical personnel to move around the room. Extraneous equipment should be removed from the room to maximize the available space. The procedural case cart, surgeon console, and ancillary equipment should be positioned at the periphery of the room so that there is a clear pathway to the patient surgical bed once the patient is in the room.

The da Vinci robot stands about 6 feet tall and weighs in at a daunting 567 kg; indeed it is a very large device. Careful preoperative placement planning of the ventilator tube, monitoring electrodes, and lines has to be specifically defined in pediatric operations because of their influence on the likelihood of robot adaptation for small children.

The best way to define the pediatric operating room is to allow the operating room table to move around the robot. Even the anesthesiologist has the choice of moving their equipment, adapting the setup to patient weight and height as well as the table. After anesthesiological preparation, the operating table may be unlocked, to allow patient rotation toward the robot (Fig. 3.8).

Maneuvering of robotic arms and insertion of robotic instruments into cannulae require a longer docking time in pediatric robotic surgery with respect to adult surgery. The external robotic arms must move without colliding with each other or with the operating room table [21].

3.4.1 Patient Positioning

Proper patient positioning on the operating table is essential to achieve optimal surgical results [22]. The specific robotic intervention determines how the patient will be positioned. Each robotic procedure requires different positioning and positional aids, and it is important for the perioperative nurse to understand the safety considerations of patient positioning during robotic procedures. The goals of positioning are to maintain circulation; protect muscles, nerves, and bony prominences from pressure injury; in general protect the patient from injury; provide adequate exposure of the operative site; maintain a functional airway; and provide the anesthesiologist adequate access to IV lines and monitoring equipment [23]. In pediatric robotic surgery, the extreme positioning usually adopted in adults to gain maximum exposure to the surgical site [23] is not required in children. Briefly:

1. Steep Trendelenburg when the patient is in the lithotomy position is used in robotic pelvic procedures and distal colorectal surgery. This position helps displace the patient's abdominal viscera cephalad, which improves the surgeon's ability to see the anatomy in the lower abdomen and pelvis.
2. The reverse Trendelenburg position is used during upper abdominal surgery procedures such as robotic cholecystectomy, gastrectomy, and Nissen fundoplication. This position provides the surgical team with adequate visibility of the surgical site by shifting the abdominal contents toward the pelvis.
3. The semilateral position is most often used during robotic procedures of the kidney and adrenal glands.

3.4.2 Pediatric Surgical Team

Robotic systems require a dedicated team with special training. The pediatric surgical team includes the pediatric surgeon, pediatric surgical assistant(s), anesthesiologists, pediatric nurse, and surgical technician. Each member must be knowledgeable in robotic assisted surgery and communication between each of these individuals is vital for successful outcomes. It is generally recommended to have a dedicated team to work through the learning curve and if possible all pediatric robotic cases [12, 24, 25]. The surgeon will lead the team and should not only master driving the robot, but also become familiar with the setup, basic operation of the system, and troubleshooting. The circulating nurse and surgical technician are critical for operating the robot and should become experts on system startup, draping, docking, instruments, troubleshooting, exchanging instruments, and turnover. The surgical assistant should have similar knowledge, but will also need to understand the basics of laparoscopic surgery and be comfortable assisting with trocar placement, clipping, suction, irrigation, retraction, and cutting [24, 25].

Once the operating room is staged and the equipment is positioned, the surgical team can prepare the system [14].

1. System cables, optical channels, focus control, and power cables are connected and the system is turned on. The system will then perform a self-test. During this time, no attempt to manipulate the system should be attempted or a fault may be triggered.
2. Instrument and camera arms are positioned so they have adequate room to move.
3. The homing sequence is initiated.
4. Patient cart arms are draped; this takes a coordinated team. The drapes should not be too tight as this may decrease the range of motion of the robotic arms.
5. The endoscope is draped by connecting the camera sterile adapter to the endoscope and then the drape is taped to the sterile adapter. The light source is connected to the endoscope with the sterile light cable; a black and white balance is performed.
6. The endoscope is aligned and endoscope settings set (three-dimensional vs. two-dimensional, 0° vs. 30° up or down).
7. The "sweet spot" of the camera arm is set by aligning the trocar mount with the center of the patient cart column and extending the camera arm.

A well-trained and collaborative surgical team is crucial for operating room dynamics and likely contributes to positive patient outcomes.

3.5 System Shutdown

Once the robotic assisted surgery is completed, all of the instruments are removed first, followed by the endoscope. The arms are disconnected from the trocars and the patient cart is undocked from the patient. Finally, the sterile accessories and drapes are removed and the system is cleaned.

As more companies bring additional robots and instruments to the market in coming years, we can anticipate that there will be improvements in miniaturization of robotic instruments that will allow for even more optimal working conditions in the limited space typical of pediatric patients.

References

1. Ng AT, Tam PC. Current status of robot-assisted surgery. Hong Kong Med J. 2014;20:241–50.
2. Moorthy K, Munz Y, Dosis A, Hernandez J, Martin S, Bello F, Rockall T, Darzi A. Dexterity enhancement with robotic surgery. Surg Endosc. 2004;18:790–5.
3. Byrn JC, Schluender S, Divino CM, Conrad J, Gurland B, Shlasko E, Szold A. Three-dimensional imaging improves surgical performance for both novice and experienced operators using the da Vinci robot system. Am J Surg. 2007;193:519–22.
4. van der Schatte Olivier RH, van't Hullenaar CDP, Ruurda JP, Broeders IAMJ. Ergonomics, user comfort, and performance in standard and robot-assisted laparoscopic surgery. Surg Endosc. 2009;23(6):1365–71.
5. Hubert N, Gilles M, Desbrosses K, Meyer JP, Felblinger J, Hubert J. Ergonomic assessment of the surgeon's physical work- load during standard and robotic assisted laparoscopic procedures. Int J Med Robot. 2013;9:142–7.
6. Lee EC, Rafiq A, Merrell R, Ackerman R, Denderlein JT. Ergonomics and human factors in endoscopic surgery: a comparision of manual vs telerobotic simulation systems. Surg Endosc. 2005;19:1064–70.
7. van Haasteren G, Levine S, Hayes W. Pediatric robotic surgery: early assessment. Pediatrics. 2009;124:1642–9.
8. Sinha CK, Haddad M. Robot-assisted surgery in children: current status. J Robot Surg. 2008;1:243–6.
9. Cundy TP, Marcus HJ, Hughes-Hallett A, Khurana S, Darzi A. Robotic surgery in children: adopt now, await, or dismiss? Pediatr Surg Int. 2015;31:1119–25.
10. Nezhat C, Lakhi N. Learning experiences in robotic-assisted laparoscopic surgery. Best Pract Res Clin Obstet Gynaecol. 2015;35:20–9. pii: S1521-6934(15)00221-7
11. Catchpole K, Perkins C, Bresee C, et al. Safety, efficiency and learning curves in robotic surgery: a human factors analysis. Surg Endosc. 2015;30(9):3749–61.
12. Higuchi TT, Gettman MT. Robotic instrumentation, personnel and operating room. In: Li-Ming S, editor. Setup Atlas of robotic urologic surgery. Current clinical urology. NY: Humana Press; 2011. p. 15–30.
13. Narula VK, Melvin SM. Robotic surgical systems. In: Patel VR, editor. Robotic urologic surgery. London: Springer-Verlag; 2007. p. 5–1.
14. Bhandari A, Hemal A, Menon M. Instrumentation, sterilization, and preparation of robot. Indian J Urol. 2005;21:83–5.
15. Szold A, Bergamaschi R, Broeders I, Dankelman J, Forgione A, Langø T, et al. European Association of Endoscopic Surgeons (EAES) consensus statement on the use of robotics in general surgery. Surg Endosc. 2015;29:253–88.
16. Pelizzo G, Nakib G, Romano P, Avolio L, Mencherini S, Zambaiti E, et al. Five millimetre-instruments in paediatric robotic surgery: advantages and shortcomings. Minim Invasive Ther Allied Technol. 2015;24:148–53.
17. Nakib G, Calcaterra V, Scorletti F, Romano P, Goruppi I, Mencherini S, et al. Robotic assisted surgery in pediatric gynecology: promising innovation in mini invasive surgical procedures. J Pediatr Adolesc Gynecol. 2013;26:e5–7.
18. Ahn N, Signor G, Singh TP, Stain S, Whyte C. Robotic single- and multisite cholecystectomy in children. J Laparoendosc Adv Surg Tech A. 2015; 25:1033–5.
19. Jones VS. Robotic-assisted single-site cholecystectomy in children. J Pediatr Surg. 2015;50:1842–5.
20. Morelli L, Guadagni S, Di Franco G, Palmeri M, Di Candio G, Mosca F. Da Vinci single site© surgical platform in clinical practice: a systematic review. Int J Med Robot. 2015;12(4):724–34. doi:10.1002/rcs.1713.
21. Meehan JJ. Robotic surgery in small children: is there room for this? J Laparoendosc Adv Surg Tech. 2009;19:707–12.
22. Chang C, Steinberg Z, Shah A, Gundeti MS. Patient positioning and port placement for robot-assisted surgery. J Endourol. 2014;28:631–8.
23. Hortman C, Chung S. Positioning considerations in robotic surgery. AORN J. 2015;102:434–9.
24. Gettman MT, Blute ML, Peschel R, Bartsch G. Current status of robotics in urologic laparoscopy. Eur Urol. 2003;43:106–12.
25. Gettman MT, Cadeddu JA. Robotics in urologic surgery. In: Graham SD, Keane TE, Glenn JF, editors. Glenn's urologic surgery. Philadelphia: Lippincott Williams & Wilkins; 2004. p. 1027–33.

Shifting from Conventional Minimally Invasive Surgery to Robotic Surgery

4

Mario Lima, Tommaso Gargano, Michela Maffi, Giovanni Ruggeri, and Michele Libri

4.1 Introduction

Robotic surgery has been introduced into clinical practice in the late 1990s to overcome well-recognized limitations of the conventional minimally invasive approach, including two-dimensional imaging, restricted range of motion of the instruments, hand tremors, and poor ergonomic positioning of the surgeon. Since then, robotic surgical systems have rapidly evolved and are used for an increasing number of complex minimally invasive surgical procedures [1–6]. Historically, new surgical techniques have had a more difficult and slower acceptance by the pediatric surgical community compared to the adults' one. Indeed, small spaces and anesthesiological management have limited the use of these technologies. In the pediatric age, robotic surgery has been accepted and utilized by a small number of pediatric surgeons around the world. Since the first reported case in a child in April 2001, the use of robotic technology has rapidly expanded within pediatric surgery. During the last decade, it has successfully been applied to a large variety of gastrointestinal, genitourinary, and thoracic procedures in infants and children, thus demonstrating the safety and feasibility of this approach. The number of pediatric robotic procedures performed per year using this emerging method is growing rapidly, with no evidence that this will change in the future. The early functional outcomes of robotic procedures are promising; however at present, most of the comparative studies are from single institutions, and lack a high level of evidence. Although increasing numbers of larger pediatric robotic surgery case series have been published over the years, authors mainly focused on the comparison with open surgery. However, in order to identify potential advantages of a particular type of robotic procedure over the corresponding conventional laparoscopic or thoracoscopic approach, comparative studies providing evidence-based information are needed [6–10]. Performing robotic surgery in pediatric patients requires a complete new redesigned concept of the surgical techniques and modifications in the surgical operating room. The introduction of this innovative technology brings new advances in instrumental maneuverability, and better optics. However, robotic surgery also brings new challenges and limitations that will require improvement in the future. The successful transition from laparoscopy to robotic surgery requires some steps. These include developing a specific robotic team that should be well informed on setting up the robot and can deal with intraoperative problems. Another task of the team is to ensure that the surgeon has spent sufficient time on the robot to be familiar and proficient, and to help in the selection of

M. Lima (✉) • T. Gargano • M. Maffi
G. Ruggeri • M. Libri
Pediatric Surgery, Bologna University,
Via Massarenti 11, Bologna 40138, Italy
e-mail: mario.lima@unibo.it

G. Mattioli, P. Petralia (eds.), *Pediatric Robotic Surgery*, DOI 10.1007/978-3-319-41863-6_4

patients, thus avoiding difficult cases in the beginning. During the first procedures it is important to have sufficient time so that no one is rushed or harassed by lack of time, and, of course, to make sure that a proctor is present. Finally, when the surgical session is over, a debriefing with the whole team will minimize problems, develop enthusiasm for this new technology, and allow checklists and protocols to be developed. With these simple steps, this transition can be performed relatively painlessly [11].

4.2 Historical Aspects

The origin of robotic surgery is rooted in the strengths and weaknesses of its predecessors. Minimally invasive surgery began in 1987 with the first laparoscopic cholecystectomy. Since then, the list of procedures performed laparoscopically has grown with technological improvements and advances in the technical skills of surgeons. The advantages of minimally invasive surgery are very popular among surgeons, patients, and insurance companies. The motivation to develop surgical robots is rooted in the desire to overcome the limitations of current laparoscopic technologies and to expand the benefits of minimally invasive surgery. Robot, taken from the Czech robota, meaning forced labor, has evolved in meaning from dumb machines that perform menial, repetitive tasks to the highly intelligent anthropomorphic robots of popular culture. Although today's robots are still unintelligent machines, great strides have been made in expanding their utility. Today robots are computer-assisted systems used to perform highly specific, highly precise, and dangerous tasks in industry and research previously not possible with a human workforce. Robotics, however, has been slow to enter the field of medicine. Voice-activated robotic arms routinely maneuver endoscopic cameras, and complex master-slave robotic systems are currently Food and Drug Administration approved, marketed, and used for a variety of surgical procedures. The robot was initially looked upon as a tool to help the surgeon make a transition from open to laparoscopic surgery. The robotic technology was introduced as a solution to minimize the shortcomings of laparoscopy. Currently, the most frequent procedures performed with robotic assistance in children are fundoplication for gastroesophageal reflux and pyeloplasty for hydronephrosis. Furthermore, robotic surgery is not alone among other new surgical advances that can be offered to patients. In fact, there are new ways to approach surgical problems such as single-incision laparoscopic surgery, single-port access, and natural orifice transluminal endoscopic surgery [9].

4.3 Robotic Impact

Robotic surgery is an endoscopic procedure, only with an added layer of technology. Robotic surgery, as conventional minimally invasive surgery, is not a technique; it is a tool to an end. It provides undoubted technical advantages to both surgeons and patients. Improved visualization and greater dexterity are two major features of robotic technology. The benefits seem more evident where a fine dissection and complex surgical reconstruction are required. However, its use in various complex surgical reconstructive procedures has shown that the robot has broader applications. It has brought the technical skills of minimally invasive surgery within the realm of a greater number of surgeons. The major advantages of robotic surgery over conventional laparoscopy are [1, 2] the following:

- Better visualization: Three-dimensional versus two-dimensional imaging of the operative field. Currently, there is an 8 mm diameter HD camera in the market that is a better suitable size and more convenient for pediatric patients.
- Mechanical improvements: Intuitive instruments with less fulcrum effect than laparoscopic instruments. Robotic instruments have also seven degrees of freedom, similar to the human arm and hand, while rigid conventional instruments have four degrees of freedom. Instruments can be flexible; they articulate and they can move like (or better than) human hand and finger joints as what is called wristing.

- Stabilization of instruments within the surgical field: In conventional laparoscopy, small movements by the surgeon are amplified (including errors or hand tremor). Robotic surgery minimizes surgeon's hand tremor.
- Improved ergonomics for the operating surgeon: The surgeon can be seated with telerobotic systems. Additionally, all surgeons can perform robot-assisted procedures in a seated position, rather than standing at the operating table.

The limitations of robotic technology include [7, 8] the following:

- Increased costs and operating room time: The high cost of purchasing and maintaining the instruments of the robotic system is one of its many disadvantages.
- Additional surgical training: The current robotic system is still sizeable and requires a team of trained staff to set it up over a lengthy time period. The availability of the robotic systems to only a limited number of centers reduces surgical training opportunities.
- Bulkiness of the devices.
- Instrumentation limitations (e.g., lack of a robotic suction and irrigation device, size, cost).
- Lack of tactile sensation or haptics: It is the most tangible impact of the robotic technology. The lack of haptic feedback is compensated with a 3D vision of the surgical field and this technology may well be introduced in the near future.
- Risk of mechanical failure: Robotic surgical systems are designed with features intended to minimize the potential effects of mechanical failures on patients. Such features include system redundancy, so-called graceful performance degradation or failure, fault tolerance, just-in-time maintenance, and system alerting. Thus, there are several mechanical checks and balances built into current robotic surgical systems so that the risk of mechanical failure is minimized.
- Limited number of energy sources (less than with conventional laparoscopy).
- Not designed for abdominal surgery involving more than two quadrants (in these cases the device needs to be re-docked and repositioned).

4.4 Robotic Planning

Hospital administrators and pediatric surgeons must define the reasons for developing a robotic surgical program. The potential is greatest when the surgical team and hospital administration can work together for patient care and institutional advancement. In developing a robotic program and timeline, it is important to collect the necessary data, including the potential increase in referrals as well as savings from reduced hospital lengths of stay and faster recovery. During this phase, it is important not to forget the cost of the yearly service contract for the robotics system as well as instruments and disposables for each case. When negotiating with hospital administrators, it is important to show them that robotics will add a dimension that will benefit the hospital through patient care. In addition to potential benefits to patients, programmatic growth potential and institutional recognition should be emphasized. In academic institutions, there is much greater opportunity for collaborative work. The intellectual process associated with a robotic program can promote scientific publishing. New programs may be developed within these working interest groups, and realistic timelines should be strictly enforced. This is a potentially great source for resident training, offering many areas for research projects. It is important for new robotics programs to provide educational programs within the community. Successful robotic surgical outcomes are directly related to the competence of the surgical team. This is particularly true in robotic surgery where the surgeon is not next to the patient and the assistant is on the bedside to carry out critical tasks. It is helpful to communicate with a technician or mentor involved directly in the field to provide guidance in the training period. The most important characteristics in developing a robotic program are intellectual curiosity, and a high-level dedication of surgeons involved in the program. Meticulous intraoperative data collection allows teams to track their progress. It should be remembered that successful programs develop slowly and iteratively. Every advancement requires critical analysis and quality review by team leaders. It is important to move to the next step only when the previous one has been mastered. With these few maxims in mind, most modern hospitals can field a robotic team and program with excellent patient care results. In addition, robotic surgery can be combined with new concepts such as virtual reality or augmented reality, which provide valuable preoperative or intraoperative information for the surgeon [10–12].

4.5 Robotic Surgical Team

As for conventional laparoscopy, the successful implementation of robotic surgery is more efficient with the establishment of a trained pediatric surgical team including bedside assistants, circulating nurses, and scrub technicians who are familiar with the setup, use, and turnover of the specific equipment. Robotic team should include anesthesia staff, surgical room nurses, surgical technicians, pediatric surgeons, nurse coordinator, and the robotic company agent. With ever-changing technologies in the field of minimally invasive surgery, such as robotics, there is now the need to train the surgeon to the next degree. Both conventional training and robotic training play an important role in improving operative skills of surgeon. Training by simulation, whether virtual, hybrid, or real, allows the surgeon to rehearse, learn, improve, or maintain their skills in a safe and stress-free environment. During the preliminary stage, adequate training is essential to accomplish a successful robotic program. Team training is the most important early step [10]. A carefully planned protocol or objective-based curriculum should be followed for the best results. Training should be designed to expand prior clinical experiences and training beginning by setup, draping, and both electrical and mechanical troubleshooting. The surgeon sits at a specialized control center known as a console where he or she controls the camera, robotic arms, and other equipment. An assistant sits at the patient's bedside and uses laparoscopic tools through ports to provide suction, change robotic tools, make adjustments to the robotic arms as needed, and introduce stitches. A scrub technician sits on the other side of the patient to provide tools and sutures and to make adjustments to the robotic arms. The anesthesiologist remains at the patient's head, providing anesthesia and monitoring the patient's heart and lungs [13–18].

4.6 Robotic Training and Surgical Education

The necessity of robotic surgical training during residency is a matter of debate among surgical educators. While surgical educators in resident training centers in which robotic surgery has been adopted are still charged with the responsibility of teaching residents the surgical management, they now face a new challenge of how to teach a resident to assist at and perform a surgery when not physically standing at the operating room table. Although the robotic system is relatively user friendly, mastering its use and performing specific procedures with it require commitment on the part of physicians and operating room staff. Incorporating robotic training into any residency program poses significant challenges: above all, resident involvement should not have a negative effect on the outcome. Traditionally, this was ensured by the teaching surgeon's constant presence and direct instruction during surgery. With the robotic system, the surgeon sits separately at a console and the first assistant is at the table side. Hence, the assistant is the only doctor in primary contact with the patient. In the future, surgical training simulators or a pilot/copilot arrangement may play a larger role in the teaching process, but for now this technology is not available. It is therefore essential that robotic surgical educators have a comfort level both with performing the surgical procedure and communicating with the assistant to teach the procedure. There is no doubt that robotic training is necessary and important for future of the residents. Three steps are essential to training residents to acquire new skills with novel technology as robotic surgery. The first is perceptual awareness that incorporates the cognitive understanding of the operation and being able to visualize the entire operation in one's mind. The second step is guided learning, during which the resident learns how to perform the segmental steps of the operation under the watchful guidance and supervision of an instructor. The final step is the autonomous stage, in which skills are refined, leading to precision and efficiency [19]. Robotic surgical systems are now routinely used in minimally invasive general surgery, pediatric surgery, gynecology, urology, cardiothoracic surgery, and otorhinolaryngology. Robotic devices continue to evolve and as they become less expensive and more widely disseminated will likely become more frequently utilized in surgical procedures. Despite many technologic leaps, surgical training has stayed more or less unchanged for more than a century. Surgeons in training have always had to gain operative experience through "supervised trial and error" on real patients. This approach makes surgical training completely dependent on the actual caseload, prolongs surgical training, and compromises patients' safety. Robotic surgery creates a new medium for acquisition of surgical skills through simulation of all procedures that can be done via the robot. Surgeons can use surgical robots to practice operations on three-dimensional, virtual-reality visual simulations. Image-guided simulations will allow surgeons to practice procedures on three-dimensional reconstructions of the anatomy of the actual patients who they plan to operate on the next day. Nowadays, the robotic training is given on a specific simulator for robotic surgery. It is a portable, stand-alone robotic surgery simulator that teaches novice surgeons the motor and cognitive skills required for operating the da Vinci surgical robot. It uses virtual reality to introduce the user to the fundamentals of robot-assisted surgery. It boasts a multilevel curriculum, designed with various levels of difficulty that takes the user through and teaches the required skills for effectively advancing robotic surgery abilities [15–19]. The learning curve for gaining technical skills in the traditional laparoscopic surgery entails a longer and more difficult process when the learning process is compared to robotic surgery. This learning process requires much more dexterity to work with rigid instruments working into the surgical field on a flat screen with a loss of the deep sensation. Junior residents learn faster and perform more advanced surgical skills with the robotic technology than with traditional laparoscopic surgery. Some laboratory simulation studies indicate that enabling benefit may pertain mostly to novice surgeons. When evaluating technically challenging tasks such as suturing, novice surgeons experienced an early and persistent enabling effect with robotic assisted laparoscopy, while experienced laparoscopic surgeons demonstrated equal proficiency in both robotic and conventional laparoscopic surgery. Robotic assistance for laparoscopy appears to eliminate the early learning curve for novices but may not provide advantages for experienced laparoscopic surgeons. As the field of robotic surgery continues to grow, continuing medical education programs that address the robotic learning for residents and practicing surgeons need to be developed [13–15].

The core objectives of the robotic surgery training are:

- To become familiar with the function and the ergonomics of robotic system (components and instrumentation)
- To do proper operative room setup
- To learn scientific port position to do proper docking
- To become familiar with the techniques of surgical dissection, intracorporeal suturing, and knot tying

4.7 Robotic Setup

Robotic room setup is critical for better efficiency. The robotic equipment consists of three major components: console, robotic cart, and tower control. Instead of standing at the operating room table, the surgeon operates seated at a console with a three-dimensional vision system from where his or her movements are scaled, filtered, and translated via electromechanical robotic arms into precise, real-time movements of articulated surgical instruments working inside the patient's body, thereby extending the surgeon's capabilities. The console is ergonomically comfortable, and it is located in the surgical room. Surgeon and the console are located out of the sterile field. The surgeon has control of the robotic instruments, camera, and position of the robotic arms. Additional equipment such as self-tying knots, multifire staple devices, or suction-irrigation catheter requires support by the assistant. The robotic cart has four fully retractable and mobile arms, which can be controlled and used by the surgeon once the arms are docked and activated in the robotic ports on the patient. Adequate positioning of the robotic cart is very important because it has to be located aligned to the organ target. Since there is no option to move the robotic cart while performing surgery, the patient position, robotic arms, and instruments should be secured by the surgeon before sitting in the console. Furthermore the equipment is rather bulky and pediatric surgical rooms are usually small in size, so it is recommended to look for the best location to allocate the robotic equipment and keep the designed layout of the room in the surgeon's preference card so everyone in the surgical room is aware how to position the equipment and patient before patient arrives to the room. The tower control holds and controls the optics, gas insufflator, and software program to run the robotic equipment. Robotic instruments have a limited life span of 10 uses in 8 mm and 20 uses in 5 mm platform. Port position in a pediatric patient is different when it is compared to the traditional laparoscopic port placement. Port location has to be distant from each other, so each instrument has enough space for adequate instrumental maneuverability. Each lateral port with the camera port should be aligned toward the target organ. One big difference is that with laparoscopy the surgeon is standing and views the surgical field on a two-dimensional monitor positioned above the patient while the camera is manipulated by an assistant. In the robotic system, as mentioned, the surgeon is sitting and uses the 3D images from a camera controlled by the surgeon himself or herself. Another difference is that laparoscopy uses handheld and nonarticulating instruments [11, 12].

4.8 Discussion and Conclusions

Robotic surgery represents the new step in the evolution of minimally invasive surgery that permits the surgeon to explore the patient's internal spaces with very little trauma. Robotic system makes complex laparoscopic skills easier to perform and will therefore increase a surgeon's minimally invasive armamentarium. In comparison with conventional laparoscopic surgery, robotic surgery provides numerous benefits, such as magnified three-dimensional visualization, articulated instruments, tremor filtering, motion scaling, or ergonomic position. Robotic surgery is suitable for the practice of pediatrics, which necessitates fine dissections and sutures in narrow anatomical spaces. However, improvements are still possible such as miniaturization of the system and instruments or enhancement of a tactile feedback. Robotic assistance allows the transition from open to laparoscopic procedure without difficulty, making easier the dissection and intracorporeal suturing. This is due to the intuitive characteristics of robotic technology. Training is certainly another important topic for discussion. Despite technological improvements, training is still a major issue in the field of minimally invasive surgery. Several publications discuss the benefits of robotic surgery over laparoscopic skills. Robotic procedure needs a low learning curve for a minimal invasive reconstructive surgery. The top of the learning curve is reached after about 10–20 procedures performed for the same pathology. The acquisition of robotic skills is more rapid and less difficult in comparison with laparoscopic skills. Most authors agree that robotic surgery is able to improve performance of traditional minimally invasive surgery, resulting in faster procedures and higher precision. Laparoscopic experience is a plus but not a "must" even if it helps the surgeon in performing difficult procedures [20]. Many principles of laparoscopic surgery are applicable to robotic surgery. Thus, a solid background in laparoscopy is helpful before embarking on robotic surgery. Although it is difficult to quantify how laparoscopic experience helps with the transition to robotic surgery, we believe that a good laparoscopic foundation is helpful for robotic surgery. Surgeons with experience in conventional laparoscopy have already dealt with visual limitations and the critical and important sensory loss. Moreover, although innovative instrumentation can be used in a wide range of situations, difficulties may arise. In fact pediatric surgeons treat pathologies of different origin affecting all organs. Surgery may therefore be used in thoracic, abdominal, and retroperitoneal procedures. Each condition requires dedicated instruments and surgical experience. Therefore, it is important for young pediatric surgeons to understand and be aware of these challenges as well as the complications unique to laparoscopy before performing robotic surgery [17]. The initial results of robotic surgery in the field of pediatrics are encouraging. The success rates of robotic procedures seem identical to those of conventional laparoscopy. However, there is no randomized study currently available for children in the literature. The published studies are essentially studies with an evidence level of III or level IV according to the Oxford Centre for Evidence-Based Medicine [5]. After the initial excitement surrounding robotic technology, laparoscopic experts seemed to agree that robotic systems are only beneficial in a limited number of surgical procedures. These operations have in common the need to perform precise maneuvers in a confined space without ample movements of the robotic arms [2]. Although still in its infancy, robotic surgery has already proven itself to be of great value, particularly in areas inaccessible to conventional laparoscopic procedures. It remains to be seen, however, if robotic systems will replace conventional laparoscopic instruments in less technically demanding procedures. In any case, robotic technology is set to revolutionize surgery by improving and expanding laparoscopic procedures, advancing surgical technology, and bringing surgery into the digital age. Although feasibility has largely been shown, more prospective randomized trials evaluating efficacy and safety must be undertaken. Further research must evaluate cost-effectiveness or a true benefit over conventional therapy for robotic surgery to take full root. Robotic technology with its inherent advantages has levelled the playing field and made it available to a large number of patients. Only the operating time is generally longer than for standard laparoscopic and open procedures. But, on the other hand, in some procedures blood loss is less, conversion rates are lower, and hospital stay is shorter. The main check to robotic surgery development is the high cost of purchase (approximately 1 million dollars), maintenance (about 10% of purchase cost each year), and consumables (about $2000 per instrument). The cost/benefit ratio remains to be validated. The issues surrounding the costs of robotic assisted laparoscopic surgery are complex. One must take into account costs to the hospital, costs to the patient, and costs to society. These include direct and indirect costs of surgery including equipment, operating time, recovery room time, length of hospital stay, nursing, anesthesia, physician fee, outpatient care, and lost wages, for example. Further prospective and comparative studies, especially comparisons between robotic and laparoscopic approaches, are necessary to confirm these preliminary results. Economic analyses are also indispensable to ensure the viability of robotic technology [9, 10]. To evaluate the future role of the robotic technique for visceral surgery, high-quality prospective randomized trials are urgently needed. To that effect, surgeons should definitely have mastered the learning curve. But already the existing evidence indicates that robotic surgery will have a permanent future role in visceral surgery. Therefore visceral surgeons should actively contribute to further development of robotic surgery and initiate high-quality comparative studies in this area. Pediatric surgeons must be actively involved in the evolution of robotics to ensure a suitable and reasoned use of this new technology for their young patients [20, 21].

References

1. Panait L, Shetty S, Shewokis PA, Sanchez JA. Do laparoscopic skills transfer to robotic surgery? J Surg Res. 2014;187:53–8.
2. Chaussy Y, Becmeur F, Lardy H, Aubert D. Robot-assisted surgery: current status evaluation in abdominal and urological pediatric surgery. J Laparoendosc Adv Surg Tech A. 2013;23(6):530–8.
3. Peters CA. Robotic assisted surgery in pediatric urology. Ped EndoSurg Innov Tech. 2003;7(4):403–13.
4. Monn MF, Bahler CD, Schneider EB, Whittam BM, Misseri R, Rink RC, Sundaram CP. Trends in robot-assisted laparoscopic Pyeloplasty in pediatric patients. Urology. 2013;81(6):1336–41.
5. Friedmacher F, Till H. Robotic-assisted procedures in pediatric surgery: a critical appraisal of the current best evidence in comparison to conventional minimally invasive surgery. J of Laparoendosc Adv Surg Tech. 2015;25:1–8.
6. Meehan JJ, Sandler A. Pediatric robotic surgery: a single-institutional review of the first 100 consecutive cases. Surg Endosc. 2008;22(1):177–82.
7. Hassan SO, Dudhia J, Syed LH, Patel K, Farshidpour M, Cunningham SC, Kowdley GC. Conventional laparoscopic vs robotic training: which is better for naive users? A randomized prospective crossover study. J Surg Educ. 2015;72(4):592–9.
8. Ferguson JL, Beste TM, Nelson KH, Daucher JA. Making the transition from standard gynecologic laparoscopy to robotic laparoscopy. JSLS. 2004;8:326–8.
9. Lanfranco AR, Castellanos AE, Desai JP, Meyers WC. Robotic surgery. A current perspective. Ann Surg. 2004;239(1):14–21.
10. De Lambert G, Fourcade L, Centi J, Fredon F, Braik K, Szwarc C, Longis B, Lardy H. How to successfully implement a robotic pediatric surgery program: lessons learned after 96 procedures. Surg Endosc. 2013;27:2137–44.
11. Camps JI. The use of robotics in pediatric surgery: my initial experience. Pediatr Surg Int. 2011;27:991–6.
12. Luebbe BN, Woo R, Wolf SA, Irish MS. Robotically assisted minimally invasive surgery in a pediatric population: initial experience, technical considerations, and description of the da Vinci surgical system. Ped EndoSurg Innov Tech. 2003;7(4):385–402.
13. Passerotti CC, Franco F, Bissoli JCC, Tiseo B, Oliveira CM, Buchalla CAO, Innoue GNC, Sencan A, Sencan A, Ruscitto do Pardo R, Nguyen HT. Comparison of the learning curves and frustration level in performing laparoscopic and robotic training skills by expert and novices. Int Urol Nephrol. 2015;47:1075–84.
14. Tasian GE, Wiebe DJ, Casale P. Learning curve of robotic assisted Pyeloplasty for pediatric urology fellows. J Urol. 2013;190:1622–7.
15. Cundy TP, Marcus HJ, Hughes-Hallett A, Najmaldin AS, Yang G-Z, Darzi A. International attitudes of early adopters to current and future robotic technologies in pediatric surgery. J Pediatr Surg. 2014;49:1522–6.
16. Tzemanaki A, Walters P, Graham Pipe A, Melhuish C, Dogramadzi S. An anthropomorphic design for a minimally invasive surgical system based on a survey of surgical technologies, techniques and training. Int J Med Robot. 2014;10:368–78.
17. Patel SR, Hedican SP, Bishoff JT, Shichman SJ, Link RE, Stuart WJ, Nakada SY. Skill based mentored laparoscopy course participation leads to laparoscopic practice expansion and assists in transition to robotic surgery. J Urol. 2011;186:1997–2000.
18. Chandra V, Nehra D, Parent R, Woo R, Reyes R, Hernandez-Boussard T, Dutta S. A comparison of laparoscopic and robotic assisted suturing performance by experts and novices. Surgery. 2010;147(6):830–9.
19. Sachdeva AK, Buyske J, Dunnington GL, Sanfey HA, Mellinger JD, Scott DJ, Satava R, Fried GM, Jacobs LM, Burns KJ. A new paradigm for surgical procedural training. Curr Probl Surg. 2011;48(12):854–968.
20. Kim I-k, Kang J, Park YA, Kim NK, Sohn S-K, Lee KY. Is prior laparoscopy experience required for adaptation to robotic rectal surgery?: feasibility of one-step transition from open to robotic surgery. Int J Color Dis. 2014;29:693–9.
21. Di Gregorio M, Botnaru A, Bairy L, Lorge F. Passing from open to robotic surgery for dismembered pyeloplasty: a single centre experience. Springerplus. 2014;3:580.

5 Paediatric Robotic Surgery: Complications

Kelvin Y. Wang, Naved Alizai, and Azad Najmaldin

5.1 Introduction

Robotic surgery has been introduced to extend the capabilities of surgeons and address the difficulties and morbidities encountered with laparoscopic surgery (minimal access surgery). The application of robotics to the fields of urological, gastrointestinal, thoracic and trans-oral surgery in children has become increasingly popular since Meininger et al. reported the first case of paediatric robotic Nissen's fundoplication in 2001 [1]. Although great advantages are conferred to the operating surgeon through 3D panoramic high resolution view with depth perception, increased magnification, ability to directly control a stable visual field, increased freedom of movement provided by the multi-jointed instruments, motion scaling and remote nature of operating, robotic surgery in children presents a specific set of associated complications. Most of these are minor and do not significantly alter the outcome. Other complications are similar to those learnt during open and conventional laparoscopic techniques. Prevention is better than cure, and most complications can be avoided by the *alert* and *trained* robotic surgeon.

K.Y. Wang, M.R.C.S.(Eng) (✉) • N. Alizai, F.R.C.S.
A. Najmaldin, F.R.C.S.(Eng), F.R.C.S.(Edin)
Leeds General Infirmary, Leeds Teaching Hospitals NHS Trust, Leeds LS1 3EX, UK
e-mail: Kelvin.wang@nhs.net

A systematic review comprising 2393 robotic procedures spanning several specialties demonstrated an overall rate of conversion to open procedure of 2.5% [2], in comparison with figures of 2.3–7.4% for laparoscopic and thoracoscopic surgery in children [3, 4]. Information allowing direct comparison of complication rates between robot-assisted surgery and laparoscopic/thoracoscopic approach is limited, owing to differences between authors in categorising complications, as well as the subjectivity associated to defining exactly what comprises a surgical complication. Nonetheless, in a multicentre series of 858 paediatric patients undergoing robot-assisted urological surgery, grade III and IVa (Clavien classification) perioperative complication rates were 4.8% and 0.1%, respectively, and grade II complications was 8.2% [5]. The overall complication rate quoted for laparoscopic and thoracoscopic procedures in a series of 2352 children was 3.6% [3].

In this chapter, we aim to discuss the challenges and complications which arise when performing robotic surgery on the paediatric population, and their management.

5.2 Preoperative Considerations

As for open technique and conventional laparoscopic surgery, consideration should be given to the following patient-specific factors:

G. Mattioli, P. Petralia (eds.), *Pediatric Robotic Surgery*, DOI 10.1007/978-3-319-41863-6_5

- Patient selection
- Indications for surgery
- Previous surgery and scarring
- Appropriate written consent including details of the technique, duration of surgery, possibility of conversion and potential complications
- Previous medical history, co-morbidity and risk factors

5.2.1 Theatre Set-Up

While dedicated or even purpose-designed robotic theatres are the best options, the performance of robotic surgery has to be integrated into existing structures in the majority of hospitals. Once the child is transferred onto the operating table, the first task is to ensure the correct positioning of patient, slave cart and equipment tower to optimise surgical access, while maintaining good anaesthetic access, especially to the airway, monitors and intravenous lines (Fig. 5.1). Such a balance will evidently become harder to achieve in small children and neonates, thus highlighting the importance of good communication between the surgeon, anaesthetist and theatre team in patient safety and outcomes [6].

Positioning of the patient, surgeon, theatre team and equipment is dependent on the planned surgical approach—whether trans-oral, intrathoracic, transperitoneal or extraperitoneal. In a 14 year retrospective study of FDA data, improper patient positioning was found to be responsible for 17 (4.1%) of 410 reported cases of iatrogenic injury secondary to robotic procedures [7]. Particular attention should also be given to pressure points, especially if a long operating time is anticipated.

5.2.2 Anaesthesia and Robotic Surgery

Currently, robotic surgery can be performed only under general anaesthesia with endotracheal intubation, controlled ventilation and full muscle relaxation. Patient's movement secondary to inadequate paralysis during robotic surgery may prove dangerous. This is because the functioning arms are fixed to the partially concealed patient, with the surgeon, and to some extent the assistant and anaesthetist, operating remotely. Further, a poorly paralysed patient is impossible to insufflate adequately. Consequently, a safe,

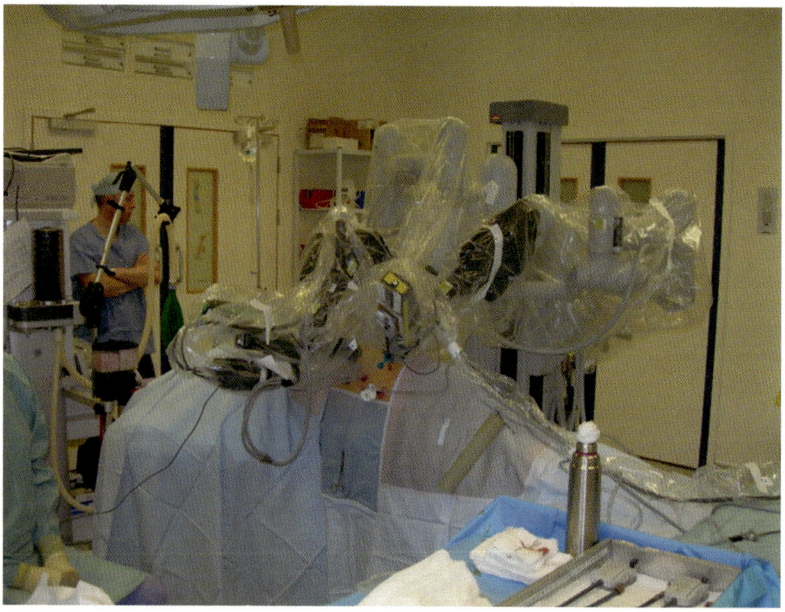

Fig. 5.1 Theatre set-up for a left pyeloplasty: note the position of patient, robotic arms, and anaesthetist. Reproduced with permission from Cundy et al. [2]

effective and successful operating space becomes unachievable.

Gaseous distension of the gastrointestinal tract is another significant problem in robotic surgery and can be a major cause of conversion, complication and failure. This is particularly so in small children and neonates where the operating space is limited and currently available robotic instruments (8 and 12 mm telescopes; 5 and 8 mm metal ports and instruments) are relatively large. Therefore, efforts should be made to minimise the use of gas induction through a mask, as well as nitrous oxide and drugs which can cause intestinal dilatation.

5.2.3 Docking

"Docking" describes the assembly of robotic arms onto the slave cart. Familiarity with hardware and arm movements, along with a well-rehearsed docking routine reduce the total anaesthetic time and minimise risks of iatrogenic injuries and complications. Appropriately docked arms optimise robot and instrument function, prevent the clashing of arms/instruments, and improve access for the surgeon, assistant(s) and anaesthetist. Using the standard Da Vinci system with three port set-up, Najmaldin and Antao reported their learning curve (first 50 paediatric cases) mean docking time of 12 min [8]. In non-complicated cases, their figure has now reduced to 4.8 min. Other authors working with adult populations quote a median docking time of 10 min, with emphasis on surgeon experience as the most important factor in reducing docking times [9, 10]. It would seem reasonable to suspect that experienced surgeons and theatre teams well-versed in docking are also able to de-assemble the robotic arms (undock) efficiently. This is particularly important in situations where time is of the essence—essentially major haemorrhage necessitating conversion.

Some authors regard the size and scale of existing instruments as a source of challenge and potential complications when operating in small children and neonates. Compared to the 3 mm instruments now routinely used in a number of advanced laparoscopic procedures, the variety of 5 and 8 mm instruments commercially available for the Da Vinci system offer less room for manoeuvre in small operative fields, where workspace is already at a premium [11].

5.3 Intraoperative Complications

5.3.1 Establishing Pneumoperitoneum and Port Placement

As in laparoscopic surgery, the establishment of a pneumoperitoneum in robotic surgery is a potential source of intraoperative complication, namely bleeding and injury to hollow viscus. The three traditional methods of creating a pneumoperitoneum and accessing the peritoneal cavity are: the open "Hasson" technique, use of Veress needle and direct insertion of trocar. All have advantages and disadvantages, with the open technique being the most popular amongst the paediatric surgeons [12, 13]. Passerotti et al. reported a complication rate of 0.8% associated with open Hasson technique compared to 2.3% when using the Veress needle, in a series of paediatric urology cases spanning one decade [14]. However, it is interesting to note that in a meta-analysis comparing the methods of peritoneal entry, no single method was found to be superior to others by way of safety and complication rate [15]. In a series of 472 paediatric robotic abdominal procedures, the authors have had no significant injuries related to use of trocar.

Irrespective of the methods of accessing the peritoneal cavity and creation of a pneumoperitoneum, the importance of careful planning and appropriate placement of camera and instrument ports cannot be over-emphasised (Fig. 5.2). This approach will minimise the risks of iatrogenic injury, allow effective economy of movement, and reduce the possibility of requiring additional ports intraoperatively.

In general, the position of the primary (telescope) and working ports are similar to that of conventional laparoscopy. However, an extra

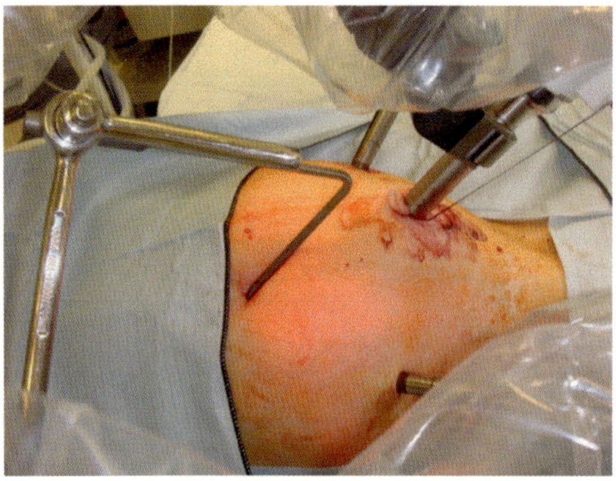

Fig. 5.2 Position of ports with a retractor in situ for robotic liver surgery in a small child

1–2 cm distance between the telescope, working/accessory ports and target organ will improve access and minimise risks of arm/instrument clashing. Care must be taken to avoid inadvertent injury to the abdominal wall vessels and intra-abdominal organs as one would in all minimal access procedures [16].

In abdomens which have undergone previous surgery or where one suspects peritoneal adhesions, an open technique to insert ports should be considered. Subsequent adhesiolysis using conventional laparoscopic or robotic methods may be required.

The 5 mm endoscope for the Da Vinci system is now no longer available due to limitations of depth perception and lack of 3D vision. Due to the size disparity, a 12 mm telescope provides a noticeably clearer picture than the 8.5 mm scope. An angled scope is more versatile than a 0 degree scope. The choice of telescopes is dependent on the surgeon's preference, availability of different sized devices, size of the patient and nature of the procedure to be executed.

Management of access-related vascular and visceral injury depends on the location and extent of injury, surgeon's experience and whether the injuries are detected intra- or post-operatively. In cases of access-related abdominal or thoracic wall bleeding, diathermy coagulation is often sufficient, with suture repair (ligature) being seldom required. Bleeding from the camera port may necessitate relocation of the telescope to an existing instrument port or a different position, with subsequent intervention carried out via the remaining port(s).

Blood emerging from the Veress needle should alert the surgeon of the likely breach of a major vessel, in which case conversion to a laparotomy should be considered. While preparing for laparotomy leaving the Veress needle in situ yields two main benefits: firstly serving as a "guidewire" to the point of injury and secondly, providing a "plug" to the damaged vessel [17]. The same is true for trocar-induced major bleeds.

Minor intra-abdominal haemorrhage can be managed safely using the robotic instruments. The management of significant visceral haemorrhage, however, is dependent on the surgeon's experience, accessibility of haemorrhage site, size of the patient and whether the patient is haemodynamically stable. When in doubt, conversion to an open technique must be considered swiftly. While undocking and preparing for a laparotomy, a pneumoperitoneum should be maintained and ports are left in situ. A visible bleeding point should be compressed or grasped using one or more suitable conventional laparoscopy instruments through the existing or additional ports. Blind diathermy coagulation, suturing or clipping must be avoided.

If access-related bowel injury is suspected, suture repair or resection can safely be accomplished using the robotic instruments, following a thorough inspection.

As for conventional laparoscopy and thoracoscopy, other complications secondary to access include gas embolus [18], subcutaneous or tissue plane carbon dioxide emphysema [19], acidosis, difficulties with ventilation and cardiovascular collapse.

5.3.2 Haptics, Tissue Handling and Damage

Since its inception in late 1990s, the lack of haptic feedback in robotic surgery has consistently been highlighted as a main drawback compared to traditional open (full haptic), and laparoscopic and thoracoscopic (reduced haptic) surgery. The absence of haptics, or tactile feedback, may influence the outcomes of robot-assisted procedures through use of excessive force, inadvertent tissue injury and suboptimal suture tension [20]. Recent reports, however, suggest experienced robotic surgeons are able to compensate significantly for loss of haptic feedback, and that various non-tactile sensory cues are central to this adaptive process [21, 22]. Using the frequency of in vivo suture damage in a series of robot-assisted pyeloplasties in children as a parameter of intraoperative complication, Cundy et al. concluded that experience-related perceptual skills that compensate for haptic loss are likely to be acquirable [22]. In recent years, significant efforts have been invested into application of kinaesthetic technology to robotic surgery, and the advent of systems incorporating haptic feedback could be in the next decade [23].

As with laparoscopic surgery, the fundamentals of safe electrocautery operation must be respected. During monopolar coagulation or cutting, all conducting parts of the working instruments are kept under direct view. This should minimise the risks of accidental collateral damage. Cases of aberrant electrosurgical arcing, and failure of insulating sheaths belonging to monopolar instruments leading to major arterial damage during robot-assisted surgery have previously been reported [24]. Such are reminders to be extra vigilant when employing diathermy in any capacity.

Injury caused by traction/retraction and grasper instruments represents other sources of intraoperative tissue damage at both macroscopic and microscopic (cellular) levels. There is a well-defined relationship between mechanical disruption of tissues and surgical stress [25], which is closely related to systemic inflammatory response syndrome (SIRS), sepsis, organ dysfunction, and ultimately, poor patient outcomes. The choice of instruments, especially the graspers, should be geared toward being as least traumatic as possible. Chang et al. express their preference for the PreCise™ bipolar forceps over Maryland and Debakey forceps for paediatric robotic procedures, citing their ability for gentle tissue handling [12]. Total duration of tissue handling should also be minimised, as it has been shown that this can result in a greater degree of histological change [26]. Traction injury and injury secondary to instrument exchange account for 0.5% of complications in robot-assisted paediatric urology procedures [5].

Published multi-institutional and unified multi-specialty data on the prevalence of intraoperative bowel and vascular injury in paediatric robotic surgery is limited. In a comprehensive multi-institutional paediatric robotic urology study, Dangle et al. (2015) reported rates of 0.3% for intraoperative vascular injury and 0.1% for injury to other viscera [5]. Smaller single institutional studies in robot-assisted paediatric general surgery and urology have quoted intraoperative rates of haemorrhage as 0–9% [27–29]. In our series of 472 infants and children (weight range 4.1–97 kg) who underwent robotic surgery for variety of gastrointestinal, hepatobiliary and urological conditions, we have had no major intraoperative vascular or intestinal injuries.

As already discussed, the importance of training, patient selection, dedicated theatre(s), an experienced theatre team, well-planned placement of trocars and ports, and appropriate use of instruments, diathermy as well as other energy sources cannot be over-emphasised. Minor bleeding is managed easily using diathermy—monopolar or bipolar, sealing devices, clips, suture ligature or suturing techniques. The management of major bleeds are dependent on circumstances and surgeon's experience. Intraoperative bowel injuries are usually amenable to a straightforward repair using a non-absorbable suture with robotic instruments. However, where injury is extensive or is implicated by ischaemia, resection with or without stoma formation should be considered.

The large majority of procedures can be completed despite intraoperative complication, but in uncertain situations or when the patient becomes haemodynamically unstable, the robotic procedure should be converted to an open technique.

5.3.3 Robotic System Failure

A number of technological pitfalls are associated with the use of robotic operating systems. In a reported series of 10,000 robotic surgery adverse events, Alemzadeh et al. found 75.9% were due to issues with hardware, software or a combination [7]. The most common type of system malfunction was detachment of instrument pieces into the patient's body (14.7%) accounting for one death. This was followed by electrosurgical complications (10.5%), unintended movement of instruments (10.1%, two deaths) and imaging/other software errors (7.4%) [7]. The overall device failure rate is reported to be 0.4–10.9% [30–32]. The authors have never witnessed intraoperative detachment of instrument pieces or injuries secondary to unintended robotic instrument movements in their series of several hundred cases of paediatric robotic procedures over a 10 year period. It has also been reported that the rates of system malfunction is reduced over time, an attribute of the theatre team learning process [31].

Most system malfunctions can be bypassed during the course of surgery (76%) [31], although this is not always the case. Solutions come under four main categories: postponement of procedure, system reset, replacement of device and conversion. If system failure is detected preoperatively the surgeon may exercise the following choices: postpone the procedure all together, or carry out the procedure using a laparoscope or an open technique. Such circumstances are to be discussed with patients and families preoperatively. Zorn et al. proposes a policy to ensure system functionality prior to induction in order to prevent futile anaesthesia [32]. System reset is mostly used as a solution in cases of software malfunction (43.1%) and video/imaging failure (19.3%) [7].

5.3.4 Conversion

As previously highlighted, the overall rate of conversion to an open technique in robotic-assisted paediatric surgery is 2.5% [2], compared to 2.3–7.4% in laparoscopic and thoracoscopic surgery in children [3, 4]. The frequency of conversion during robot-assisted operations varies between specialties; the lowest reported rates are in urology (1.5%), with gastrointestinal and thoracic procedure rates being 3.9% and 10%, respectively [2]. This variation is probably experience related within the named subspecialties. In their first 267 cases of robotic urological and gastrointestinal procedures (age range 6 weeks–16 years), the authors' conversion rate was 4.4%, of which one in six were for surgical complications.

The reasons for converting can be categorised into three main groups:

1. *Surgical error and iatrogenic injury*. Potential factors leading to inadvertent intraoperative and access-related injuries include learning curve of the surgeon and theatre team, poor patient or procedure selection, inadequate instrumentation and suboptimal anaesthetic techniques (e.g. gaseous intestinal distention and poor muscle relaxation).
2. *Inherent technical difficulties* encompassing complex surgery, internal adhesions [33], abnormal anatomy and obesity [34].
3. *Robotic system failure* accounting for software and hardware malfunction. The disparity between the size of patient and size of instrument can occasionally become a problem. This is particularly so in infants and neonates, and in intra-vesical procedures.

The robotic procedure may be converted to a laparoscopic or an open operation depending on the surgeon's preference and experience, and the circumstances that lead to conversion. For example, a haemodynamically unstable situation can only be converted to an open technique, while a computer or robotic instrument failure can be converted to a laparoscopic technique. Provided the surgeon has adequate experience, the pre-existing robotic ports may be used in certain situations, but not all. As always, the possibility of conversion must be clearly noted in the preoperative decision-making process and while consenting the patient for the procedure.

5.4 Post-operative Complications

Post-operative complications can be subdivided into those applicable to all robot-assisted surgery in general, and those which are specialty specific.

They range from trivial and self-limiting Clavien grade I complications to grade V (death of a patient). For the most part, generic complications we discuss in this section can be managed identically to those occurring after conventional laparoscopic surgery and in some instances, open technique surgery.

5.4.1 Post-operative Bleeding and Intestinal Injury

As with all surgical procedures, conventional open or laparoscopic, these complications can happen as the consequences of unrecognised intraoperative injuries. Bleeding and perforation of viscera can present late with hypotension, tachycardia or anaemia, or signs of intra-abdominal infection (peritonism and systemic sepsis), respectively. These may result in serious morbidity or even death, so the importance of appropriate post-operative observation and early management of suspected injury cannot be stressed enough. Insufflation pressure may slow the speed of mild to moderate bleeding or leak from a small hollow viscus perforation as such that they can easily be missed at the time of surgery. Therefore, a thorough inspection of the operative field with a lowered insufflation pressure at the end of all robotic (and conventional laparoscopic) procedures may prove helpful and reassuring. Other than direct inadvertent intraoperative trauma, as outlined above, late complications could also arise from inappropriately applied sutures or clips, as well as ischaemia secondary to poor dissection or thermal injuries.

In the aforementioned series of children, the authors have not experienced any instances of missed or late post-operative robot-related bleeding or perforation.

Most patients with a suspected late complication can be managed expectantly after assessment. It is worth noting that residual CO_2 pneumoperitoneum and surgical emphysema may persist for a number of days and plain film X-rays in this period are misleading [35, 36]. Re-do robotic exploration or conventional laparoscopy are valid options, and are dependent on the individual circumstances and clinician's expertise. Open technique re-do surgery is an alternative approach.

5.4.2 Post-operative Ileus

Nearly all children exhibit a mild to moderate degree of ileus following routine robotic abdominal surgery. The degree of distension can be alarming at times, but rarely a source of pain or distress. Dangle et al. reported a prevalence of approximately 1% for robotic urological procedures, equating to 20% of all recorded Clavien grade I complications [5]. An increased and more protracted episode of ileus is expected with gastrointestinal and contaminated procedures.

In children, the vast majority settle spontaneously within 12–36 h of minimal, if any, treatment. A delayed fluid and food intake for 24 h or less may be required in some. Insertion of a nasogastric tube or blood tests for measurement of electrolytes are almost never required following straightforward and routine surgery.

However, the possibility of bleeding and perforation presenting post-operatively should be considered in all children who suffer:

- Ileus and abnormal vital signs (unexpected tachycardia, high temperature or hypotension)
- Ileus and significant abdominal pain
- Deteriorating or significant ileus not responding to simple measures beyond 36 h

5.4.3 Wound Infection

As with all paediatric minimal access procedures, post-operative wound infection is rare. Hermsen et al. (2010) have reported 5.9% as an overall figure for port site infection in adults [37]. A much higher rate is evident in gastrointestinal procedures, six times greater when compared to prostate and genitourinary procedures [37]. Prophylactic antibiotics may be used if contamination is suspected.

5.4.4 Port Site Hernia

Port site hernia is a rare complication following laparoscopic and robot-assisted surgery. In paediatric laparoscopic and robotic urology, the incidence is reported to be 0.5–3.2% [38, 39]. Literature demonstrates statistically higher rates of port site hernia in young children and infants, due to the smallness of bowel calibre relative to the standard sized laparoscopic ports [39, 40]. The importance of residual intra-peritoneal carbon dioxide in herniating intra-abdominal contents during the post-operative period has also been highlighted [39]. Surgical repair is expected in all, but the nature and timing of surgery undertaken are dependent on individual cases.

To reduce the risks of post-operative port site herniation, we recommend:

- Using small sized ports (5 mm) in infants, if possible.
- Closing (in layers) all port sites which are 5 mm or greater in infants, and 8–12 mm in older children.
- Firstly removing the working instruments and ports under direct vision, followed by the telescope port, if port site closure is not possible.

Applying this regimen, the authors have had no reported cases of robotic port site hernia in several hundred infants and children.

5.4.5 Specialty Complications of Robotic Surgery

To date, urology forms the majority of experience in robot-assisted paediatric surgery, comprising 60% of all reported cases between 2001 and 2012 [2]. Of these, over three-quarters were robot-assisted pyeloplasty and ureteric reimplantation procedures. Migration of ureteric stent is the most common significant post-operative complication (1.6–5%) reported in paediatric robotic urology [41–43]. Urine leak, infection and urinoma formation are the second commonest reported complications following pyeloplasty (1.5%) [41], reimplantation of ureter and nephrectomy. These complications are not necessarily robot specific and should be managed expectantly. Post-pyeloplasty recurrent obstruction is reported to be around 0–3%, figures which compare favourably to those of laparoscopic and open techniques [41, 44]. Many authors are proponents of the robot-assisted re-do pyeloplasty (secondary pyeloplasty) due to the relative ease of negotiating adhesions, fine manipulation and re-do anastomosis compared to a laparoscopic or even an open approach [41, 43, 45].

The role of robotics in general surgery is less well defined, with robot-assisted fundoplication for gastric reflux being the commonest reported procedure to 2012—approximately one-third of the total robotic procedures reported in children [2]. In a series of 57 robotic paediatric fundoplications, Cundy et al. reported three instances of Clavien grade III complications, including two cases of wrap failure requiring re-do fundoplication [46]. The authors were able to successfully complete both re-do cases robotically. Toolboom et al. (2016) reported a 2% incidence of oesophageal perforation and 4% for gastric perforation in 45 patients undergoing robotic fundoplication [47].

5.5 Summary

The risks of intra- and post-operative complications in paediatric robotic surgery are low but can be further lessened by:

- Appropriate training of surgeons and theatre team
- Proper patient selection
- Good instrumentation
- Appropriate anaesthetic techniques (full muscle relaxation and avoiding mechanically or pharmacologically induced gaseous distension of the gastrointestinal tract)
- Routine use of open technique insertion of the telescope port
- Insertion of working ports under vision
- Insertion, movement and removal of all instruments and sharp objects/needles under vision

- Application of sound principles of surgery including manipulation, dissection, clipping and suturing
- Understanding safe usage of electro coagulation and other energy sources
- Understanding and appreciation of the lack of tactile feedback (haptics) in robotic surgery
- Final inspection of the operative field for several minutes
- Closure of port sites in layers (5–12 mm ports in infants and 8–12 mm ports in older children)
- Appropriate post-operative observation, management and follow-up

Conclusion

Paediatric robotic surgery is still in its infancy. A recurring theme from our review of literature is that most authors have identified initial complication rates as a product of the initial learning curve, and many have reported improvements with experience. As with all aspects of medicine and surgery, underreporting of adverse events remains an issue [48]. Despite this, there appears to be little disagreement that telerobotic surgery is safe and will be the centre of future paediatric urological, gastrointestinal and thoracic surgery.

References

1. Meininger DD, Byhahn C, Heller K, Gutt CN, Westphal K. Totally endoscopic Nissen fundoplication with a robotic system in a child. Surg Endosc. 2001;15(11):1360.
2. Cundy TP, Shetty K, Clark J, Chang TP, Sriskandarajah K, Gattas NE, Najmaldin A, Yang GZ, Darzi A. The first decade of robotic surgery in children. J Pediatr Surg. 2013;48(4):858–65.
3. Adikibi BT, Mackinlay GA, Clark MC, Duthie GH, Munro FD. The risks of minimal access surgery in children: an aid to consent. J Pediatr Surg. 2012;47(3):601–5.
4. te Velde EA, Bax NM, Tytgat SH, de Jong JR, Travassos DV, Kramer WL, van der Zee DC. Minimally invasive pediatric surgery: increasing implementation in daily practice and resident's training. Surg Endosc. 2008;22(1):163–6.
5. Dangle PP, Akhavan A, Odeleye M, Avery D, Lendvay T, Koh CJ, Elder JS, Noh PH, Bansal D, Schulte M, MacDonald J, Shukla A, Kim C, Herbst K, Corbett S, Kearns J, Kunnavakkam R, Gundeti MS. Ninety-day perioperative complications of pediatric robotic urological surgery: a multi-institutional study. J Pediatr Urol. 2016;12(2):102.e1–6.
6. Hsu RL, Kaye AD, Urman RD. Anesthetic challenges in robotic-assisted urologic surgery. Rev Urol. 2013;15(4):178–84.
7. Alemzadeh H, Raman J, Leveson N, Kalbarczyk Z, Iyer RK. Adverse events in robotic surgery: a retrospective study of 14 years of FDA data. PLoS One. 2016;11(4):e0151470.
8. Najmaldin A, Antao B. Early experience of telerobotic surgery in children. Int J Med Robot. 2007;3(3):199–202.
9. Iranmanesh P, Morel P, Wagner OJ, Inan I, Pugin F, Hagen ME. Set-up and docking of the da Vinci surgical system: prospective analysis of initial experience. Int J Med Robot. 2010;6(1):57–60.
10. Iranmanesh P, Morel P, Buchs NC, Pugin F, Volonte F, Kreaden US, Hagen ME. Docking of the da Vinci Si Surgical System® with single-site technology. Int J Med Robot. 2013;9(1):12–6.
11. Bruns NE, Soldes OS, Ponsky TA. Robotic surgery may not "Make the Cut" in pediatrics. Front Pediatr. 2015;3:10.
12. Chang C, Steinberg Z, Shah A, Gundeti MS. Patient positioning and port placement for Robotic-Assisted Surgery. J Endourol. 2014;28(6):631–8.
13. Chao SYC, Tan HL. General principles of laparoscopic access. In: Spitz L, Coran A, editors. Operative paediatric surgery. 7th ed. New York: CRC Press; 2014. p. 333–6.
14. Passerotti CC, Nguyen HT, Retik AB, Peters CA. Patterns and predictors of laparoscopic complications in pediatric urology: the role of ongoing surgical volume and access techniques. J Urol. 2008;180(2):681–5.
15. Ahmad G, O'Flynn H, Duffy JMN, Phillips K, Watson A. Laparoscopic entry techniques. Cochrane Database of Systematic Reviews 2012, Issue 2. Art. No.: CD006583.
16. Epstein J, Arora A, Ellis H. Surface anatomy of the inferior epigastric artery in relation to laparoscopic injury. Clin Anat. 2004;17(5):400–8.
17. Usal H, Sayad P, Hayek N, Hallak A, Huie F, Ferzli G. Major vascular injuries during laparoscopic cholecystectomy. An institutional review of experience with 2589 procedures and literature review. Surg Endosc. 1998;12(7):960–2.
18. Mattei P, Tyler DC. Carbon dioxide embolism during laparoscopic cholecystectomy due to a patent paraumbilical vein. J Pediatr Surg. 2007;42(3):570–2.
19. Ott DE. Subcutaneous emphysema—beyond the pneumoperitoneum. JSLS. 2014;18(1):1–7.
20. Wagner CR, Howe RD. Force feedback benefit depends on experience in multiple degree of freedom robotic surgery task. IEEE Trans Robot. 2007;23(6):1235–40.
21. Meccariello G, Faedi F, AlGhamdi S, Montevecchi F, Firinu E, Zanotti C, Cavaliere D, Gunelli R, Taurchini M,

Amadori A, Vicini C. An experimental study about haptic feedback in robotic surgery: may visual feedback substitute tactile feedback? J Robot Surg. 2016;10(1):57–61.
22. Cundy TP, Gattas NE, Yang GZ, Darzi A, Najmaldin AS. Experience related factors compensate for haptic loss in robot-assisted laparoscopic surgery. J Endourol. 2014;28(5):532–8.
23. Okamura AM. Haptic feedback in robot-assisted minimally invasive surgery. Curr Opin Urol. 2009; 19(1):102–7.
24. Cormier B, Nezhat F, Sternchos J, Sonoda Y, Leitao MM Jr. Electrocautery-associated vascular injury during robotic-assisted surgery. Obstet Gynecol. 120(2 Pt 2): 491–3.
25. Miyake H, Kawabata G, Gotoh A, Fujisawa M, Okada H, Arakawa S, Kamidono S, Hara I. Comparison of surgical stress between laparoscopy and open surgery in the field of urology by measurement of humoral mediators. Int J Urol. 2002;9(6):329–33.
26. Marucci DD, Shakeshaft AJ, Cartmill JA, Cox MR, Adams SG, Martin CJ. Grasper trauma during laparoscopic cholecystectomy. Aust N Z J Surg. 2000;70(8):578–81.
27. Bansal D, Defoor WR Jr, Reddy PP, Minevich EA, Noh PH. Complications of robotic surgery in pediatric urology: a single institution experience. Urology. 2013;82(4):917–20.
28. Camps JI. The use of robotics in pediatric surgery: my initial experience. Pediatr Surg Int. 2011;27(9):991–6.
29. Marhuenda C, Giné C, Asensio M, Guillén G, Martínez Ibáñez V. Robotic surgery: first pediatric series in Spain. Cir Pediatr. 2011;24(2):90–2.
30. Andonian S, Okeke Z, Okeke DA, Rastinehad A, Vanderbrink BA, Richstone L, Lee BR. Device failures associated with patient injuries during robot-assisted laparoscopic surgeries: a comprehensive review of FDA MAUDE database. Can J Urol. 2008;15(1):3912–6.
31. Nayyar R, Gupta NP. Critical appraisal of technical problems with robotic urological surgery. BJU Int. 2010;105(12):1710–3.
32. Zorn KC, Gofrit ON, Orvieto MA, Mikhail AA, Galocy RM, Shalhav AL, Zagaja GP. Da Vinci robot error and failure rates: single institution experience on a single three-arm robot unit of more than 700 consecutive robot-assisted laparoscopic radical prostatectomies. J Endourol. 2007;21(11):1341–4.
33. Bhama AR, Wafa AM, Ferraro J, Collins SD, Mullard AJ, Vandewarker JF, Krapohl G, Byrn JC, Cleary RK. Comparison of risk factors for unplanned conversion from laparoscopic and robotic to open colorectal surgery using the Michigan Surgical Quality Collaborative (MSQC) Database. J Gastrointest Surg. 2016;20(6):1223–30.
34. Jiménez Rodríguez RM, De la Portilla De Juan F, Díaz Pavón JM, Rodríguez Rodríguez A, Prendes Sillero E, Cadet Dussort JM, Padillo J. Analysis of conversion factors in robotic-assisted rectal cancer surgery. Int J Color Dis. 2014;29(6):701–8.
35. Draper K, Jefson R, Jongeward R Jr, McLeod M. Duration of postlaparoscopic pneumoperitoneum. Surg Endosc. 1997;11(8):809–11.
36. Smith KS, Wilson TC, Luces L, Stevenson AA, Hajhosseini B, Siram SM. Pneumoperitoneum 48 days after laparoscopic hysterectomy. JSLS. 2013;17(4):661–4.
37. Hermsen ED, Hinze T, Sayles H, Sholtz L, Rupp ME. Incidence of surgical site infection associated with robotic surgery. Infect Control Hosp Epidemiol. 2010;31(8):822–7.
38. Tapscott A, Kim SS, White S, Graves R, Kraft K, Casale P. Port-site complications after pediatric urologic robotic surgery. J Robot Surg. 2009;3:187.
39. Cost NG, Lee J, Snodgrass WT, Harrison CB, Wilcox DT, Baker LA. Hernia after pediatric urological laparoscopy. J Urol. 2010;183(3):1163–7.
40. Paya K, Wurm J, Fakhari M, Felder-Puig R, Puig S. Trocar-site hernia as a typical postoperative complication of minimally invasive surgery among preschool children. Surg Endosc. 2008;22(12):2724–7.
41. Mufarrij PW, Woods M, Shah OD, Palese MA, Berger AD, Thomas R, Stifelman MD. Robotic dismembered pyeloplasty: a 6-year, multi-institutional experience. J Urol. 2008;180(4):1391–6.
42. Gupta NP, Nayyar R, Hemal AK, Mukherjee S, Kumar R, Dogra PN. Outcome analysis of robotic pyeloplasty: a large single-centre experience. BJU Int. 2010;105(7):980–3.
43. Minnillo BJ, Cruz JA, Sayao RH, Passerotti CC, Houck CS, Meier PM, Borer JG, Diamond DA, Retik AB, Nguyen HT. Long-term experience and outcomes of robotic assisted laparoscopic pyeloplasty in children and young adults. J Urol. 2011;185(4):1455–60.
44. Schwentner C, Pelzer A, Neururer R, Springer B, Horninger W, Bartsch G, Peschel R. Robotic Anderson-Hynes pyeloplasty: 5-year experience of one centre. BJU Int. 2007;100(4):880–5.
45. Hemal AK, Mishra S, Mukharjee S, Suryavanshi M. Robot assisted laparoscopic pyeloplasty in patients of ureteropelvic junction obstruction with previously failed open surgical repair. Int J Urol. 2008;15(8):744–6.
46. Cundy TP, Rowland SP, Gattas NE, White AD, Najmaldin AS. The learning curve of robot-assisted laparoscopic fundoplication in children: a prospective evaluation and CUSUM analysis. Int J Med Robot. 2015;11(2):141–9.
47. Tolboom RC, Draaisma WA, Broeders IA. Evaluation of conventional laparoscopic versus robot-assisted laparoscopic redo hiatal hernia and antireflux surgery: a cohort study. J Robot Surg. 2016;10(1):33–9.
48. Cooper MA, Ibrahim A, Lyu H, Makary MA. Underreporting of robotic surgery complications. J Healthc Qual. 2015;37(2):133–8.

6 Paediatric Anaesthesia in Laparoscopic and Robotic Surgery

Nicola Disma, Rachele Bonfiglio, and Giovanni Montobbio

Video-assisted surgery was born at the beginning of the century and more widely diffused from the 1960s, principally to respond to the need to perform surgeries applying less invasive methodologies. In the following years, thanks to increasingly technologically advanced equipment, there has been an expansion of clinical indications, until you get to its daily use in paediatrics, in children as infants.

From the anaesthesiologist's point of view, we have to consider that the video-assisted surgery involves a large number of physiological modifications mainly related to cardio-respiratory dynamics and due to the patient's health status, the patient's position on the operating room table and the insufflation of gas in the abdominal cavity. For all this reasons, it is important that the anaesthesiologist knows all the physio-pathological changes during laparoscopic surgery in order to prevent them with the careful application of vital signs monitoring, especially in children in order to deliver the best anaesthetic care and promote patient safety [1].

N. Disma (✉) • R. Bonfiglio • G. Montobbio
Department of Pediatric Anesthesia, Giannina Gaslini Institute, Genoa, Italy
e-mail: nicoladisma@tin.it

6.1 Laparoscopic Surgery

6.1.1 Advantages

Laparoscopic surgery is nowadays considered a safe and well-tolerated approach, widely applied to most of the paediatric surgical patients and it has many advantages if compared to "open surgery":

- Smaller surgical incisions with better cosmetic results and therefore greater patient acceptance
- Reduced post-operative pain with less need for analgesic drugs
- Magnified view of the surgical field that allow improved visualization of some difficult areas (pelvis, subphrenic spaces and thoracic apices)
- Fewer post-operative respiratory complications
- Fewer wound complications and fewer adhesions
- A short period of post-operative ileus
- Less fluid loss
- Earlier post-operative mobilization
- Quicker recovery from surgery
- A short hospital stay with benefits both to the work of parents and the child's absence from school

G. Mattioli, P. Petralia (eds.), *Pediatric Robotic Surgery*, DOI 10.1007/978-3-319-41863-6_6

6.1.2 Disadvantages

While the length of hospital stay decreased, other surgical time increases in inverse proportion to the experience of the surgeon performing the procedure. Laparoscopic surgery is particularly difficult in infants because of the smaller operative field: we have instruments with limited degrees of freedom, two-dimensional vision with an assistant-dependent unstable video camera platform and amplification of natural tremor [2, 3]. In addition, surgical equipment has very high costs.

6.2 Robotic Surgery

6.2.1 Advantages

Robotic-assisted surgery is an evolutionary step in the advancement of minimally invasive surgical procedures. Nowadays there are two surgical robotic systems commercially available: the Zeus® surgical system and the da Vinci® surgical system, and they both offer further advantages over the laparoscopic technique [4, 5]:

- High-quality vision
- Improved operative field visibility, thanks to a three-dimensional stereoscopic view similar to open surgery that allows a more natural orientation between the structures of thoracic/abdominal cavity
- A magnification of the operating field on the surgeon's console of 10 times the natural vision (da Vinci® Surgical System) for a better visibility of difficult-to-reach areas
- Instruments with 7 degrees of motion to mimic human dexterity and improved control of fine movements
- Improved ergonomic position of the surgeon
- A safety feature built into the system: an infrared sensor crossing the plane of the viewer; the console will not move any of the robotic surgical arms unless the surgeon is in position to view the surgical field [6] (Fig. 6.1).

All these elements appear to enhance surgical precision [7].

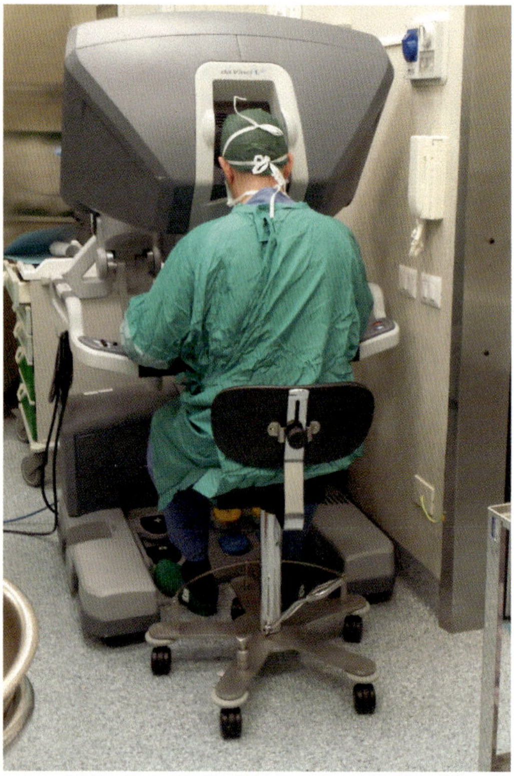

Fig. 6.1 Giannina Gaslini Institute-Genova

6.2.2 Disadvantages

One of the biggest disadvantages which severely limits the choice of this technique compared to laparoscopic one consists in a longer surgical time compared to the first due to two principal reasons: first, the time required for the positioning of the robot's mechanical arms (Fig. 6.2); second, longer operating time especially in the early stages of the learning curve. A drawback of the system is that it does not give the surgeon tactile feedback (ability to sense changes in tissue density or elasticity), although there is some sense of force feedback. Not the last to be considered is that several pieces of equipment require a large amount of precious operating room space because of the large size of robot itself and the positioning of the robotic arms in order to avoid collision with its own arms, assistants and/or the patient. Cost may also be another problem. The relatively limited selection of instruments and the size of the device

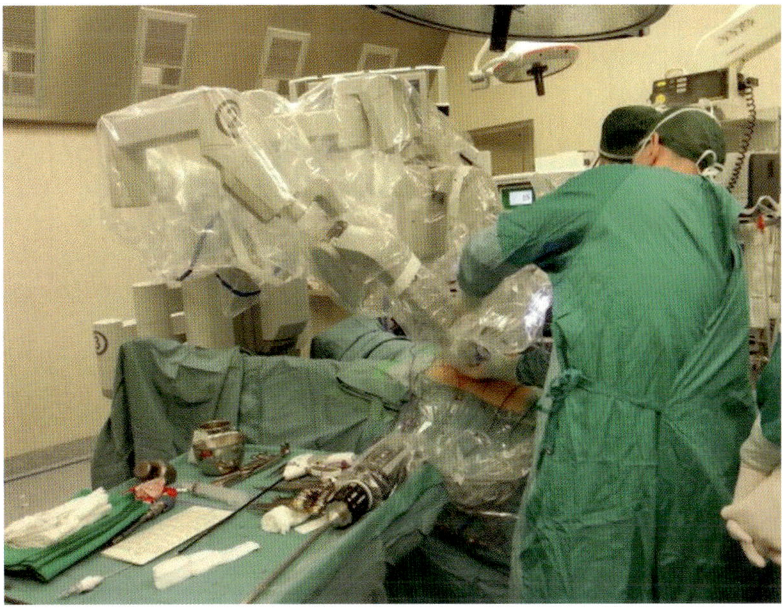

Fig. 6.2 Giannina Gaslini Institute-Genova

port sites, which should be separated by a minimal distance of 46 cm, are emphasized as limitations for its use in small children [8].

6.3 Indications

Most of the video-assisted surgical procedures are similar to that performed in "open". What changes is only the method to access to the surgical area.

Nowadays there are a lot of procedures performed using the laparoscopic method:

- On the digestive system:
  - Nissen fundoplication
  - Gastrostomy
  - Cholecystectomy
  - Appendectomy
  - Treatment of Hirschsprung's disease
  - Intestinal perforations
- On the genitourinary tract:
  - Varicocele
  - Nephrectomy
  - Orchiectomy
  - Ureterolitotomia
- In the abdomen:
  - Splenectomy
  - Adrenalectomy
  - Exploratory laparoscopy
- In the thorax:
  - Lobectomies
  - Biopsies of mediastinal mass
  - Oesophageal surgery

Robotic surgery has its own strengths particularly in paediatric urologic surgery whenever the operational field is limited owing to the small abdominal cavity of children.

6.4 Contraindications

The child who undergoes video-assisted intervention must be in physical condition to withstand the cardio-respiratory changes associated with this method. This shows a whole series of contraindications associated with the clinical condition of the child:

- Severe congenital heart disease not surgically treated
- Impaired cardiac function (EF <60%)
- Pulmonary hypertension
- Acute and chronic broncho-pulmonary diseases
- Coagulopathy

There is also a whole range of surgical contraindications related to infectious, anatomical or systemic problems, in the presence of which is better to prefer an open surgical technique.

6.5 Pathophysiology

6.5.1 Pneumoperitoneum

Laparoscopy requires the formation of a working area within the peritoneal cavity. This is achieved by the insufflation of a gas that distends the peritoneal space. This produces an increase in intra-abdominal pressure (IAP) which is dependent on the compliance of the abdominal cavity and the volume of gas insufflated.

Over the past years, many gases have been tested and today the carbon dioxide (CO_2) is the agent of choice. CO_2 is very soluble in the blood (minimizing the risk of air embolism), is colourless, is easily eliminated by the pulmonary circulation, is non-toxic, non-flammable (so it does not interfere with the electrocautery) and it has a low cost. At the same time, however, CO_2 causes peritoneal irritation (with subsequent pain) and therefore it is easily diffusible; then, during laparoscopic surgery, in addition to the pressure effects caused by the increase of the IAP and the effects related to the position of the patient on the operating room table, we have to consider the pharmacological effects related to absorption of this gas.

6.5.2 Pharmacological Effects of CO_2

Carbon dioxide is easily diffusible through the peritoneal membrane and reaches the lung through the portal and systemic venous circulation. It is estimated that during laparoscopic surgery the load of CO_2 to dispose increases from 7 to 30%; this leads quickly to hypercapnic acidosis because of the inability of the organism to respond to an acute increase of CO_2: renal compensation indeed, high efficiency, takes hours to activate, otherwise the cell buffers, much quicker to intervene, have limited efficiency. The CO_2 overload is then accumulated in the body into three compartments: alveolar-blood, muscles and bones.

The effects of hypercapnia will mainly affect the CNS and cardiovascular system causing vasodilatation (increased cerebral blood flow) with increased intracranial pressure from one side and reflected catecholamines hypersecretion with an increased cardiac output on the other. At extreme levels CO_2 causes, on the contrary, cardio depression.

6.5.3 Cardiovascular Effects

The haemodynamic effects of PN are the consequence of several factors: hypercapnia, increased IAP, patient volaemia and position of the patient on the operating room table during the procedure.

At an early stage of creation of the PN, at IAP values less than 7 mmHg (right atrial pressure), there is an increase in cardiac output for squeezing of the venous vessels in the splanchnic circulation and increasing of venous return. When the IAP exceeds 15 mmHg, the consequent compression of the inferior vena cava reduces preload and thus the cardiac output.

In both cases there is an increase in systemic vascular resistance due to the release of catecholamines and vasoactive hormones (vasopressin) induced by hypercapnia, thanks to the Mean Arterial Pressure (MAP) which remains in the normal range. In addition we have to consider that, while the *trendelenburg* (head-down) position promotes venous return, the anti-trendelenburg (head-up) favours the decrease in cardiac output, as well as hypovolaemia accentuates the effects of the pneumoperitoneum while hypervolaemia seems to prevent them.

Recent studies agree to observe that, up to 12 mmHg of IAP in anti-Trendelenburg, there are not significant haemodynamic changes.

In neonates and children under 4 months of age, an IAP of greater than 15 mmHg may seriously impair cardiac output due to a decrease in contractility and compliance of the left ventricle. An IAP of no more than 6–8 mmHg was recommended in this age group [9].

Comparing studies of Mattioli & Co [10] with those of Meininger & Co [11] we can see as the total intravenous anaesthesia provides a greater haemodynamic stability than inhaled (in the first the heart rate does not change).

6.5.4 Respiratory Effects

During laparoscopic procedures, the increase in IAP enhances the cranial displacement of the diaphragm, which is even more exacerbated by the cephalad shift of the abdominal organs in a head-down position. This may lead to a dramatic reduction in lung volumes, static compliance and functional residual capacity (FRC) below the closing volume, which predisposes to airway closure, atelectasis and to an increase of peak airway pressure, plateau pressure, intrathoracic pressure and in the dead space to tidal volume ratio [12, 13].

The increase of dead space is due to the decrease in cardiac output that reduces lung perfusion in the normally well-perfused areas (II and III West's zone) and to the reduction in lung compliance that entails a redistribution of the gaseous flow to areas not perfused (and more distensible).

Direct consequence of all these changes is an alteration of the ventilation/perfusion ratio resulting in hypoxia and/or opening of a right-left intrapulmonary shunt.

These effects are all more pronounced in children, and they are maximized in newborns and infants in which, despite the consumption of oxygen is greater, respiratory reserves are significantly reduced. These conditions are exacerbated by the Trendelenburg position and mitigated by anti-Trendelenburg.

A fundamental element in the determinism of the respiratory effects during laparoscopy is the CO_2 portion absorbed. It depends on the extent and perfusion of the absorbent surface, but especially on the diffusibility of CO_2 which increases in direct proportion to the pressure of insufflation and duration of its application. It is seen that, on average, in an organism with normal ventilatory function, during a long laparoscopy, ventilation alone is no longer sufficient for disposal of excess CO_2 rate, which accumulates in muscles and bones. It is possible to delete it only in the postoperative in a gradual manner.

Particular attention should be given to children younger than 4 years in which, given the lower distance between absorbent membrane and capillaries, and given the high absorption surface in relation to body weight, the CO_2 absorption takes place in a much more rapid and increased way if compared to the adult.

6.5.5 Effects on Renal Function

At levels of IAP > 15 mmHg hourly diuresis contraction occurs for decrease in renal plasma flow and glomerular filtration fraction. All this is accompanied by an increase of the enzyme N-acetyl-glucosaminidase in urine that is then used as diagnostic marker of proximal tubule damage.

These effects have been attributed to multiple causes: reduced cardiac output, compression of the renal parenchyma and renal vessels, temperature, CO_2 insufflated, increased ADH and plasma renin activity. These changes have proven to be all transient, returning to normal within a few hours after the end of surgery.

6.5.6 Effects on Other Organs

The PN decrease portal vein flow, hepatic vein flow, total hepatic blood flow and flow through the hepatic microcirculation but there are not changes in hepatic arterial flow.

The PN decreases gastric pH, mesenteric blood flow and gastrointestinal microcirculation blood flow.

6.6 Anaesthesia

6.6.1 Preparation

The pre-anaesthesia assessment does not differ from that for the general paediatric surgery and laparoscopic surgery. Consequently, children should continue medications, as for other surgical operations.

6.6.2 Positioning on the Operating Room Table

The correct positioning of the patient on the operating room table is a crucial time for various reasons: it allows the surgeon an optimum exposure of the area to approach surgically and minimizes the risk of causing internal organ injury during insertion of trocars and surgical instruments. Retroperitoneal organs interventions and procedures in the chest require a lateral position, for the upper abdomen is preferred instead the supine position in anti-Trendelenburg, procedures in the pelvis are usually done in the lithotomy and steep Trendelenburg positions.

When the patient is positioned, we have to consider that the operating room table can be modified in the course of intervention: generally it starts in supine position for the creation of the PN, then later, the surgeon decides what kind of inclination to give to the operating room table; so we need to pay attention to the haemodynamic and respiratory consequences subsequent to the Trendelenburg or anti-Trendelenburg position. Many laparoscopic surgical procedures require extreme patient positioning in order to take advantage of gravitational effects that allows movement of obstructing organs from the surgical field. Since extreme positioning often increases the risk of patient sliding off on the operating room table, restraints must be used.

6.6.3 Monitoring

What kind of intraoperative monitoring to prefer depends on the preoperative clinical condition of the child and the type of surgery that must be applied.

In case of minor surgery and ASA I/II risk standard monitoring is required: ECG, non-invasive blood pressure, pulse oximetry, capnography, inspiratory peak airway pressure, naso-pharyngeal temperature, inspiratory oxygen fraction and diuresis. Generally in laparoscopic interventions performed on adults the $ETCO_2$ is considered essential reference value to change the parameters of minute ventilation according to the levels of CO_2 absorbed.

In children suffering from conditions that cause an altered ventilation/perfusion ratio, in infants (that have reduced functional residual capacity and increased alveolar dead space), in all that condition in which the dead space is increased by an excessive IAP or when there is a collapse of cardiac output, $ETCO_2$ is not considered a reliable indicator because it is still far from the real values of $PaCO_2$, so it is essential that, for very long interventions or major surgery, in which large haemodynamic alterations are envisaged, we provide for an invasive blood pressure monitoring that also allows us to perform serial blood gas controls [14].

6.6.4 Anaesthetic Technique

The anaesthetic technique of choice for laparoscopic interventions in children is general anaesthesia with tracheal intubation.

After inhaled or intravenous induction, first step is finding a suitable gauge venous access preferably in upper limbs because the increase in IAP delays the effect of drugs administrated through the venous circulation in the lower limbs.

Anaesthesia can be induced and maintained by inhalation or intravenously, usually we prefer the latter as it allows a greater cardiovascular stability.

Adequate analgesia must be provided to block painful stimuli from the operative field. The opioid of choice is remifentanil due to its unique pharmacokinetic properties. Metabolism of remifentanil is independent of the liver and kidney function with a short, context-sensitive half-life, and it does not accumulate within the body even during prolonged procedures.

The use of nitrous oxide is not recommended since it causes dilation of the intestinal loops with risk of bowel perforation during insertion of surgical instruments and, given its high diffusibility, it could cause combustion when using electrosurgical units. This risks are more theoretical than real.

Adequate ventilation is essential during laparoscopy in order to allow the disposal of CO_2 absorbed during the PN through modification and adaptation of ventilatory parameters. Important is that the tube is cuffed in order to prevent air leaks with impossibility in reaching an adequate tidal volume because of the increasing inspiratory peak air pressure during the PN. The position of the tracheal tube must be rechecked after positioning on the table and after the creation of the PN because of the cephalic dislocation of the diaphragm during PN (especially in infants).

In the case of extremely short procedures and patients with absence of cardio-respiratory problems we can consider to use also the laryngeal mask [15].

In urgency and in operations on the high abdomen it is recommended to place a nasogastric tube for the risk of regurgitation associated with increased abdominal pressure and to allow better surgical view.

For long interventions we can consider the use of a muscle relaxant in order to reduce the peak inspiratory pressure at constant current volume.

During the course of the intervention the ventilatory parameters should be modified (by acting mainly on the respiratory rate) in order to maintain a normocapnia. It is estimated that to achieve this aim the ventilation should be increased by 30% compared to the physiological values. It is recommended to use a protective tidal volume keeping the Peak Inspiratory Pressure < 20 cm H_2O, and apply an End Expiratory Pressure (PEEP) of 3–5 cm H_2O.

A PEEP of 5 cm H_2O is the limit below which we can have advantages in oxygenation without significant haemodynamic alterations [16]: with a PEEP of 5 cm H_2O we can observe an increase in arterial oxygenation due to the increase in functional residual capacity and tidal volume, an improvement in lung compliance and in the ventilation/perfusion ratio due to the expansion and stabilization of the partially collapsed alveoli [17].

During laparoscopy, mean airway pressure and dynamic compliance were significantly higher during PCV with 5 cm H_2O of PEEP compared with that in VCV with 5 cm H_2O of PEEP. As there were no differences in other ventilatory parameters and oxygen saturation, both VCV and PCV can be used safely in children undergoing laparoscopic surgery [18].

Another aspect of great importance is the control of body temperature as the cold gas insufflated into the peritoneum lowers the core temperature: so we have to pay attention and use heated fluid, thermal mattresses with coverage of exposed areas and heating/humidification of inspired gases [19].

6.6.5 Post Operatory Treatment

For post-operative pain control is useful to infiltrate surgical incisions with local anaesthetic, associated with the administration of paracetamol, NSAIDs and an opiate.

A useful trick is to make sure that the surgeon removes from the abdominal cavity as much CO_2 as possible to limit its irritating effect due to the formation of carbonic acid: CO_2 left over in the peritoneum, as well as pain, may impair the ventilatory mechanics immobilizing the diaphragm (effect of no less importance since the moment that the breathing in children is mainly diaphragmatic) and cause nausea and vomiting.

Younger patients, generally, can be safely extubated in the operating room after the resolution of neuromuscular blockade but, in case of impaired ventilation, they require a greater and more prolonged post-operative observation: it is at this stage, in fact, that we have the elimination of CO_2 accumulated in the bones and muscles during surgery, and in cases of impaired ventilation we have to expect that the patient will take longer time to reach the normocapnia.

6.6.6 Complications

It is crucial for the anaesthesiologist to recognize early complications that this type of surgery can lead.

The most frequent complications are related to CO_2 diffusion: subcutaneus emphysema, pneumomediastinum and pneumothorax. The more the subcutaneous emphysema is extended much higher will be the values of $PaCO_2$ and lower pH.

Other complications include vascular or visceral lesions caused by the insertion of trocars. Generally vascular lesions affect the aortic bifurcation or the iliac vessels and occur with haemorrhagic shock.

A very rare but serious complication is the air embolism: the gas bubbles enter the bloodstream through the small open vessels and reach the right ventricle through the inferior vena cava. This can lead to right heart failure that is manifested by a sudden and significant reduction of $EtCO_2$.

6.7 Peculiarities

6.7.1 Laparoscopic Surgery

In preschool children and in newborns the distance between the anterior abdominal wall and the abdominal organs is reduced: surgeons should be careful to avoid perforation of internal organs during the insertion of trocars.

The presence of a limited abdominal space forces to create the PN very slowly with proportional gas volumes: it is recommended to use an IAP not exceeding 10–12 mmHg.

The thin abdominal wall of child does not allow a tight fit between the drilled holes and the tools introduced in the abdominal cavity. This causes a gradual escape of gas with progressive decline of the IAP and increased risk of subcutaneous emphysema development.

At the end of the surgical procedure, before extracting trocars, the IAP should be reduced to 5 mmHg to exclude the possible presence of bleeding.

6.7.2 Robotic Surgery

The da Vinci® system is composed of three distinct components: a control console where the surgeon sits to view and control in real time from a remote location the robot, the electrocautery, ultrasonic instruments and alternate between robotic arms as the need arises; a computer/visualization tower which contains video equipment to record and display images of the surgical site on two-dimensional monitors (while the surgeon sees the operating field in 3D) for the convenience of the rest of the operating room team; and the robot itself which consist of three or four arms (the central arm holds the stereoscopic camera while a right and left arm perform manipulations through interchangeable instruments) (Fig. 6.3).

In most cases, two surgeons perform the operation. Beside the surgeon at the console, the other skilled assistant at the table side places the trocars and connects them with the robotic arms,

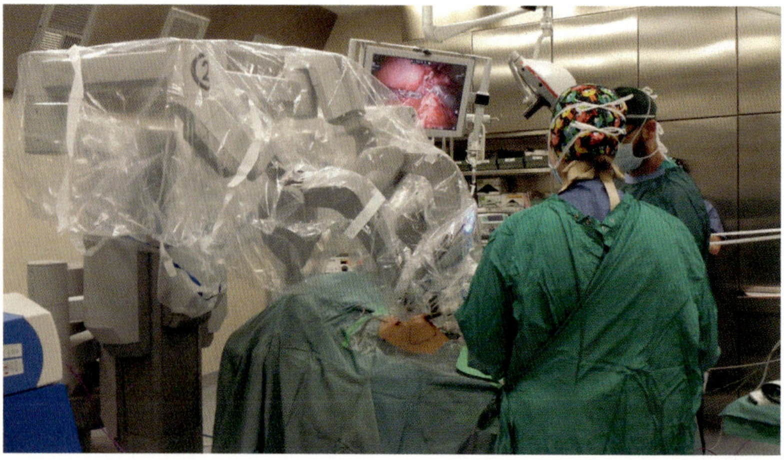

Fig. 6.3 Giannina Gaslini Institute-Genova

changes the robotic instruments and manipulates additional endoscopic instruments.

The Zeus® system is very similar but it uses a voice activated camera, the robotic arms are attached to the operating room table and the robotic arm only allows for five degrees of motion versus the seven degrees of motion in the da Vinci® system.

Patient safety during robotic surgery requires advance planning. Although robotic technology offers distinct advantages to the paediatric surgeon, paediatric anaesthesiologists need to face many difficulties [20].

First of all, access to the patient is severely limited, making preparation, team work and open communication between the anaesthesiologist and surgeon essential.

Robotic surgery with the da Vinci® system does not allow for changes in patient position on the operating room table once the robot has been docked. Anaesthesiologist need to be aware that robotic equipment can interfere with patient access and prepare accordingly. In the case of an airway emergency or cardiac arrest, resuscitating the patient requires disengaging the robotic instruments before backing the cart away from the operating room table [21].

The operating room team must be prepared and organized in case of emergency scenarios since the moment that removing the robot from the operating field to gain access to the patient requires considerable timing. Anaesthesiologists must therefore pay close attention to the initial positioning of the patient on the operating room table (it is imperative to ensure the patient is properly positioned with pressure points adequately padded prior to draping and docking the robot to avoid tissue and nerve impingement), to the setting up of the monitoring and to provide all intravenous lines of extensions that allow to reach the patient despite the robot's presence: it is mandatory that the robot is docked only after the patient has been optimally positioned for surgery.

Finally we have to consider that, until surgeons become accustomed to robotic technology, prolonged operative time with CO_2 peritoneal insufflation will exaggerate negative physiologic cardio-respiratory effects: decreased lung volumes, impaired ventilation, increased CO_2 absorption (with acidosis and risk of air embolism), decreased venous return which may result in lower extremity oedema and in a 50% reduction in cardiac index [22].

References

1. Lee JR. Anesthetic consideration for robotic surgery. Korean J Anaesthesiol. 2014;66:3–11.
2. Lorincz A, Langenburg S, Klein MD. Robotics and pediatric surgeon. Curr Opin Pediatr. 2003;15:262–6.
3. Giri S, Sarkar DK. Current status of robotic surgery. Indian J Surg. 2012;74:242–7.
4. Heller K, Gutt C, Schaeff B, et al. Use of the robot system da Vinci for laparoscopic repair of gastro-oesophageal reflux in children. Eur J Pediatr Surg. 2002;12:239–42.
5. Meiniger D, Byhahn C, Markus BH, et al. Roboterassistierte, endoskopiscke Fundolpikatio nach Nissen bei Kindern. Der Anaesthetist. 2001;50:271–5.
6. Michael J. Sullivan, Elizabeth A. M. Frost & Michael W Lew. Anesthetic care of the patient for robotic surgery. Middle East J Anaesthesiol. 2008;19(5):967–82.
7. Gutt CN, Markus B, Kim ZG, et al. Early experiences of robotic surgery in children. Surg Endosc. 2002;16:1083–6.
8. Van Haasteren G, Levine S, Hayes W. Pediatric robot surgery: early assessment. Pediatrics. 2009;124:1642.
9. Sfez M. Laparoscopic surgery in pediatrics: the point of view of the anesthetist. Cah Anesthesiol. 1993;41:237–44.
10. Mattioli G, Montobbio G, Pini Prato A, et al. Anesthesiologic aspects of laparoscopic fundoplication for gastroesophageal reflux in children with cronic respiratory and gastroenterological symptoms. Surg Endosc. 2003;17:559–66.
11. Meininger D, Byhahn C, Mierdl S, et al. Hemodynamic and respiratory effects of robot-assisted laparoscopic fundoplication in children. World J Surg. 2005;29:615–20.
12. Safran DB, Orlando R. Physiologic effects of pneumoperitoneum. Am J Surg. 1994;167:281–6.
13. Nishio I, Noguchi J, Konishi M, et al. The effects of anesthetic technoques and insufflating gases on ventilation during laparoscopi. Masui. 1993;42(6):862.
14. Wedgewood J, Doyle E. Anaesthesia and laparoscopic surgery in children. Paediatr Anaesth. 2001;11:391–9.
15. Mironov PI, Estekhin AM, Mirasov AA. Anaesthetic maintenance with laryngeal mask for a laparoscopic surgery in pediatric patients. Anesteziol Reanimatol. 2013;1:10–4.
16. Meininger D, Byhahn C, Mierdl S, Westphal K, Zwissler B. Positive end-expiratory pressure improves arterial oxygenation during prolonged pneumoperitoneum. Acta Anaesthesiol Scand. 2006;49:778–83.

17. Hazebroek EJ, Haitsma JJ, Lachmann B, Bonjer HJ. Mechanical ventilation with positive end-expiratory pressure preserves arterial oxygenation during prolonged pneumoperitoneum. Surg Endosc. 2002;16:865–9.
18. Kim JY, Shin CS, Lee KC, Chang YJ, Kwak HJ. Effect of pressure-versus volume-controlled ventilation on the Ventilatory and hemodynamic parameters during laparoscopic appendectomy in children: a prospective, randomized study. J Laparoendosc Adv Surg Tech A. 2011;21(7):655–821.
19. Kaynan AM, Winfield HN. Thermostasis during laparoscopic urologic surgery. J Endourol. 2002;16:465–70.
20. Mariano ER, Furukawa L, Woo RK. Anesthetic concerns for robot-assisted laparoscopy in an infant – case report. Anesth Analg. 2004;99:1665–7.
21. Parr KG, Talamini MA. Anesthetic implications of the addition of an operative robot for endoscopic surgery: a case report. J Clin Anesth. 2002;14:228–33.
22. Joris JL, Noirot DP, Legrand MJ, et al. Haemodynamic changes during laparoscopic cholecystectomy. Anesth Analg. 1993;76:1067–71.

Part 2

Urology

7 Pediatric Robotic Pyeloplasty

Kunj Sheth and Craig A. Peters

7.1 Introduction

For the treatment of ureteropelvic junction (UPJ) obstruction, the gold standard dismembered pyeloplasty has reported success rates greater than 90%. However, attempts to modify this traditionally open procedure have evolved in recent years. The first laparoscopic pyeloplasty reported in 1993 [1, 2] was soon followed in the pediatric population in 1995 [3]. The minimally invasive approach allowed for similar success rates with improved postoperative pain and decreased hospital stay [4–10]. Nonetheless, due to the steep learning curve for intracorporeal suturing, the adoption of laparoscopic pyeloplasty was slow. This soon changed with the introduction of the da Vinci Surgical system (Intuitive Surgical, Sunnyvale, CA) in 2000. Robotic assistance specifically allows for improved surgical precision and technical dexterity for reconstructive surgery with 3D visualization [11] in a minimally invasive context. In the adult population the use of robotic pyeloplasty has now surpassed that of open pyeloplasty [12], and as the number of children's hospitals with access to the da Vinci system grows, we expect to see this progression in the pediatric population as well.

K. Sheth, M.D.
Department of Urology, University of Texas Southwestern, Dallas, TX, USA

C.A. Peters, M.D. (✉)
Pediatric Urology, Children's Medical Center Dallas, University of Texas Southwestern, Dallas, TX, USA
e-mail: craig.peters@childrens.com

7.2 Preoperative Workup

With the prominent use of prenatal ultrasound, the diagnosis of UPJ obstruction is often incidental. While serial ultrasounds can be used to monitor the degree of hydronephrosis, voiding cystourethrogram (VCUG) and renal nuclear medicine scans (DMSA or MAG3) are helpful in the diagnostic workup. An intraoperative retrograde pyelogram provides a clear anatomical picture in patients in undergoing pyeloplasty, and is recommended to most clearly define surgical anatomy. This is specifically important in cases of retrocaval ureters or low appearing UPJ obstruction, which may actually represent a mid-ureteral stricture.

The use of prophylactic antibiotics is debated in these patients as some are asymptomatic while others present with infection. Indications for surgery include febrile urinary tract infections (UTIs), associated flank pain, decreased differential function (<40%), or a >10% change in the differential function. The issue of non-resolving hydronephrosis is a relative indication that varies on a case-by-case basis.

All patients undergoing robotic pyeloplasty receive a limited bowel preparation the day before surgery. Patients are instructed to only

G. Mattioli, P. Petralia (eds.), *Pediatric Robotic Surgery*, DOI 10.1007/978-3-319-41863-6_7

drink clear liquids the day before surgery. In addition, younger patients under 5 years are given a single dulcolax suppository, while older patients are given oral dulcolax or senna to reduce bowel distention.

7.3 Setup

Ureteral stent placement can be performed either retrograde or antegrade during the procedure. If retrograde placement is selected, the patient undergoes a cystoscopy and a retrograde pyelogram. Although it is preferable to place the stent with the proximal coil at the level of the UPJ to prevent decompression of the renal pelvis, in practice this can be difficult. Alternatively, a wire can be placed at the time of cystoscopy and used for retrograde stent placement after identification of the renal pelvis. Once the stent is in place, the attached string is secured to the patient's inner thigh. A Foley catheter is then placed for bladder drainage, and the patient is positioned for the robotic portion of the case.

Straight-arm positioning is used to allow for unrestricted access to the abdominal wall with ample robotic arm clearance. Similar to the flank technique, the affected side is elevated 30–45° with a gel roll or towel. An axillary roll can be used on the contralateral side to relieve any undue strain and the patient's arms are kept straight [13]. A folded towel passes under the lower back and over each arm, secured with tape.

The table is then rotated to allow the abdomen to be flat during trocar placement. Port placement varies based on laterality of pyeloplasty, but is essentially a mirror image (Fig. 7.1). The camera port is placed at the umbilicus using the modified Hassan technique [14]. The two working ports (5 mm or 8 mm size) are then placed, one midline roughly half the distance between the umbilicus and the xiphoid, and the other about 2/3 the distance between the umbilicus and ipsilateral anterior superior iliac spine. The second port can be adjusted medially and inferiorly for smaller children as needed (Fig. 7.2). The key to port placement is identifying the approximate location of the UPJ, which can vary by renal pelvis size, and drawing an imaginary line to the umbilicus. If a second imaginary line was drawn between the two working ports, they should cross at a right angle, and the two ports should be equidistant from the line, allowing for maximal robotic efficiency and movement. For right-sided pyeloplasty,

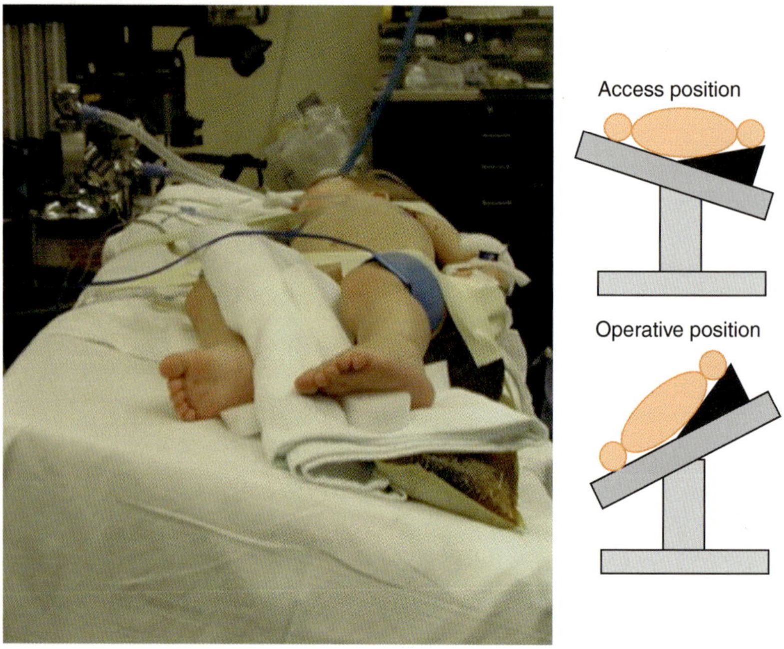

Fig. 7.1 Positioning of the patient on the operating room table using an ipsilateral wedge and maintaining the arms at the side allows the table to be rotated to the degree needed for effective exposure. *Blue* towels and tape are used to secure the chest arms and thighs. The diagrams demonstrate positioning of the patient with the abdomen flat for access and in the ipsilateral elevated position for the operation

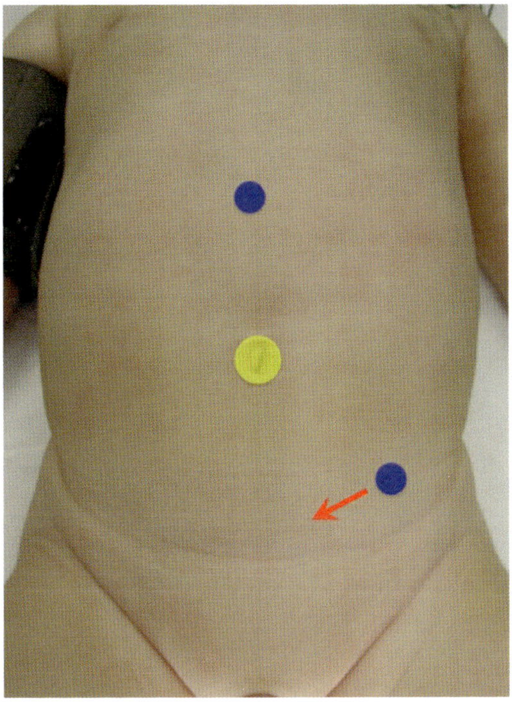

Fig. 7.2 Port placement for a left-sided pyeloplasty with the camera placed in the umbilicus (*yellow circle*), superior working port in the midline between the umbilicus and the xiphoid process (*blue circle*), and an ipsilateral lower quadrant working port (*blue circle*). The inferior working port should be moved medially and inferiorly for smaller patients or a larger renal pelvis

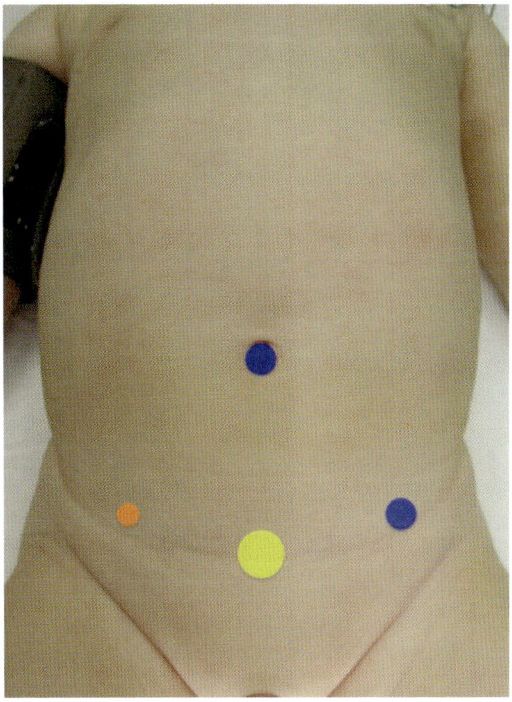

Fig. 7.3 Port placement for the HIdES technique to keep all ports below the clothing line except for the umbilical port. The color-coding corresponds to that in Fig. 7.2. A smaller assistant port may be placed in the opposite end of the inferior line of ports

an additional 3.5 mm or 5 mm port is used by some for liver retraction, but the author has rarely needed this.

The HIdES (hidden incision endoscopic surgery) technique has also been used for robotic pyeloplasty [15], allowing all port sides to be hidden at the level of a Pfannenstiel incision and thus eliminating visibility in even a swimsuit. In this technique a gel bump is placed on the operative side and the operative side arm is tucked while the contralateral arm is extended. An infraumbilical incision is made through which a 5 mm laparoscope is introduced in the surgeon's preferred manner. Under direct visualization, the camera port, assistant port, and working port are all placed at the level of the Pfannenstiel incision. Thereafter the initial infraumbilical port is exchanged for a robotic working trocar (Fig. 7.3).

Once all ports are in place, the abdomen is examined for any bleeding or injuries during initial port placement. The table is rotated while observing the renal pelvis until the exposure is optimized. This allows for medial displacement of the small bowel, optimizing visualization. The da Vinci robot is then docked. Initially, a hook cautery or hot scissors are placed in the dominant hand and the Maryland or DeBakey forces are placed in the nondominant hand.

7.4 Transperitoneal Approach

The majority of pediatric cases are approached transperitoneally, and the ureter can be identified in the transmesenteric or a retrocolic fashion. When feasible, the transmesenteric approach is preferred as it allows for minimal anatomical disruption, decreased bowel dissection, and expedited access to the ureter. The ideal patient population

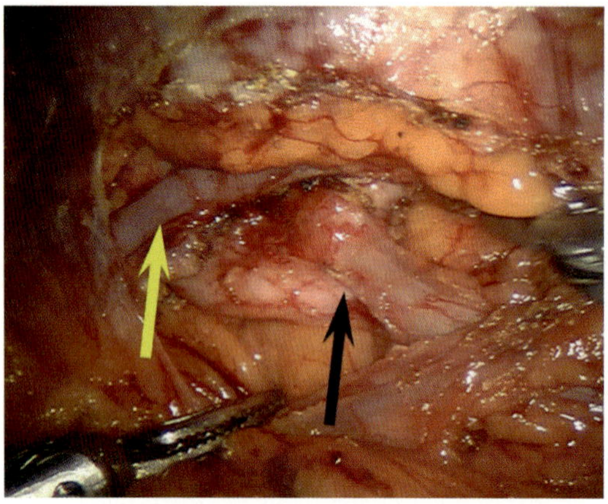

Fig. 7.4 Operative view of a transmesenteric approach to the ureteropelvic junction on the *left*. The *black arrow* indicates the UPJ. The *yellow arrow* indicates one of the main renal vessels

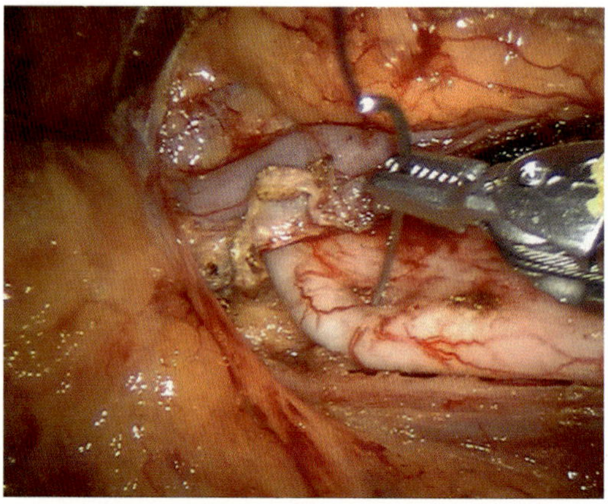

Fig. 7.5 Placement of the hitch stitch through the renal pelvis using a 3-0 PDS suture passed through the abdominal wall. The hitch stitch should be placed on the medial most aspect of the renal pelvis to maintain orientation

for this technique is infants and thin children, with left-sided UPJO. If planning for a transmesenteric approach, keep in mind not to position the patient too steeply in the flank position, as this may allow the left colon to drape over the surgical site. Upon identification of the UPJ, a mesenteric window is formed and through it, the renal pelvis and proximal ureter are mobilized (Fig. 7.4).

The retrocolic approach is necessary in older and heavier children as well as patients undergoing right pyeloplasty. In this approach the ascending or descending colon is mobilized medially from the flexure to the iliac vessels along the white line of Toldt to identify the UPJ. Thereafter, the proximal ureter, UPJ, and renal pelvis are mobilized to proceed with a dismembered pyeloplasty.

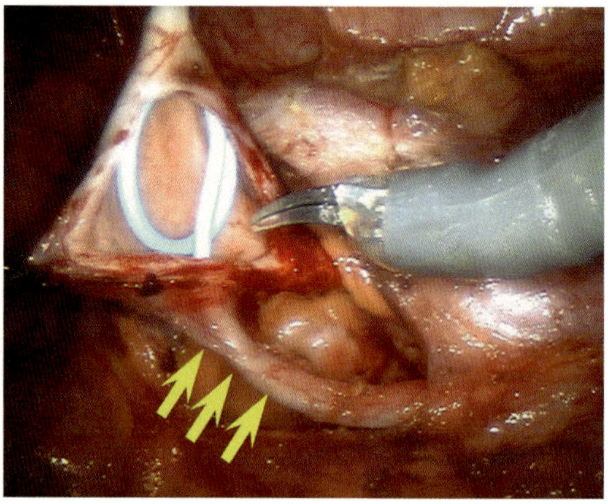

Fig. 7.6 Partial transection of the renal pelvis on the anterior aspect, showing the coil of the pre-placed ureteral stent. *Yellow arrows* indicate the proximal portion of the ureter

7.5 Surgical Steps

Upon mobilization of the UPJ, a "hitch" stitch is placed in the renal pelvis. This critical step allows for appropriate retraction and exposure of the renal pelvis, facilitating dissection, and providing stabilization during the anastomosis. The "hitch" stitch can be placed in one of two ways—directly through the abdominal wall with a 3-0 or 4-0 PDS stitch secured externally or sewn to the abdominal wall with the appropriate tension after passing a 3-0 or 4-0 vicryl stitch through one of the trocars (Fig. 7.5). The former allows for variability in tension, but cannot be used in larger patients with thicker abdominal walls. During placement, it is important to place the stitch high enough in the pelvis to avoid any interference with the pyelotomy, and when applying tension, care must be taken to not tear the renal pelvis.

Once the renal pelvis is secured, it is transected proximal to the UPJ and a segment of renal pelvis is left on the proximal ureter (Fig. 7.6). This segment serves as a handle, allowing manipulation of the ureter without harming the ureteral tissue itself. Using this flap

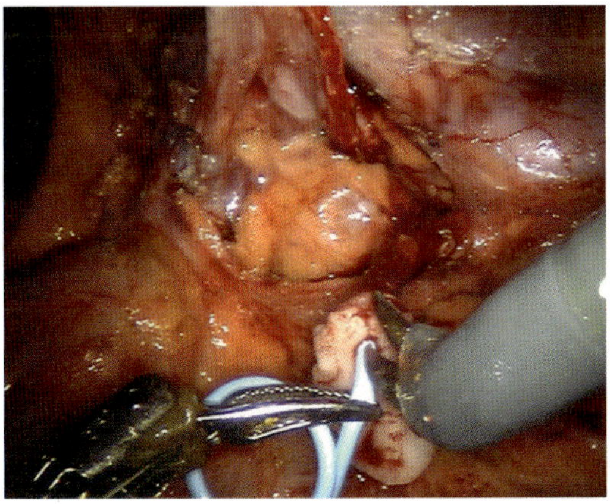

Fig. 7.7 Spatulation of the lateral aspect of the ureter can be facilitated by aligning the ureter with the position of the scissors. The double-J stent can be used to move the ureter into position

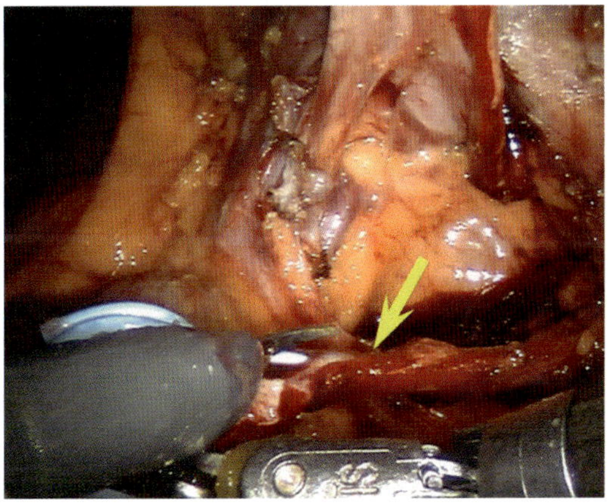

Fig. 7.8 Spatulation of the ureter may also be accomplished by moving the scissors to the left hand and aligning the ureter with the instrument

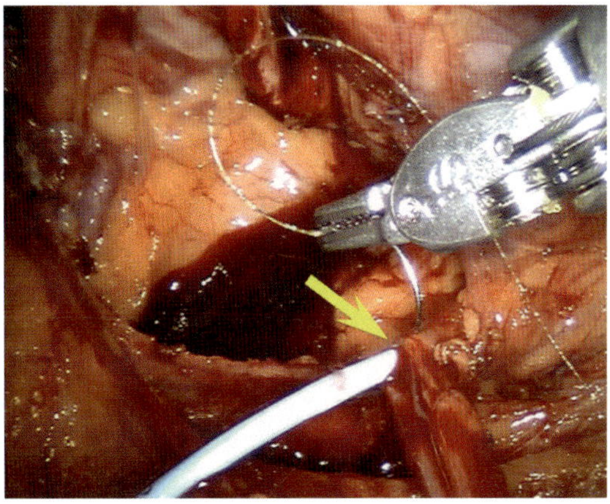

Fig. 7.9 Placement of the initial stitch of the anastomosis at the vertex of the speculation using a 5-0 Monocryl suture

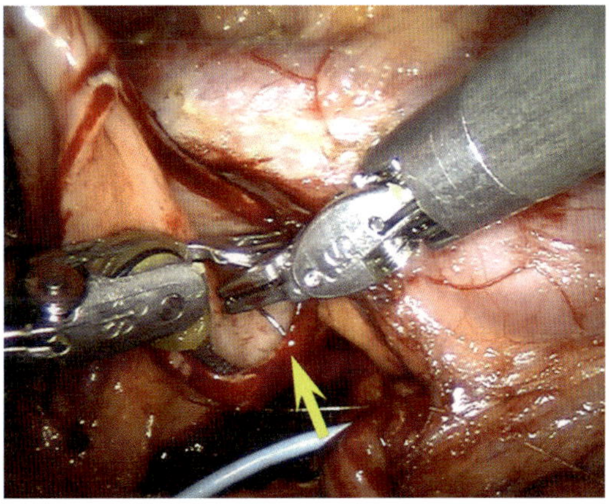

Fig. 7.10 Placement of the first stitch in the inferior aspect of the pelvis from the inside out

of tissue the ureter is spatulated along the lateral aspect for about 1.5–2 cm until healthy tissue is encountered and the ureteral lumen opens up (Figs. 7.7 and 7.8). In the presence of a crossing vessel, the ureter must be transposed anteriorly to prevent any further obstruction after the anastomosis is complete. The renal pelvis is later resected after partial completion of the reanastomosis. Care should be taken to not over-excise the renal pelvis during this step.

Although the anastomosis can be completed by a running or interrupted technique, we prefer a running stitch as this provides for even suture tension, decreases time to perform the anastomosis, and minimizes instrument changes. The type of suture used for the anastomosis is variable, each with its own set of pros and cons. A monofilament suture, such as monocryl or PDS, glides through the tissues very easily. In contrast, vicryl is easier to handle, but often saws through the delicate UPJ tissue. It is possible that adding oil or wax may help soften a vicryl suture. We prefer monocryl among the monofilament suture as it dissolves more rapidly than PDS. The stitch is cut to about 12–14 cm to optimize the balance between sufficient length and excessive redundant suture.

The initial stitch is placed at the lower vertex of the ureteral spatulation and run up the posterior aspect of the new ureteropelvic junction (Figs. 7.9 and 7.10). Care should be taken to not leave any

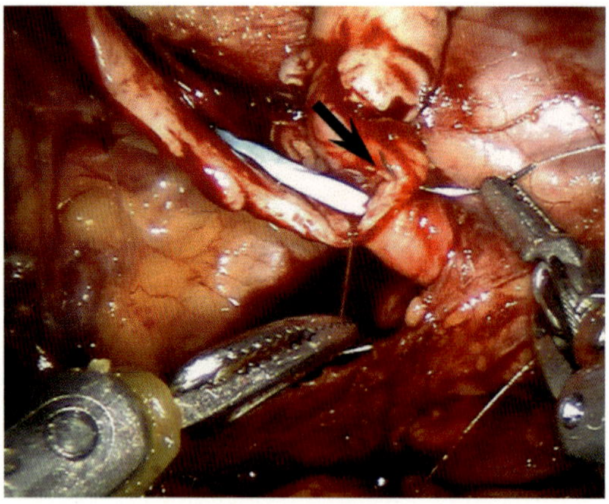

Fig. 7.11 The second side of the anastomosis is performed with a running suture from the inferior aspect moving superiorly. The *black arrow* indicates positioning of the needle in the ureteral wall. The tail of the suture on the opposite side is used for exposure and traction

tension on the anastomosis, further mobilizing the ureter if necessary, and to only touch the anastomotic line with the needle. Once the first half of the anastomosis is complete, the stent is placed in the appropriate position. If a retrograde stent was placed during cystoscopy or advanced over a preplaced wire, the proximal coil is advanced into the renal pelvis such that it can maintain its position.

Otherwise, antegrade stent placement is performed via a 14-gauge angiocatheter. The guiding needle is passed through the anterior abdominal wall. Upon removing the needle a guide-wire with a preloaded stent is passed into the abdomen and directed into the proximal ureter towards the bladder. As this is being done blind, if any resistance is noted, an angled guidewire may be needed to avoid perforation of the ureter. Once the majority of the stent has been passed and only the proximal coil is left, the wire is removed and the coil positioned in the renal pelvis. Flexible cystoscopy can be performed at the bedside to confirm placement in the bladder while the anastomosis is being completed. Running the suture from the apex of the spatulation superiorly prevents any mismatch of pelvic and ureteral tissue (Fig. 7.11). Upon completion, it is important to evaluate for any bleeding or kinking of the new anastomosis. After checking for any inadvertent injuries or bleeding, the robot is disengaged, the ports are removed, and all incisions are closed with application of local anesthetic.

7.6 Retroperitoneal Approach

While the retroperitoneal approach mirrors the open pyeloplasty techniques and avoids entry into the peritoneum, it is technically challenging in pediatric patients due to the small retroperitoneal working space. This approach was first described laparoscopically by Yeung et al. in 2001 [16], but difficulty completing the anastomosis laparoscopically did lead to higher conversion rates [6]. Robotic implementation of the retroperitoneal approach has been described by Olsen et al. with successful outcomes [17, 18]. Upon reaching the UPJ, the steps are similar to the transperitoneal approach, but initial setup, preparation, and dissection differ.

Port placement is completed in 100° lateral semiprone position. Initially a 15 mm incision is made 1–3 cm below the tip of the 12th rib allowing entrance into the retroperitoneum with blunt dissection. A 200–400 ml balloon is used to further develop this space and create room for placement of two 8 mm trocars and a 5 mm assistance port. The two working ports are placed at the lateral aspect of the latissimus dorsi muscle two fingerbreadths above the iliac crest and beneath the costal margin at the anterior axillary line. The assistant port is optional and placed in the iliac fossa. All ports are placed with direct palpation to avoid any peritoneal injuries. Thereafter the 12 mm balloon-tipped port is passed into the original 15 mm incision and secured with closure of the surrounding fascia.

The robot is then docked at a 45–60° angle, and dissection is again performed with a hot scissors or hook cautery in the dominant hand and a Maryland or DeBakey forceps in the nondominant hand. However, in this approach the Gerota's fascia is incised to identify the UPJ (Fig. 7.12) and complete dissection of the lower pole is vital to identify a crossing vessel. In our own experience as well as in reported experiences, incomplete dissection can lead to failed repair. Two holding stitches are placed, one at the proximal

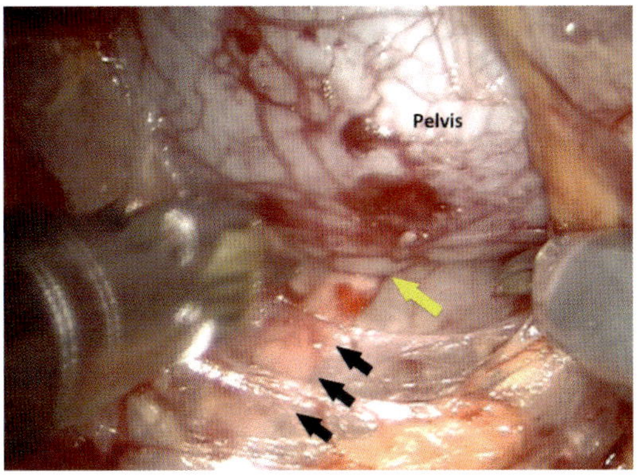

Fig. 7.12 Operative view of the renal pelvis and UPJ through a retroperitoneal approach. The *yellow arrow* indicates the actual UPJ and the *black arrows* demonstrate the ureter. (Image courtesy of Dr. L. Henning Olsen)

ureter and one at the renal pelvis, and the remainder of the surgery follows the same principles as the transperitoneal technique.

7.7 Alternative Reconstructive Techniques

While the Anderson-Hynes dismembered pyeloplasty is the preferred technique and gold standard for UPJ repair, certain clinical scenarios demand modifications and alterations during repair. These techniques were initially described for open pyeloplasty and can be adapted in the robotic approach.

7.7.1 Foley Y-V Plasty

This technique is especially useful in a high insertion of the ureter or in cases of significant UPJ scarring limiting renal pelvis mobilization and/or higher ureteral insertion when no accessory vessels are present. Starting with the apex of the V at the UPJ, the lines are extended over the medial dependent aspect of the renal pelvis. Thereafter the incision is carried along the lateral aspect of the proximal ureter well into the normal ureteral tissue, forming the Y portion. The apex of the pelvic flap is then stitched to the distal most part of the ureterotomy, and the posterior walls are re-approximated followed by the anterior walls.

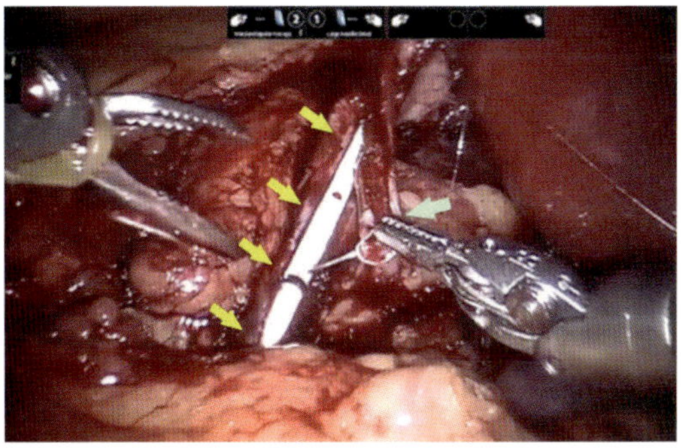

Fig. 7.13 Operative view of a spiral flap pyeloplasty in a patient with a long proximal ureteral stenosis. The flap (*light green arrow*) has been mobilized from the dilated renal pelvis and is being swung down onto the spatulated stenotic segment (*yellow arrows*) with an indwelling ureteral stent

7.7.2 Spiral Flap

For cases of severe hydronephrosis with a long stenotic ureteral segment and dependent UPJ, a spiral flap can be performed to allow tension-free anastomosis. The base of the spiral is placed obliquely on the dependent aspect of the renal pelvis and lateral to the UPJ between the ureteral insertion and renal parenchyma. The medial line of the spiral is then carried down through the UPJ to normal ureter so the length is determined by the extent of the strictured segment, but the ratio of flap length to width cannot exceed a 3:1 ratio. Upon creation of the flap the apex is rotated down to the distal end of the ureterotomy and the remaining anastomosis follows over an indwelling stent (Fig. 7.13).

7.7.3 Modified Bypass Procedure

The modified bypass procedure is an alternative technique for long dysplastic upper ureteral segments. For the classic dismembered technique, the kidney can be completely mobilized to decrease the distance between the ureter and renal pelvis, but a horizontal incision of the lower pelvis with a side-to-side anastomosis can provide additional length, lending to a tension-free anastomosis [19].

7.7.4 Ureterocalicostomy

If none of these techniques are sufficient to allow a tension-free anastomosis between a severely small and scarred renal pelvis and scarred ureter, a ureterocalicostomy must be considered. In this technique a lower pole nephrotomy is performed and the proximal ureter is spatulated laterally. The anastomosis is then performed between the lower pole calyx and proximal ureter over a stent with strong consideration given to leaving a nephrostomy tube. When possible the renal capsule is closed over the parenchyma, being careful not to extrinsically compress the new lumen. Furthermore, a graft of perinephric fat or omentum can be used to cover and protect the anastomosis.

7.8 Special Considerations: Vascular Hitch

In older children presenting with UPJ obstruction, an extrinsic lower pole crossing vessel is often the cause of obstruction as opposed to an intrinsic UPJ anomaly. While the gold standard has remained a dismembered pyeloplasty, Hellstrom et al. described an alternative technique where the lower pole vessels were dissected off the UPJ and anchored in a more cranial position on the anterior pelvic wall with permanent sutures [20]. After multiple modifications, this technique was first described laparoscopically in 2008 by Gundeti et al. [21]. In this technique after mobilization of the lower pole vessels, the "shoe-shine" maneuver is used to determine sufficient mobility of the anterior pelvis to form a tunnel around the vessels. Using a 4-0 PDS suture, 2–3 interrupted stitches are placed in the anterior pelvis securing the vessels [22]. Although success has been reported with this technique laparoscopically, many question the ability to identify which patients are truly obstructed due to a crossing vessel with no intrinsic component. Miranda et al. has reported the use of intraoperative ureteral opening pressure measurements to confirm a true extrinsic compression prior to performing vascular hitch procedure [23]. Another intraoperative test described is a diuretic test to identify those patients with a nonobstructing crossing vessel [24]. Outcomes in these reports have been promising, but the key is appropriate patient selection. Re-operation in these patients is challenging, as the renal artery is densely adherent to the renal pelvis.

7.9 Postoperative Care

Postoperatively, patients are admitted for overnight observation and diet is advanced as tolerated. Patients usually have a voiding trial the following morning and are usually discharged home on POD1 after transition to oral medications. The stent is kept in place for 2 weeks with easy office removal if an extraction string was left, but otherwise an anesthetic is necessary for cystoscopy and stent removal. After stent removal an ultrasound is performed in 4 weeks and patients are kept on prophylactic antibiotics until that time. If ultrasound shows good decompression of the renal pelvis, a repeat ultrasound is performed in 3 months and no functional studies are obtained unless the patient had decreased (<40%) differential function preoperatively. In cases of stable hydronephrosis on postop imaging, a repeat ultrasound is done in another 4–6 weeks, and if no further improvement is seen a MAG3 renal scan is performed. Lastly, if the 4-week ultrasound shows significant worsening of hydronephrosis, an immediate MAG3 renal scan is performed to guide further management.

7.10 Outcomes

Although a few studies have evaluated the efficacy of robotic pyeloplasty in the pediatric population, the data is limited with no formal prospective trials. Nonetheless, outcomes have been similar to open surgery with high success rates of 94–100% [25]. Initial studies have shown no differences between open and robotic pyeloplasty [26]. Over a 7-year time curve Minnillo et al. demonstrated a gradual improvement in both operative time and hospital stay with robotic pyeloplasty, while maintaining a complication rate similar to open surgery. This improvement signifies the robotic learning curve and emphasizes the importance of a dedicated trained team for robotic surgery [27]. The use of retrograde versus antegrade stent placement has long been debated, but Silva et al. has argued the case for stentless repair in a cohort of 25 patients with 100% success [28].

Re-intervention rates are reported as 2–4% and complication rates vary from 8 to 18% [25], the majority of which are minor in character. Intraoperative complications usually deal with laparoscopic access and inadvertent bowel injury, and should be prevented when possible, but if they occur the key is early recognition. It is important to keep all working instruments in the visual field at all times, especially when using cautery. In the advent of bowel injury, careful examination and cleaning followed by repair, usually with an imbricating figure-of-eight stitch is usually sufficient, but if there is any question a general surgery consultation is appropriate. Bleeding from vascular injury is rare, but in such an instance similar techniques to open surgery can be used for vascular control with compression and occasional suture ligation.

Postoperatively, complications are relatively unusual. In the acute setting, a bowel ileus or bowel injury is the greatest concern. While ileus can be managed conservatively, it is important to always consider a bowel injury, moving to CT with oral contrast if there is strong suspicion, and upon diagnosis laparoscopic versus open exploration. Additionally a urine leak can present with ileus and urinary ascites, usually manifesting by no spontaneous voiding upon removal of Foley catheter. These can usually be managed conservatively with replacement Foley catheter for 3–5 days. Later complications include persistent hydronephrosis secondary to anastomotic stricture after initial stent removal. Conservative management with placement of a double-J stent for 6 weeks is an initial option, but if the issue persists a reoperation may be necessary, often also robotically [29]. Numbers are limited with most pediatric series reporting less than ten patients and a lower success rate varying from 78–90% [25].

Conclusions

Overall, the introduction of da Vinci to the pediatric population has significantly changed the feasibility of minimally invasive surgery for UPJ obstruction. Success and complication rates mirror that of open pyeloplasty with potential for less operative time, hospital stay, and potential narcotic use. Various techniques for port placement and approach to the UPJ are available, and the decision has to be made on a case-by-case basis.

References

1. Kavoussi LR, Peters CA. Laparoscopic pyeloplasty. J Urol. 1993;150(6):1891–4.
2. Schuessler WW, Grune MT, Tecuanhuey LV, Preminger GM. Laparoscopic dismembered pyeloplasty. J Urol. 1993;150(6):1795–9.
3. Peters CA, Schlussel RN, Retik AB. Pediatric laparoscopic dismembered pyeloplasty. J Urol. 1995;153(6):1962–5.
4. Tan HL. Laparoscopic Anderson-Hynes dismembered pyeloplasty in children. J Urol. 1999;162(3 Pt 2):1045–7. discussion 1048
5. Klingler HC, Remzi M, Janetschek G, Kratzik C, Marberger MJ. Comparison of open versus laparoscopic pyeloplasty techniques in treatment of uretero-pelvic junction obstruction. Eur Urol. 2003;44(3):340–5.
6. El-Ghoneimi A, Farhat W, Bolduc S, Bagli D, McLorie G, Aigrain Y, Khoury A. Laparoscopic dismembered pyeloplasty by a retroperitoneal approach in children. BJU Int. 2003;92(1):104–8.
7. Reddy M, Nerli RB, Bashetty R, Ravish IR. Laparoscopic dismembered pyeloplasty in children. J Urol. 2005;174(2):700–2.
8. Braga LH, Pippi-Salle J, Lorenzo AJ, Bagli D, Khoury AE, Farhat WA. Pediatric laparoscopic pyeloplasty in a referral center: lessons learned. J Endourol. 2007;21(7):738–42.
9. Ravish IR, Nerli RB, Reddy MN, Amarkhed SS. Laparoscopic pyeloplasty compared with open pyeloplasty in children. Journal of endourology/Endourological Society. 2007;21(8):897–902.
10. Piaggio LA, Franc-Guimond J, Noh PH, Wehry M, Figueroa TE, Barthold J, Gonzalez R. Transperitoneal laparoscopic pyeloplasty for primary repair of ureteropelvic junction obstruction in infants and children: comparison with open surgery. J Urol. 2007;178(4 Pt 2):1579–83.
11. Atug F, Woods M, Burgess SV, Castle EP, Thomas R. Robotic assisted laparoscopic pyeloplasty in children. J Urol. 2005;174(4 Pt 1):1440–2.

12. Monn MF, Bahler CD, Schneider EB, Sundaram CP. Emerging trends in robotic pyeloplasty for the management of ureteropelvic junction obstruction in adults. J Urol. 2013;189(4):1352–7.
13. Chandrasoma S, Kokorowski P, Peters C, Koh C. Straight-arm positioning and port placement for pediatric robotic-assisted laparoscopic renal surgery. J Robotic Surg. 2010;4(1):29–32.
14. Poppas DP, Bleustein CB, Peters CA. Box stitch modification of Hasson technique for pediatric laparoscopy. J Endourol. 1999;13(6):447–50.
15. Gargollo PC. Hidden incision endoscopic surgery: description of technique, parental satisfaction and applications. J Urol. 2011;185(4):1425–31.
16. Yeung CK, Tam YH, Sihoe JD, Lee KH, Liu KW. Retroperitoneoscopic dismembered pyeloplasty for pelvi-ureteric junction obstruction in infants and children. BJU Int. 2001;87(6):509–13.
17. Olsen LH, Jorgensen TM. Computer assisted pyeloplasty in children: the retroperitoneal approach. J Urol. 2004;171(6 Pt 2):2629–31.
18. Olsen LH, Rawashdeh YF, Jorgensen TM. Pediatric robot assisted retroperitoneoscopic pyeloplasty: a 5-year experience. J Urol. 2007;178(5):2137–41. discussion 2141
19. Mesrobian HG. Bypass pyeloplasty: description of a procedure and initial results. J Pediatr Urol. 2009;5(1):34–6.
20. Hellstrom J, Giertz G, Lindblom K. Pathogenesis and treatment of hydronephrosis. J Belge Urol. 1951;20(1):1–6.
21. Gundeti MS, Reynolds WS, Duffy PG, Mushtaq I. Further experience with the vascular hitch (laparoscopic transposition of lower pole crossing vessels): an alternate treatment for pediatric ureterovascular ureteropelvic junction obstruction. J Urol. 2008;180(4 Suppl):1832–1836; discussion 1836.
22. Sakoda A, Cherian A, Mushtaq I. Laparoscopic transposition of lower pole crossing vessels ('vascular hitch') in pure extrinsic pelvi-ureteric junction (PUJ) obstruction in children. BJU Int. 2011;108(8):1364–8.
23. Miranda ML, Pereira LH, Cavalaro MA, Pegolo PC, de Oliveira-Filho AG, Bustorff-Silva JM. Laparoscopic transposition of lower pole crossing vessels (vascular hitch) in children with Pelviureteric junction obstruction: how to be sure of the success of the procedure? J Laparoendosc Adv Surg Tech A. 2015;25(10):847–51.
24. Chiarenza SF, Bleve C, Fasoli L, Battaglino F, Bucci V, Novek S, Zolpi E. Ureteropelvic junction obstruction in children by polar vessels. Is laparoscopic vascular hitching procedure a good solution? Single center experience on 35 consecutive patients. J Pediatr Surg. 2015;
25. Autorino R, Eden C, El-Ghoneimi A, Guazzoni G, Buffi N, Peters CA, Stein RJ, Gettman M. Robot-assisted and laparoscopic repair of ureteropelvic junction obstruction: a systematic review and meta-analysis. Eur Urol. 2014;65(2):430–52.
26. Franco I, Dyer LL, Zelkovic P. Laparoscopic pyeloplasty in the pediatric patient: hand sewn anastomosis versus robotic assisted anastomosis--is there a difference? J Urol. 2007;178(4 Pt 1):1483–6.
27. Minnillo BJ, Cruz JA, Sayao RH, Passerotti CC, Houck CS, Meier PM, Borer JG, Diamond DA, Retik AB, Nguyen HT. Long-term experience and outcomes of robotic assisted laparoscopic pyeloplasty in children and young adults. J Urol. 2011;185(4):1455–60.
28. Silva MV, Levy AC, Finkelstein JB, Van Batavia JP, Casale P. Is peri-operative urethral catheter drainage enough? The case for stentless pediatric robotic pyeloplasty. J Pediatr Urol. 2015;11(4):175.e1–5.
29. Davis TD, Burns AS, Corbett ST, Peters CA. Reoperative robotic pyeloplasty in children. J Pediatr Urol. 2016; 12(6):394.e1–394.

8 Ureteral Reimplantation

Alexander C. Small, Michael J. Lipsky,
Julia B. Finkelstein, and Pasquale Casale

8.1 Introduction

Minimally invasive techniques are increasingly utilized for complex reconstructive surgeries in the field of pediatric urology. Compared to open procedures, laparoscopic approaches can result in lower morbidity, decreased postoperative pain, lower analgesic requirements, accelerated postoperative recovery, and shorter hospital stays [1, 2]. The steep learning curve and technical difficulty with suturing associated with standard laparoscopy limited the widespread adoption of laparoscopic ureteral reimplantation among reconstructive urologists. However, many of these challenges were overcome with the introduction of robot-assisted laparoscopic surgery [3].

Robotic surgery has demonstrated advantages over both open and conventional laparoscopic surgery [4]. The Intuitive Surgical daVinci Surgical System has features designed to enhance surgeon performance including tremor filtration, motion scaling, and wristed instrumentation [5]. These innovations can measurably increase dexterity by up to 50% compared to standard laparoscopy [6] and have allowed reconstructive surgeons to tackle complex procedures that would not have been previously possible with a conventional laparoscopic approach [7].

Since the introduction of the Da Vinci surgical system in 2000, robotic surgery has gained popularity. This is especially true within the field of pediatric urology where robotic approaches are utilized for upper and lower urinary tract reconstructive procedures including nephrectomy, pyeloplasty, ureteral reconstruction, and bladder augmentation. The rate of pediatric urologic procedures using the surgical robot dramatically increased by 17% per year from 2008 to 2013 [8].

Vesicoureteral reflux (VUR) represents the abnormal retrograde flow of urine from the bladder into the ureters and kidneys due to incompetent closure of the ureterovesical junction (UVJ). It affects approximately 1% of all newborns [9]. These children typically present with hydronephrosis, urinary tract infections, and/or pyelonephritis and are predisposed to developing permanent renal scars [10]. Mild and moderate VUR (grade I, II, and III) spontaneously resolves in 49–72% of cases and can often be treated conservatively. Meanwhile, high-grade VUR (grade IV or V) resolves in less than 30% of cases and requires surgery [11].

A.C. Small, M.D. • M.J. Lipsky, M.D.
J.B. Finkelstein, M.D.
Department of Urology, Morgan Stanley Children's Hospital, Columbia University Medical Center, New York, NY 10032, USA

P. Casale, M.D. (✉)
Department of Urology, Morgan Stanley Children's Hospital, Columbia University Medical Center, New York, NY 10032, USA

Pediatric Urology, Morgan Stanley Children's Hospital, Columbia University Medical Center, 3959 Broadway, 11th Floor, New York, NY 10032, USA
e-mail: pc2581@cumc.columbia.edu

G. Mattioli, P. Petralia (eds.), *Pediatric Robotic Surgery*, DOI 10.1007/978-3-319-41863-6_8

Ureteral reimplantation aims to correct the abnormal refluxing UVJ. Open ureteral reimplantation (OUR) represents the gold standard of surgical treatment. However, advances in surgical technology have made minimally invasive approaches viable options for ureteral reimplantation. Laparoscopic ureteral reimplantation (LUR) was introduced in a porcine model in 1993 and first implemented in humans in 1994 [12, 13]. LUR was not widely adopted due to technical difficulties. The challenges of LUR were overcome a decade later with the introduction of RALUR. The first series of RALUR procedures were published in 2004 and 2005 by Peters and colleagues [14, 15]. Enhanced visualization, easier intracorporeal suturing, and excellent cosmesis have made this procedure appealing. While nationally the total number of ureteral reimplantations has been declining, the proportion of RALUR is on the rise. In one population study, 14,581 ureteral reimplantations were performed between 2000 and 2012 with an increase of the proportion of RALUR procedures from 0.3 to 6.3% during this time [16].

This chapter will discuss the role of ureteral reimplantation and the evolving body of evidence supporting the expansion of the robotic approach to this procedure.

8.2 Indications for Ureteral Reimplantation

8.2.1 Clinical Indications

There are a number of clinical indications to perform ureteral reimplantation, particularly in the pediatric population. The most common indication for reimplantation is VUR. Conservative management options include observation and antibiotic prophylaxis, while interventional approaches include endoscopic injection of UVJ bulking agents and definitive surgical management with ureteral reimplantation. The VUR guidelines of the American Urological Association (AUA) state that curative therapy is recommended in children older than 1 year without evidence of bowel/bladder dysfunction and with recurrent infections or new radiographic renal abnormalities [17]. Similarly, the European Association of Urology (EAU) recommends surgical correction of VUR in patients with persistent high-grade reflux (grades IV/V) as well as in patients with frequent breakthrough infections or evidence of abnormal renal parenchyma [18]. In one large study of 3738 children presenting with VUR, older age, antenatal hydronephrosis, and bilateral/high-grade VUR were independent predictors of patients undergoing VUR-corrective surgery [19].

Other congenital indications include primary obstructing megaureter, ectopic ureter, and ureterocele. While primary obstructing megaureter is a rare entity, it may account for 20% of obstructive uropathy cases in neonates [20]. Surgery is not recommended as a primary therapy in the majority of cases since approximately 85% spontaneously resolve. Reimplantation is only recommended in patients with megaureters with recurrent infections, deterioration of split renal function, or significant obstruction [18]. Ureteroceles may occur in up to 1 in 500 children [21]. Management options include observation, endoscopic decompression, ureteral reimplantation, or partial nephroureterectomy. Ectopic ureteral insertion occurs less frequently than ureteroceles in approximately 1 in 2000 children. Ureteral reconstruction including reimplantation is an option in cases in which the kidney has viable function [18].

Additional conditions which may require ureteral implantation in both children and adults are ureteral trauma and stricture disease. The guidelines on urological trauma recommend repairing ureteral injuries distal to the iliac vessels with ureteral reimplantation or primary repair over a stent [22]. Finally, severe distal ureteral strictures may be managed with robotic reimplantation.

8.2.2 Factors Influencing Approach

The decision whether to perform an open or robotic reimplant is multifactorial. Considerations include patient size, prior abdominal or pelvic surgeries, as well as patient comorbidities. Patient size is of utmost importance in pediatrics, especially in infants where working space is limited. The smaller space may cause problems with port site placement and collisions of robotic instruments [23]. The impact of patient weight on the success of robotic surgery has been assessed in multiple studies. Ballouhey in 2015 conducted a multi-institutional study analyzing the success rates of multiple different types of robotic procedures in children above and below 15 kg [24]. Among 178 procedures, the most common were pyeloplasty, partial nephrectomy, and fundoplication. There were no differences in operating time, length of hospital stay, or postoperative complication rate among the two groups. The authors concluded that robotic surgery is feasible in patients less than 15 kg, but cautious adjustments may need to be made in smaller children. In another analysis of 45 robotic general surgery procedures in children less than 10 kg, the overall completion rate was 89% [25]. For children 3 kg and greater, the intra-abdominal instrument maneuverability was adequate, but, for children less than 3 kg, there was significant difficulty due to space limitations. While weight may act as a surrogate for overall working space, body dimensions may be a more accurate way to identify patients suitable for robotic surgery. In a prospective study, our group measured the distance between anterior superior iliac spines (ASIS) as well as pubis to xiphoid distance (PXD) in 45 infants aged 3–12 months. When the inter-ASIS distance was less than 13 cm and/or PXD was less than 15 cm, there were a significantly higher number of robotic instrument collisions [23].

In addition to patient size, prior abdominal or pelvic surgeries and comorbidities must be considered. While prior abdominal surgery is not an absolute contraindication to robotic surgery, there may be adhesions in the abdomen obscuring the view into the pelvis and requiring additional time for adhesiolysis. Respiratory comorbidities are also not an absolute contraindication to the use of the robotic platform, but these patients require preoperative evaluation by anesthesia to ensure that insufflation during surgery will not compromise patient ventilation [26].

8.3 Procedure

8.3.1 Approaches

There are two approaches to RALUR that have been investigated—the intravesical/transvesical version of the Cohen cross-trigonal reimplant and the extravesical adaptation of the Lich-Gregoir procedure. The robotic implementation of the cross-trigonal procedure was first described by Olsen in 2003 utilizing a porcine model and then in children in 2005 [14, 27]. Briefly, patients are placed in the supine split-leg position. The bladder is filled with saline via a urethral catheter for easier identification during port placement. Port sites are marked just above the level of a standard pfannenstiel incision. The bladder dome is exposed via midline dissection and the 12 mm camera port is placed. At this point, the bladder is insufflated with carbon dioxide which displaces the saline and the working ports are placed. Ureteral tunnels are created and then the ureters are brought through and sutured in place with a 4-0 or 5-0 monocryl or chromic suture. After completion of the reimplantation, the ports are removed and sites are closed with pre-placed bladder sutures followed by standard fascial and skin sutures [14].

The extravesical RALUR is adapted from the open Lich-Gregoir procedure. Due to the risk of postoperative voiding dysfunction associated with bilateral OUR and early cases of bilateral RALUR, Peters initially recommended only performing unilateral RALUR [15, 28]. However, voiding complications may be prevented if the pelvic nerve plexus is identified and spared [29]. We prefer to utilize the nerve sparing extravesical approach to minimize postoperative voiding complications and will describe this below.

8.3.2 Anesthesia

General anesthesia is administered in standard fashion and the patient is intubated with an endotracheal tube for the procedure. When feasible, our pediatric anesthesia team also performs a caudal block. The utilization of regional anesthesia in combination with general anesthesia has been shown to decrease intraoperative opioid requirements in patients undergoing robotic lower urinary tract surgery compared to general anesthesia alone. In addition, patients who received caudal blocks were the least likely to require postoperative antiemetics. There was no difference between the groups in postoperative opioid use and in maximum pain scores at 6 and 24 h postoperatively [30].

8.3.3 Cystoscopy

Prior to port placement and initiation of abdominal insufflation, the patient is placed in dorsal lithotomy position and rigid cystoscopy is performed. Whistle-tip ureteral catheters are placed at this time to allow easy identification of ureteral injury during the procedure [29]. Cystoscopy is then terminated, a urethral catheter is placed and the whistle-tip catheters are secured to the urethral catheter to prevent migration.

8.3.4 Patient Positioning and Port Placement

After completion of cystoscopy, the patient is then repositioned supine and re-prepped and draped in standard surgical fashion. While most institutions utilize three ports for a transperitoneal approach, some prefer the use of an additional assistant port for suctioning and irrigation [31]. We use the three port configuration and ports are placed to allow maximal visualization during surgery. The 8.5 mm camera port is placed via a periumbilical incision and two 8 mm working ports are placed lateral to the rectus muscle at the level of the ASIS bilaterally (Fig. 8.1). No bedside assistant port is utilized. At this time, the robot is docked, the reimplantation operation begins. For younger patients, the robot is docked between the legs and in older patients the robot side-docked, pointing to the contralateral shoulder.

8.3.5 Operative Technique

Once the robot is docked, the peritoneal reflection on the bladder is incised and the space is entered just posterior to the bladder. The course

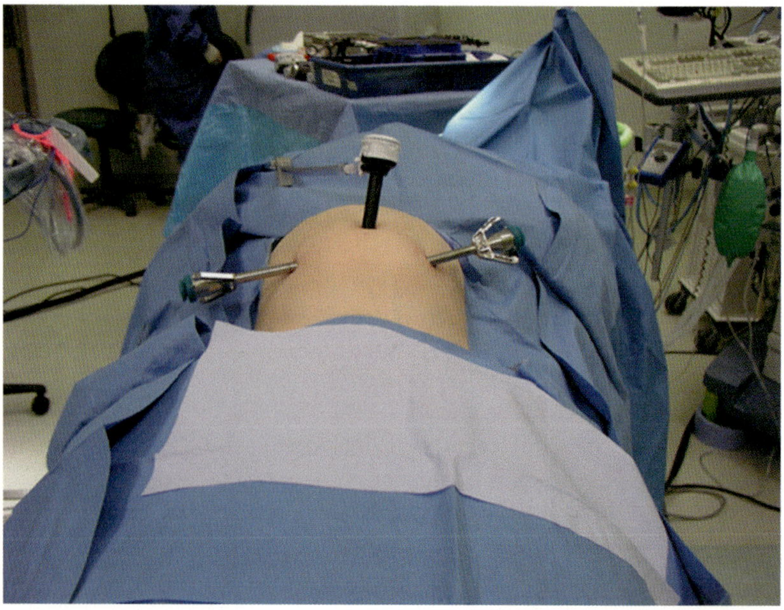

Fig. 8.1 Robotic port placement

of the ureters are identified, and they are dissected free of surrounding tissues from the point just distal to the vas deferens in boys or to above the broad ligament lateral to the uterus in girls to the level of the trigone [4]. Care must be taken to protect the pelvic plexus, which may be found caudal and medial to the ureter [29]. Some groups use hitch-stitches placed through the abdominal wall to assist with retraction [32]. We utilize a hitch stitch placed through the posterior bladder to improve visualization of the posterior bladder and the ureteral course. The detrusor tunnels are then created to 3 cm in length (Fig. 8.2). The bladder is distended and any mucosal perforations are closed with absorbable 5-0 sutures. The ureter is then placed within the detrusor tunnel and the detrusor is closed proximally to distally over the top of the ureter catching the ureteral adventitia with interrupted 3-0 or 4-0 absorbable sutures (Fig. 8.3). At this point the robot is

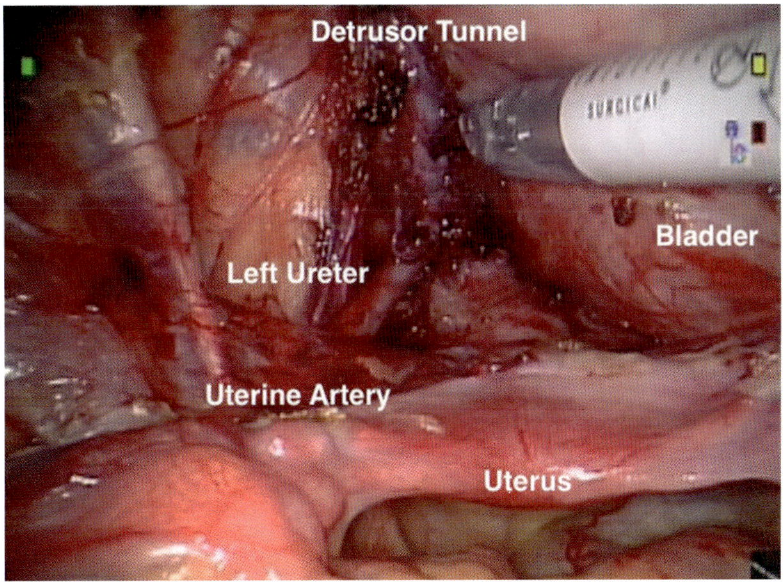

Fig. 8.2 Operative view of left ureter and detrusor tunnel

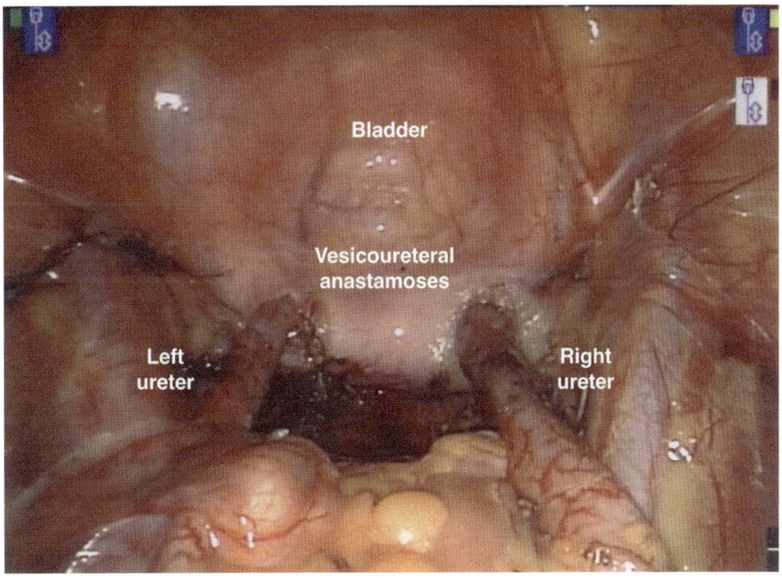

Fig. 8.3 Operative view following bilateral robotic-assisted ureteral reimplantation

undocked, the ports are removed and the standard fascial and skin closure is performed. The patient is then extubated and transferred to the recovery room with urethral catheter in place and ureteral catheters still secured.

8.3.6 Postoperative Inpatient Protocol

Patients are admitted overnight postoperatively and continued on intravenous antibiotics while the catheters remain in place. Patients are started immediately on a clear liquid diet which is then advanced as tolerated. Pain is controlled with a combination of acetaminophen as well as ketorolac with narcotic medications only being used for significant breakthrough pain. On postoperative day 1, the urethral catheter is removed along with the bilateral ureteral catheters and patients are discharged after completing a trial of void.

8.3.7 Follow-Up

Patients are seen at 3 months and 1 year postoperatively with a repeat renal ultrasounds. Postoperative voiding cystourethrogram (VCUG) is not routinely performed at our institution, and is reserved for those who have febrile UTIs [29]. This practice is in contrast to many prior studies which advocate for renal ultrasound at 1–3 months postoperatively and VCUG 3–4 months postoperatively to document any hydronephrosis and resolution of VUR. At our institution, antibiotic prophylaxis is discontinued immediately after discharge from the hospital. However, some groups continue antibiotic prophylaxis until documented resolution of VUR [33, 34].

8.4 Outcomes

8.4.1 RALUR Success Rates

Historical success rates of OUR have been 93–99% [35]. However, the definitions of success vary between studies and depend on several factors such as timing of postoperative VCUG. As discussed, LUR was not widely adopted due to technical difficulties as well as postoperative voiding dysfunction in up to 10% of patients (i.e., incontinence, delayed voiding, or incomplete emptying/retention). The body of evidence for pediatric RALUR consists of mostly single institutional case series (Table 8.1), but is evolving to show comparable success rates to OUR. Other outcome measures such as operative time, hospital length of stay, and postoperative pain have become important when comparing minimally invasive and open surgical procedures.

When Peters and Woo first described RALUR using an intravesical cross-trigonal technique, they performed the operation on six children age 5–15 years with VUR [14]. Patients were subsequently hospitalized for 2–4 days, and post-procedure VCUG showed complete reflux resolution in five patients (83% success rate). The authors noted adequate operative field size allowing good visibility of the ureters and delicate manipulation of the tissues. Their initial experience was limited, but served to generate interest in this new procedure.

In 2008, Casale and colleagues published a large case series of extravesical RALUR in 41 patients [29]. The authors hypothesized that visualization of the pelvic nerve plexus using an extravesical approach would decrease the incidence of postoperative voiding dysfunction complications. Their technique leveraged the magnified view of the surgical robot to visualize and avoid the pelvic nerve plexus along the periureteral tissues. In their series, patients were ages 16–81 months with grade ≥ III VUR. Mean operative time was 2.3 h and hospital stay was 26 h. All patients had urethral and ureteral catheters removed on postoperative day 1, with no episodes of urinary retention. VCUG performed at 3 months showed a VUR resolution rate of 98%. While the study was limited by lack of a comparative group like OUR or non-nerve sparing, it successfully demonstrated feasible technical aspects of the operation, an excellent success rate, and a low complication rate. This cohort was reevaluated in 2012 with 150 total patients and a 2-year follow-up period [36]. The success rate

Table 8.1 Studies of pediatric robotic-assisted ureteral reimplantation (RALUR)

Study	Study design (technique)	Patients (ureters)	RALUR complications	RALUR success rate	Evidence level[a]
Peters (2005) [14]	RALUR case series (intravesical)	6 (12)	1 Urine leak	83%	4
Casale (2008) [29]	RALUR case series (extravesical)	41 (82)	1 Pyelonephritis	98%	4
Sorensen (2010) [37]	RALUR vs. OUR case control (extravesical)	13 (18) vs. 26 (36)	1 Urinoma 1 Ureteral obstruction	85%	3b
Marchini (2011) [38]	RALUR vs. OUR case control (intra- and extravesical)	39 (65) vs. 39 (61)	4 Trocar-site urine leaks 2 Anastomotic leaks 1 Re-do reimplant	92% intra, 100% extra	3b
Smith (2011) [34]	RALUR vs. OUR case control (extravesical)	25 (33) vs. 25 (46)	(None)	97%	3b
Chalmers (2012) [39]	RALUR case series (extravesical)	16 (22)	(None)	88%	4
Kasturi (2012) [36]	RALUR case series (extravesical)	150 (300)	(None)	99%	4
Schomburg (2014) [42]	RALUR vs. OUR case control (extravesical)	20 (38) vs. 20 (35)	1 Urine leak 1 Ureteral stenosis	100%	3b
Akhavan (2014) [33]	RALUR case series (extravesical)	50 (78)	2 Ureteral obstruction 2 Ileus 1 Ureteral injury 1 Fluid collection	92%	4
Dangle (2014) [40]	RALUR case series (extravesical)	29 (40)	(Not reported)	80%	4
Hayashi (2014) [41]	RALUR case series (extravesical)	9 (15)	(None)	93%	4
Harel (2015) [46]	RALUR vs. OUR (extravesical)	23 (33) vs. 11 (15)	1 UTI	84%	3b
Grimsby (2015) [43]	RALUR case series (extravesical)	61 (93)	3 Ureteral obstruction 2 Anastomotic leak 1 Ileus	72%	4

Abbreviations: *OUR* open ureteral reimplantation, *RALUR* robotic-assisted laparoscopic ureteral reimplantation
[a]*Evidence levels: 1*: randomized controlled trials or meta-analyses, *2a:* Systematic reviews of cohort studies, *2b*: Individual cohort study, *2c*: Outcomes research, *3a:* Systematic review of case-control studies, *3b*: Individual case-control study, *4*: Case-series or poor quality cohort studies, *5*: Expert opinion without explicit critical appraisal

remained high with 99.3% resolution of VUR and still no patients experienced postoperative voiding dysfunction.

Sorenson and colleagues described their experience starting a pediatric robotics program in 2010 [37]. Among their first 50 robotic procedures, they focused on the outcomes of 13 RALUR procedures by comparing them to historical OUR controls. RALUR had an 85% success rate (two patients had persistent VUR) and 15% complication rate (one patient formed a urinoma and one developed ureteral obstruction, both requiring ureteral stent placement). These rates were similar to OUR controls. The total operative time for RALUR was 361 min, about 2 h longer than OUR. Akhavan updated this case series in 2012 with 50 total patients (78 ureters) [33]. The success rate rose to 92% and complication rate fell to 10%, potentially indicating an evolving learning curve for RALUR.

In 2011, Marchini compared case-matched robotic and open ureteral reimplantation using both intravesical and extravesical techniques [38]. Patients older than 4 years with bilateral VUR and bladder capacity greater than 200 cm^3 were offered intravesical ($n = 19$) or extravesical RALUR ($n = 20$). These cases were matched to 22 open intravesical reimplantations and 17 open extravesical reimplantations. Intraoperative outcomes were similar between the robotic and open groups; however, postoperative hematuria, bladder spasms, Foley catheter time, and overall hospital stay were decreased in the intravesical RALUR group. The extravesical RALUR group did not show the same benefit. Among the patients undergoing intravesical RALUR, one patient had urinary retention requiring a catheter for two extra days and four patients had bladder leaks from trocar sites that resolved after 5 days of catheterization. In the extravesical RALUR group, two patients had urinary retention and two had ureteral leaks requiring stent placement. Overall, there were no statistically significant difference in the success rates for intravesical or extravesical RALUR (92% intravesical, 100% extravesical) vs. OUR groups. This ambitious study was the first to directly compare each of the major techniques for ureteral reimplantation. Yet, it is difficult to draw firm conclusions since several sources of bias are introduced from comparing multiple groups in a retrospective fashion.

Subsequently, numerous case series have been published on pediatric RALUR. Smith and colleagues wrote a case-control series of 25 patients undergoing extravesical RALUR compared to 25 OUR patients [34]. In the RALUR group, there were no complications and there was a 97% success rate. Length of stay and morphine-equivalent analgesia were also significantly reduced after RALUR compared to OUR. Chalmers presented a case series of 16 patients who underwent RALUR and 88% had resolution of VUR [39]. Similarly, Dangle reported a success rate of 80% in 29 patients (40 ureters) and Hayashi reported success in 93% of 9 patients (15 ureters) [40, 41]. Schomburg wrote a case-control study of RALUR versus OUR in 20 patients (38 ureters) and 20 patients (35 ureters), respectively [42]. Success rates were 100% for RALUR and 95% for OUR, and complication rates were similar. The most recent case series was a multi-institutional collaboration published in 2015 by Grimsby [43]. In this cohort of 61 patients (93 ureters), there was a notably lower success rate of 72% and complication rate of 10%. Theories to explain the variable success rates across these cohorts include bias toward publication of positive studies, different definitions of procedure failure, and heterogeneous case complexity. Taken together, there are an estimated 469 patients who have undergone RALUR in the published literature with an overall success rate of 91% [43].

Studies of pediatric national databases have also provided insight into population trends and outcomes. The Pediatric Health Information System (PHIS) includes administrative data from 47 large children's hospitals in the United States. One PHIS study showed that half of these hospitals were performing robotic surgery between 2008 and 2013, including 1292 robotic urologic procedures of which 351 were ureteral reimplantations [8]. The rate of robotic urologic procedures increased by 17.4% annually and the rate of RALUR increased by 1.7% annually.

Although the most common complication of RALUR was procedure failure in ~9% of patients, a variety of other complications have been identified across these case series (Table 8.1). Patients often experience transient new onset voiding dysfunction including urinary retention, incontinence, or hesitancy which rarely requires catheterization. There is an approximately 1% rate of ureteral leak and 1% rate of ureteral obstruction, both of which can often be managed with temporary ureteral stent placement. Otherwise, there have been low <1% rates of infection, ileus, pelvic fluid collections, and ureteral injuries noted. Finally, across all genitourinary robotic procedures, there is an approximately 1.4% conversion rate to open surgery [44, 45].

With smaller incisions, robotic surgery may also be less painful than open surgery. Harel and colleagues prospectively evaluated postoperative pain scores and narcotic requirements among 23 patients undergoing RALUR compared to 11 undergoing OUR [46]. They found reduced narcotic requirements in the robotic group (0.07 mg/kg vs. 0.17 mg/kg, $p < 0.05$) with nearly half of patients in the robotic group requiring no narcotics on the first postoperative day compared to only one patient in the open surgery group. However, subjective pain scores were not significantly different between groups. Other studies, while limited by patient age and retrospective designs, have similar findings.

Cosmetic appearance of laparoscopic incisions also merits consideration, especially in children. One study showed that at the time of diagnosis of VUR, most parents prefer their children to avoid surgery and be treated with prophylactic antibiotics or endoscopic bulking agents [47]. If VUR persisted longer than 36 months, however, preference for surgery significantly increased. Another study surveyed 116 parents and patients older than 7 years on scar appearance after robotic or open surgery for ureteral reimplantation, pyeloplasty, and bladder augmentation using photographs of each [48]. For ureteral reimplantation, 85% of parents and 76% of patients preferred the appearance of robotic scars, and the majority of subjects rated scar size as important or very important as a factor affecting their decision on surgical approach. While it is certainly less crucial than overall efficacy or complication rates, scar appearance is influential for children/parents and should be discussed during preoperative counseling.

In summary, RALUR techniques have been evolving since they were first described in 2004 and the procedure has increasingly been adopted nationally. Success rates vary widely between case series from 72 to 100%, and overall average to about 91%. Success rates may differ due to publication bias, differing definitions of procedure success, and/or heterogeneous case complexities between institutions. Other benefits of the robotic approach may include decreased pain and improved cosmetic appearance.

8.4.2 Learning Curve

The learning curve for minimally invasive approaches to ureteral reimplantation can be a major barrier to its adoption. Laparoscopy and robotic surgery require surgeons to develop new technical skills and perform operations from unfamiliar perspectives. Authors have emphasized that deliberate practice using simulation and mentorship is essential to become proficient in minimally invasive surgery [49]. For some experienced laparoscopic surgeons, the learning curve for RALUR has been shown to plateau after as few as 5–7 cases [29]. Others, however, saw no decrease in operative time for RALUR after their first 13 procedures [37]. In a study of 39 RALUR patients, there were significantly more complications early in the series, prompting changes to the surgical protocol [38]. In a study on learning curve for robotic pyeloplasty, pediatric urology fellows were estimated to achieve comparable operative times to an experienced attending surgeon after 37 cases [50]. It is reasonable to assume that robotic surgical skills translate between procedures and therefore may require 30 or more procedures to achieve proficiency in RALUR. This, however, may change as robotic surgery and robotic skills training become increasingly integrated in residency education.

Institutional learning curve is also a factor. When a robotic surgery program is implemented, surgical support staff needs to become proficient with all new equipment and procedures. The University of Washington invested in a Da Vinci surgical robot in 2006, and in 2010 reported on their experience initiating a multispecialty robotics program [37]. The average case volume was 2.5 cases/month (range 0–5) over the 20 month study period. To maximize programmatic success, they recommended using a dedicated surgical team, assigning specific operative days for robotic surgery, securing administrative commitment to robotics, and partnering with other specialties to increase case volume.

8.4.3 Cost Considerations

In addition to the clinical outcomes, it is important to examine the costs associated with robotic surgery. High initial capital expenditures and recurring maintenance fees can make robotic surgery extremely expensive. Between 2005 and 2009, Rowe and colleagues compared costs among multiple pediatric urologic robotic and open procedures [51]. They surprisingly found that RAL surgery direct costs were 12% lower than those for open surgery overall ($8795 vs. $9978). The longer length of hospital stay associated with open surgery drove the higher costs. Indirect costs were estimated to be $1343 per case for robot purchase (based on approximately $1.2 million purchase cost, 10 year life span and average 67 cases per year) plus $1492 per case for robot maintenance (based on $100,000 annual service contract). When these indirect purchase and maintenance costs were included, robotic surgery costs were 17% greater than those of open surgery.

Beyond the direct costs of robotic technology, human capital is an important topic within pediatric surgery. The burden of a child's illness can result in large nonmedical costs in the form of lost wages and travel time for parents. One study of robotic versus open pediatric pyeloplasty analyzed human capital losses associated with length of hospital stay and parental work days lost [52]. Excluding amortized robot costs, the study demonstrated that robotic pyeloplasty resulted in a $929 increased cost per procedure compared to open surgery. It found a reduction in length of hospital stay by 1 day for robotic surgery, which translated to an average $90 savings of lost parental wages and $613 savings in hospitalization expenses. This suggests that cost savings from shortened hospitalizations may help offset the increased operative costs. Moreover, reducing hospital stay may allow for better allocation of limited hospital resources and bed space.

Conclusions

Robot-assisted laparoscopic surgery minimizes the challenges associated with traditional laparoscopic surgery and has become popular for complex reconstructive surgeries in pediatric urology. Ureteral reimplantation is the chief intervention for children with vesicoureteral reflux. While open surgery remains the gold standard with high success rates, minimally invasive ureteral reimplantation is increasingly utilized. Patients undergoing RALUR have been shown to benefit from decreased length of hospital stay, decreased pain medication requirements, and improved cosmesis. Success rates vary across case series, but approach the success rate of OUR. Finally, the higher initial costs associated with robotic technology may be offset by human capital gains and reduced indirect costs.

References

1. Van Batavia JP, Casale P. Robotic surgery in pediatric urology. Curr Urol Rep. 2014;15:402. doi:10.1007/s11934-014-0402-9.
2. Tobias JD. Anaesthesia for minimally invasive surgery in children. Best Pract Res Clin Anaesthesiol. 2002;16:115–30.
3. Volfson IA, Munver R, Esposito M, Dakwar G, Hanna M, Stock JA. Robot-assisted urologic surgery: safety and feasibility in the pediatric population. J Endourol. 2007;21:1315–8. doi:10.1089/end.2007.9982.
4. Tomaszewski JJ, Casella DP, Turner RM, Casale P, Ost MC. Pediatric laparoscopic and robot-assisted laparoscopic surgery: technical considerations. J Endourol. 2012;26:602–13. doi:10.1089/end.2011.0252.
5. Camarillo DB, Krummel TM, Salisbury JK. Robotic technology in surgery: past, present, and future. Am J Surg. 2004;188:2S–15S. doi:10.1016/j.amjsurg.2004.08.025.
6. Moorthy K, Munz Y, Dosis A, Hernandez J, Martin S, Bello F, Rockall T, Darzi A. Dexterity enhancement with robotic surgery. Surg Endosc. 2004;18:790–5. doi:10.1007/s00464-003-8922-2.
7. Casale P. Robotic pediatric urology. Curr Urol Rep. 2009;10:115–8.
8. Mahida JB, Cooper JN, Herz D, Diefenbach KA, Deans KJ, Minneci PC, McLeod DJ. Utilization and costs associated with robotic surgery in children. J Surg Res. 2015;199:169–76. doi:10.1016/j.jss.2015.04.087.
9. Chand DH, Rhoades T, Poe SA, Kraus S, Strife CF. Incidence and severity of vesicoureteral reflux in children related to age, gender, race and diagnosis. JURO. 2003;170:1548–50. doi:10.1097/01.ju.0000084299.55552.6c.
10. Shaikh N, Craig JC, Rovers MM, Da Dalt L, Gardikis S, Hoberman A, Montini G, Rodrigo C, Taskinen S, Tuerlinckx D, Shope T. Identification of children and adolescents at risk for renal scarring after a first urinary tract infection: a meta-analysis with individual patient data. JAMA Pediatr. 2014;168:893–900. doi:10.1001/jamapediatrics.2014.637.
11. Estrada CR, Passerotti CC, Graham DA, Peters CA, Bauer SB, Diamond DA, Cilento BG, Borer JG, Cendron M, Nelson CP, Lee RS, Zhou J, Retik AB, Nguyen HT. Nomograms for predicting annual resolution rate of primary vesicoureteral reflux: results

from 2,462 children. J Urol. 2009;182:1535–41. doi:10.1016/j.juro.2009.06.053.
12. Atala A, Kavoussi LR, Goldstein DS, Retik AB, Peters CA. Laparoscopic correction of vesicoureteral reflux. J Urol. 1993;150:748–51.
13. Ehrlich RM, Gershman A, Fuchs G. Laparoscopic vesicoureteroplasty in children: initial case reports. Urology. 1994;43:255–61.
14. Peters CA, Woo R. Intravesical robotically assisted bilateral ureteral reimplantation. J Endourol. 2005;19:618–21. doi:10.1089/end.2005.19.618; discussion 621–2
15. Peters CA. Laparoscopic and robotic approach to genitourinary anomalies in children. Urol Clin North Am. 2004;31:595–605. doi:10.1016/j.ucl.2004.04.022; xi
16. Bowen DK, Faasse MA, Liu DB, Gong EM, Lindgren BW, Johnson EK. Use of pediatric open, laparoscopic and robot-assisted laparoscopic ureteral Reimplantation in the United States: 2000 to 2012. J Urol. 2016;196:207–12. doi:10.1016/j.juro.2016.02.065.
17. Peters CA, Skoog SJ, Arant BS, Copp HL, Elder JS, Hudson RG, Khoury AE, Lorenzo AJ, Pohl HG, Shapiro E, Snodgrass WT, Diaz M. Summary of the AUA guideline on Management of Primary Vesicoureteral Reflux in children. J Urol. 2010;184:1134–44. doi:10.1016/j.juro.2010.05.065.
18. Tekgül S, Riedmiller H, Hoebeke P, Kočvara R, RJM N, Radmayr C, Stein R, Dogan HS, European Association of Urology. EAU guidelines on vesicoureteral reflux in children. Eur Urol. 2012;62:534–42. doi:10.1016/j.eururo.2012.05.059.
19. Szymanski KM, Oliveira LM, Silva A, Retik AB, Nguyen HT. Analysis of indications for ureteral reimplantation in 3738 children with vesicoureteral reflux: a single institutional cohort. J Pediatr Urol. 2011;7:601–10. doi:10.1016/j.jpurol.2011.06.002.
20. Shokeir AA, Nijman RJ. Primary megaureter: current trends in diagnosis and treatment. BJU Int. 2000;86:861–8.
21. Pohl HG, Joyce GF, Wise M, Cilento BG. Vesicoureteral reflux and ureteroceles. JURO. 2007;177:1659–66. doi:10.1016/j.juro.2007.01.059.
22. Morey AF, Brandes S, Dugi DD, Armstrong JH, Breyer BN, Broghammer JA, Erickson BA, Holzbeierlein J, Hudak SJ, Pruitt JH, Reston JT, Santucci RA, Smith TG, Wessells H, Assocation AU. Urotrauma: AUA guideline. J Urol. 2014;192:327–35. doi:10.1016/j.juro.2014.05.004.
23. Finkelstein JB, Levy AC, Silva MV, Murray L, Delaney C, Casale P. How to decide which infant can have robotic surgery? Just do the math. J Pediatr Urol. 2015;11(170):e1–4. doi:10.1016/j.jpurol.2014.11.020.
24. Ballouhey Q, Villemagne T, Cros J, Szwarc C, Braik K, Longis B, Lardy H, Fourcade L. A comparison of robotic surgery in children weighing above and below 15.0 kg: size does not affect surgery success. Surg Endosc. 2015;29:2643–50. doi:10.1007/s00464-014-3982-z.
25. Meehan JJ. Robotic surgery in small children: is there room for this? J Laparoendosc Adv Surg Tech A. 2009;19:707–12. doi:10.1089/lap.2008.0178.
26. Bannister CF, Brosius KK, Wulkan M. The effect of insufflation pressure on pulmonary mechanics in infants during laparoscopic surgical procedures. Paediatr Anaesth. 2003;13:785–9.
27. Olsen LH, Deding D, Yeung CK, Jørgensen TM. Computer assisted laparoscopic pneumovesical ureter reimplantation a.m. Cohen: initial experience in a pig model. APMIS Suppl. 2003;109:23–5.
28. Lipski BA, Mitchell ME, Burns MW. Voiding dysfunction after bilateral extravesical ureteral reimplantation. JURO. 1998;159:1019–21.
29. Casale P, Patel RP, Kolon TF. Nerve sparing robotic extravesical ureteral reimplantation. J Urol. 2008;179:1987–9. doi:10.1016/j.juro.2008.01.062; discussion 1990
30. Faasse MA, Lindgren BW, Frainey BT, Marcus CR, Szczodry DM, Glaser AP, Suresh S, Gong EM. Perioperative effects of caudal and transversus abdominis plane (TAP) blocks for children undergoing urologic robot-assisted laparoscopic surgery. J Pediatr Urol. 2015;11:121.e1–7. doi:10.1016/j.jpurol.2014.10.010.
31. Orvieto MA, Large M, Gundeti MS. Robotic paediatric urology. BJU Int. 2012;110:2–13. doi:10.1111/j.1464-410X.2011.10877.x.
32. Lendvay T. Robotic-assisted laparoscopic management of vesicoureteral reflux. Adv Urol. 2008:732942. doi:10.1155/2008/732942.
33. Akhavan A, Avery D, Lendvay TS. Robot-assisted extravesical ureteral reimplantation: outcomes and conclusions from 78 ureters. J Pediatr Urol. 2014;10:864–8. doi:10.1016/j.jpurol.2014.01.028.
34. Smith RP, Oliver JL, Peters CA. Pediatric robotic extravesical ureteral reimplantation: comparison with open surgery. J Urol. 2011;185:1876–81. doi:10.1016/j.juro.2010.12.072.
35. Weiss DA, Shukla AR. The robotic-assisted ureteral reimplantation: the evolution to a new standard. Urol Clin North Am. 2015;42:99–109. doi:10.1016/j.ucl.2014.09.010.
36. Kasturi S, Sehgal SS, Christman MS, Lambert SM, Casale P. Prospective long-term analysis of nerve-sparing extravesical robotic-assisted laparoscopic ureteral reimplantation. Urology. 2012;79:680–3. doi:10.1016/j.urology.2011.10.052.
37. Sorensen MD, Johnson MH, Delostrinos C, Bice JB, Grady RW, Lendvay TS. Initiation of a pediatric robotic surgery program: institutional challenges and realistic outcomes. Surg Endosc. 2010;24:2803–8. doi:10.1007/s00464-010-1052-8.
38. Marchini GS, Hong YK, Minnillo BJ, Diamond DA, Houck CS, Meier PM, Passerotti CC, Kaplan JR, Retik AB, Nguyen HT. Robotic assisted laparoscopic ureteral reimplantation in children: case matched comparative study with open surgical approach. J Urol. 2011;185:1870–5. doi:10.1016/j.juro.2010.12.069.

39. Chalmers D, Herbst K, Kim C. Robotic-assisted laparoscopic extravesical ureteral reimplantation: an initial experience. J Pediatr Urol. 2012;8:268–71. doi:10.1016/j.jpurol.2011.04.006.
40. Dangle PP, Shah A, Gundeti MS. Robot-assisted laparoscopic ureteric reimplantation: extravesical technique. BJU Int. 2014;114:630–2. doi:10.1111/bju.12813.
41. Hayashi Y, Mizuno K, Kurokawa S, Nakane A, Kamisawa H, Nishio H, Moritoki Y, Tozawa K, Kohri K, Kojima Y. Extravesical robot-assisted laparoscopic ureteral reimplantation for vesicoureteral reflux: initial experience in Japan with the ureteral advancement technique. Int J Urol. 2014;21:1016–21. doi:10.1111/iju.12483.
42. Schomburg JL, Haberman K, Willihnganz-Lawson KH, Shukla AR. Robot-assisted laparoscopic ureteral reimplantation: a single surgeon comparison to open surgery. J Pediatr Urol. 2014;10:875–9. doi:10.1016/j.jpurol.2014.02.013.
43. Grimsby GM, Dwyer ME, Jacobs MA, Ost MC, Schneck FX, Cannon GM, Gargollo PC. Multi-institutional review of outcomes of robot-assisted laparoscopic extravesical ureteral reimplantation. J Urol. 2015;193:1791–5. doi:10.1016/j.juro.2014.07.128.
44. Cundy TP, Shetty K, Clark J, Chang TP, Sriskandarajah K, Gattas NE, Najmaldin A, Yang G-Z, Darzi A. The first decade of robotic surgery in children. J Pediatr Surg. 2013;48:858–65. doi:10.1016/j.jpedsurg.2013.01.031.
45. Dangle PP, Akhavan A, Odeleye M, Avery D, Lendvay T, Koh CJ, Elder JS, Noh PH, Bansal D, Schulte M, MacDonald J, Shukla A, Kim C, Herbst K, Corbett S, Kearns J, Kunnavakkam R, Gundeti MS. Ninety-day perioperative complications of pediatric robotic urological surgery: a multi-institutional study. J Pediatr Urol. 2016;12(102):e1–6. doi:10.1016/j.jpurol.2015.08.015.
46. Harel M, Herbst KW, Silvis R, Makari JH, Ferrer FA, Kim C. Objective pain assessment after ureteral reimplantation: comparison of open versus robotic approach. J Pediatr Urol. 2015;11(82):e1–8. doi:10.1016/j.jpurol.2014.12.007.
47. Krill AJ, Pohl HG, Belman AB, Skoog SJ, Snodgrass WT, Rushton HG. Parental preferences in the management of vesicoureteral reflux. J Urol. 2011;186:2040–4. doi:10.1016/j.juro.2011.07.023.
48. Barbosa JA, Barayan G, Gridley CM, Sanchez DC, Passerotti CC, Houck CS, Nguyen HT. Parent and patient perceptions of robotic vs open urological surgery scars in children. J Urol. 2013;190:244–50. doi:10.1016/j.juro.2012.12.060.
49. Casale P. Laparoscopic and robotic approach to genitourinary anomalies in children. Urol Clin North Am. 2010;37:279–86. doi:10.1016/j.ucl.2010.03.005.
50. Tasian GE, Wiebe DJ, Casale P. Learning curve of robotic assisted pyeloplasty for pediatric urology fellows. J Urol. 2013;190:1622–6. doi:10.1016/j.juro.2013.02.009.
51. Rowe CK, Pierce MW, Tecci KC, Houck CS, Mandell J, Retik AB, Nguyen HT. A comparative direct cost analysis of pediatric urologic robot-assisted laparoscopic surgery versus open surgery: could robot-assisted surgery be less expensive? J Endourol. 2012;26:871–7. doi:10.1089/end.2011.0584.
52. Behan JW, Kim SS, Dorey F, De Filippo RE, Chang AY, Hardy BE, Koh CJ. Human capital gains associated with robotic assisted laparoscopic pyeloplasty in children compared to open pyeloplasty. J Urol. 2011;186:1663–7. doi:10.1016/j.juro.2011.04.019.

9 Robot Assisted Laparoscopic Bladder Augmentation in Children

William R. Boysen and Mohan S. Gundeti

9.1 Introduction

Augmentation cystoplasty (AC) has long been a staple in the management of bladder dysfunction in children, traditionally performed via an open approach. The use of various bowel segments has been described, including the stomach, small bowel, and colon, but the open ileocystoplasty remains the most popular bladder augmentation procedure [1].

Minimally invasive techniques have gained popularity among pediatric urologists in recent years, particularly with the use of robot assisted laparoscopic approaches. The first laparoscopic approach to appendicovesicostomy (APV) was described in 1993 [2], in which laparoscopy was used to mobilize the appendix and cecum with subsequent APV creation using an open transverse suprapubic incision. The robot assisted laparoscopic Mitrofanoff appendicovesicostomy (RALMA) was then described in 2004 [3], followed by a report of total intracorporeal robot assisted laparoscopic ileocystoplasty with Mitrofanoff appendicovesicostomy (RALIMA) in 2008 [4].

Given the complexity of AC and APV creation, adoption of the minimally invasive approach has been slow. Other barriers to adoption have been historical preference for the open approach and lack of standardized training in pediatric robotic surgery. However, growing case series have been published in recent years that demonstrate the safety and efficacy of RALMA [5] and RALIMA [6] as viable minimally invasive alternatives to the traditional open approach. This chapter provides an overview of our approach to RALIMA, including patient selection and workup, detailed description of technique, potential complications, and outcomes.

W.R. Boysen, M.D. • M.S. Gundeti, M.D., M.Ch., F.E.B.U., F.R.C.S. (✉)
Department of Surgery, University of Chicago Medical Center, Chicago, IL, USA
e-mail: mgundeti@surgery.bsd.uchicago.edu

9.2 Patient Selection and Preoperative Workup

Reconstruction of the lower urinary tract in children can consist of a variety of procedures, including APV formation, AC, bladder neck closure (BNC), and bladder neck reconstruction (BNR). The specific combination of procedures selected will be dictated by the individual patient's clinical scenario and indication for surgical intervention. The majority of children who require lower urinary tract reconstruction have a neurogenic bladder secondary to myelomeningocele, tethered cord, or other neurologic conditions. The bladder dysfunction associated with these conditions can include poor capacity and compliance that place the upper urinary tracts at risk of deterioration, and urinary incontinence that affects the child's socialization [7]. Though initial medical management and temporary diversion with suprapubic catheter, cutaneous vesicostomy, or clean intermittent catheterization (CIC) can be attempted, surgery is indicated in those patients who are unresponsive to

G. Mattioli, P. Petralia (eds.), *Pediatric Robotic Surgery*, DOI 10.1007/978-3-319-41863-6_9

conservative measures or who desire more definitive intervention. The goals of surgery are to preserve the upper urinary tract and achieve urinary continence.

The decision to pursue a robotic approach rather than open should be based on surgeon comfort, patient preference, and patient characteristics. Patients who have had multiple prior reconstructions are likely to require an open approach due to adhesive disease and complex anatomy. Wheelchair-bound patients with significant kyphoscoliosis also pose a challenge for the robotic approach with respect to port placement and insufflation, so the robotic approach in these patients should be attempted only once proficiency is achieved.

Preoperative workup should include videourodynamics to assess the bladder and bladder neck, as well as radiographic assessment of the upper urinary tract with renal ultrasound and possible DMSA scan to assess for renal scarring and split function. Creation of a catheterizable channel without augmentation is appropriate for patients with an adequate capacity and compliance, but who desire a catheterizable channel to facilitate CIC by patient or caregiver. Augmentation cystoplasty is indicated for patients with poor capacity and/or compliance, and is typically performed with a catheterizable channel but can be performed alone if patient or caregiver is willing and able to perform CIC per urethra. We recommend that patients and caregivers meet with a skilled nurse prior to surgery, to become acquainted with CIC.

Stoma site for planned APV is marked on the skin in the supine and standing position, to ensure ease of catheterization. The author prefers to use the right iliac fossa for ambulatory children, and the umbilicus for children who are wheelchair bound. Often the final decision is based on the orientation of the appendix mesentery.

Children can continue their normal bowel regimen and diet preoperatively. We do not perform an additional bowel preparation, based on the author's prior work demonstrating that there is no difference in hospital length of stay or complications among children undergoing open AC with or without a mechanical bowel preparation and enema [8].

We suggest diagnostic laparoscopy prior to docking the robot, especially in those who have a ventriculoperitoneal (VP) shunt. We have found that in these patients, the appendix is often atretic with poor mesentery. Scarring and abnormal appendix location (e.g., suprahepatic or retrocolic) can make mobilization challenging with the robotic approach, so this portion may need to be performed laparoscopically prior to docking the robot.

9.3 Technique

Various techniques for performing RALMA and RALIMA have been described in the literature [3, 5, 6, 9–14]. What follows is a detailed overview of our approach to these techniques. Table 9.1 provides troubleshooting and tips for challenging clinical situations.

Table 9.1 Troubleshooting and tips (adapted with permission from Murthy et al. [6])

Scenario	Tips
High BMI	• Use bariatric ports after proficiency is established
Kyphoscoliosis	• Move camera port supra-umbilically if pubo-umbilical distance is too short
Presence of VP shunt	• Perform diagnostic peritoneoscopy
	• Expect adhesions and need for adhesiolysis
	• Isolate VP shunt in Endopouch bag to decrease contamination risk
	• Appendix often found in subhepatic space
Short appendix	• Utilize cecal flap for ACE channel
Short ileal mesenteric vessels	• Begin dividing ileum on antimesenteric side, prior to dividing mesentery to better identify vessels
Fatty mesentery	• Decreasing Trendelenburg can bring the loop of ileum into the pelvis
Mesenteric orientation and twisting	• Use stay sutures on proximal and distal ends of loop, diligently monitor for twisting
	• For appendix, place stay suture on antimesenteric side of proximal edge
Bladder neck closure	• Use laparoscopy prior to docking robot to mobilize omentum from the greater curvature of the stomach to cover repair

9.3.1 Patient Positioning and Port Placement

The patient is placed in the dorsal lithotomy position with slight Trendelenburg of 10–20 °, and all pressure points are carefully padded given the relatively long duration of surgery. The patient is prepped and draped in the normal sterile fashion, and in select cases cystoscopy is performed with placement of bilateral double-J stents to aid in identifying the ureteral orifices during cystoplasty. For the experienced surgeon, ureteral stent placement can be omitted but is useful for identifying anatomy as one becomes proficient with this procedure. We no longer routinely place ureteral stents at the start of the case.

A Foley catheter is then placed in the surgical field to decompress the bladder during port placement but allow the assistant to fill the bladder during the procedure. A nasogastric or orogastric tube is placed to decompress the stomach prior to port placement. A 12 mm camera port is placed superior to the umbilicus approximately 12 cm from the pubic symphysis using an open Hasson technique. Two 8 mm robotic trocars are then placed under direct vision bilaterally at the midclavicular line at the level of the umbilicus. An assistant port is placed in the left upper quadrant to aid in retraction and allow passage of suture material. A third robotic port is placed at the right anterior axillary line for the third arm of the robot. The robot is then docked between the patient's legs [15]. Figure 9.1 shows patient positioning and port placement. If a VP shunt is present, we recommend placing the VP shunt in an endocatch bag in the subhepatic space to prevent contamination [16]. We also broaden out preoperative antibiotics to include vancomycin in patients with a VP shunt.

9.3.2 Appendiceal Harvest

The procedure begins by identifying the appendix, and a premeasured umbilical tape can be used to ensure that adequate length is present. The appendix is detached sharply from the cecum (Fig. 9.2), and the defect is closed with 3–0 Vicryl suture in

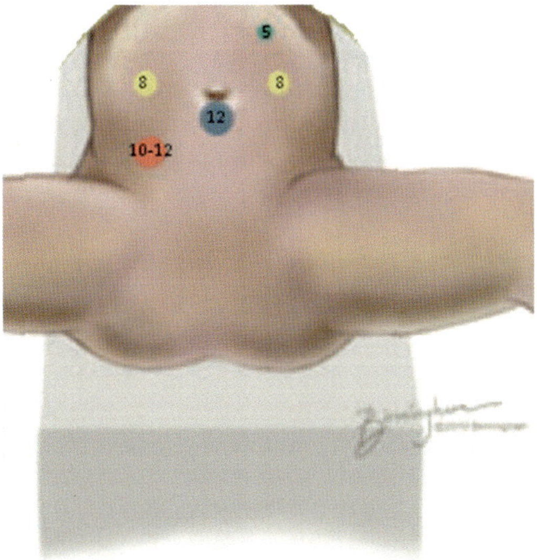

Fig. 9.1 Patient position and port placement (reproduced with permission from Gundeti et al. [10])

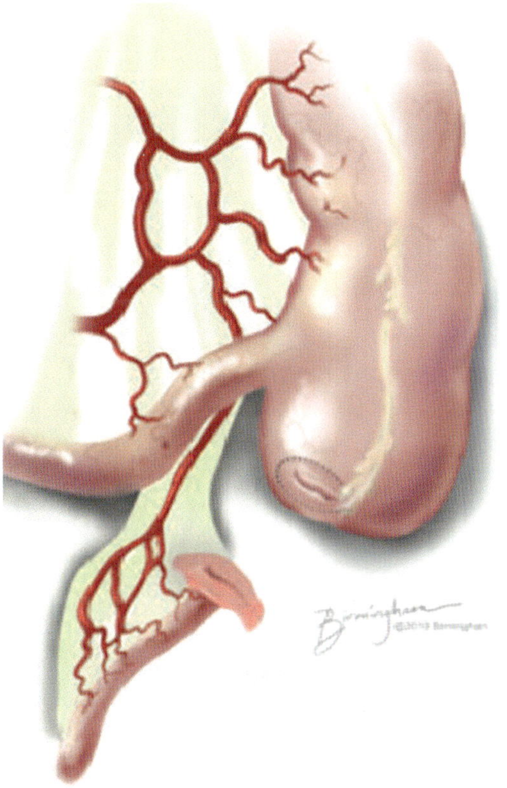

Fig. 9.2 Appendix isolation and closure of cecum (reproduced with permission from Gundeti et al. [10])

two layers. If an antegrade colonic enema (ACE) channel is planned, the proximal 1 cm of appendix is left in continuity with the cecum or a cecal flap is raised and the defect is left open until ACE is matured at completion of the procedure.

9.3.3 Ileal Loop Isolation and Bowel Anastomosis

A 20 cm segment of ileum is measured using pre-measured umbilical tape, starting approximately 20 cm proximal to the ileocecal junction. Percutaneous stay sutures can be useful for stabilizing the bowel while measuring the loop, dividing the mesentery, and completing bowel anastomosis. A 2–0 silk suture on a straight Keith needle is passed through the abdominal wall by the assistant, through the serosa of one end of the planned bowel segment, and then back out through the abdominal wall. A similar stay suture is placed for the opposite end of the bowel segment. The ends of the ileal loop can then be sharply transected using the monopolar scissor and the mesentery divided with a harmonic scalpel to ensure hemostasis. Bowel continuity is reestablished using a single-layer, full-thickness running suture (Fig. 9.3). We use a 5–0 polydioxanone II suture (PDS; Ethicon, Somerville, NJ, USA) in the pediatric population and a 4–0 PDS II in adolescent and adult patients. The third arm of the robot can be useful for retraction and stabilization during the bowel anastomosis, though in our experience the patient must be at least 5 ft tall

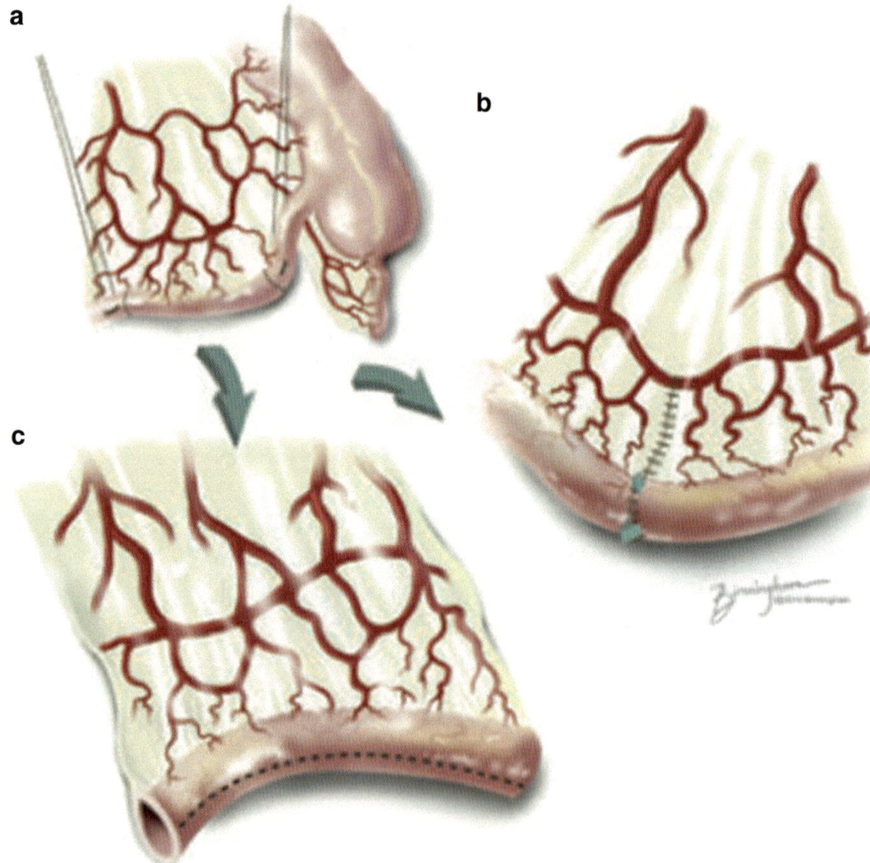

Fig. 9.3 Isolation of ileal loop, including traction sutures on ileum (**a**), ileo-ileo anastomosis with closure of mesentery (**b**), and isolation of 20 cm ileal loop (**c**) (reproduced with permission from Gundeti et al. [10])

to accommodate this additional port. The mesenteric defect is also closed.

9.3.4 Bladder Neck Closure

In select patients, BNC is indicated and can be performed concurrently with bladder augmentation. If planned, BNC should be performed at this stage in the procedure by mobilizing the bladder and releasing it from the puboprostatic ligaments. Traction on the catheter can be useful in identifying the bladder neck. The dorsal venous complex is then suture ligated and the bladder neck is divided. Care should be taken to ensure that the transection is away from the ureteral orifices. The bladder neck is then closed in two layers using a running 4–0 Vicryl suture. Prior to docking the robot, omentum can be mobilized laparoscopically if an extra layer is desired over the bladder neck closure.

9.3.5 Bladder Neck Reconstruction and Sling Placement

Bladder neck reconstruction (BNR) and sling placement can be performed as an alternative to BNC, if an outlet procedure is indicated for urinary incontinence. The described technique mimics the Leadbetter/Mitchell BNR and uses a cadaveric fascial sling. The sling is prepared on the back table by securing two 2.5 cm tunneling devices to a 10 cm × 1 cm strip of Tutoplast cadaveric fascia (IOP, Inc., Costa Mesa, CA) using 3–0 PDS II suture. A crescent-shaped incision is made posterior to the bladder to separate the bladder from the rectum in males and the vagina in females. The peritoneum is then incised near the dome of the bladder and the space of Retzius is developed. Posteriorly, the rectovesical space (boys) and vesicouterine space (girls) is developed, to facilitate passage of the tunneling devices ventrally into the space of Retzius on either side of the bladder neck.

The dorsal venous complex is then suture ligated and the anterior bladder neck is opened to unroof the proximal urethra and bladder neck to the level of the interureteric ridge. The Foley catheter can be exchanged for a smaller 5-Fr feeding tube and the urethra is retubularized in two layers using a running 5–0 PDS II suture and 4–0 PDS II suture. The bladder is filled with saline via the 5-Fr feeding tube to ensure that there is no leak. To preserve bladder capacity, a 3–4 cm strip of bladder is not excised as described in the typical open Leadbetter/Mitchell BNR.

Following BNR, the tunneling devices are identified by dissecting lateral to the urethra and the sling is wrapped tightly 360 ° around the urethra. The tunneling devices are removed and sling is secured to the pubic bone using six screws from a hernia tacker [14].

9.3.6 Detrusorotomy and Appendicovesicostomy

After filling the bladder with 60 mL of sterile saline through the Foley catheter, a 4 cm detrusorotomy is made at the dome of the bladder in the coronal plane. The bladder is often thick walled and highly vascular; the monopolar scissor or harmonic scalpel can be useful to control bleeding. The preplaced ureteral catheters are identified once cystotomy is performed to confirm that the incision is away from the ureters. If APV is the only procedure planned, anastomosis to the anterior wall of the bladder is performed. However for concurrent APV and AC, a posterior wall anastomosis is performed. A small incision is made in the posterior bladder wall and the distal appendix is pulled into the bladder. This incision is made in the midline if an umbilical stoma is planned, or the right posterior bladder if a right iliac fossa stoma is planned. A tunnel is then created in the bladder mucosa and detrusor intravesically, at least 4 cm in length. The distal 1 cm of the appendix is removed and spatulated to generate an adequate lumen, and a 5–0 PDS II suture is used to begin the appendico-vesical anastomosis. This anastomosis is then completed in a running fashion over an 8-Fr feeding tube. The appendix is then placed in the submucosal tunnel and the detrusor and mucosa are closed over top of the appendix with a running 4–0 Vicryl suture. A stay suture is placed proximally between the appendix and the proximal extent of the detrusorraphy to prevent slippage of the appendix within this tunnel. The 8-Fr feeding tube is also secured to the bladder mucosa with a 5–0 PDS II suture. The final appearance is shown in Fig. 9.4.

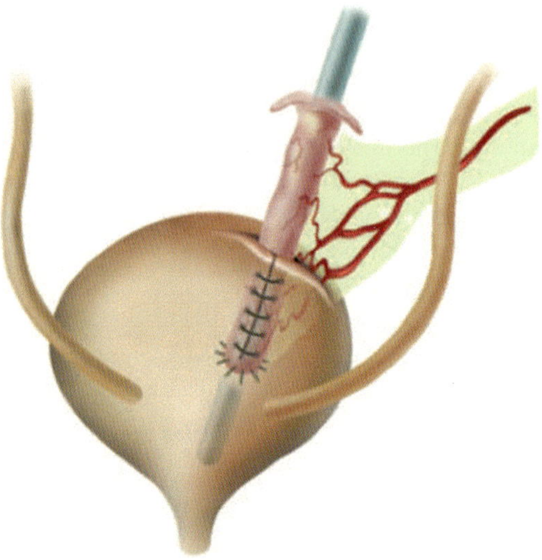

Fig. 9.4 Completed appendicovesicostomy and detrusor imbrication (reproduced with permission from Gundeti et al. [10])

9.3.7 Ileovesical Anastomosis and Suprapubic Catheter Placement

An 18-Fr suprapubic catheter is introduced percutaneously and passed through the bladder wall away from the existing cystotomy, and secured in place with a purse-string suture. In patients undergoing BNC, a second suprapubic catheter is placed to maximize postoperative drainage.

The previously isolated segment of ileum is incised along the antimesenteric border, with care taken not to twist the segment on its mesentery. The bowel patch is now anastomosed to the previously made coronal cystotomy, starting by approximating the posterior corners of the patch to the respective apices of the cystotomy. The posterior edge is then anastomosed with a running 2–0 Vicryl suture, followed by the anterior edge (Fig. 9.5). At the completion of the anastomosis, the bladder is distended with saline through the urethral catheter to ensure that urine leak is not present. The completed augmentation is shown in Fig. 9.6.

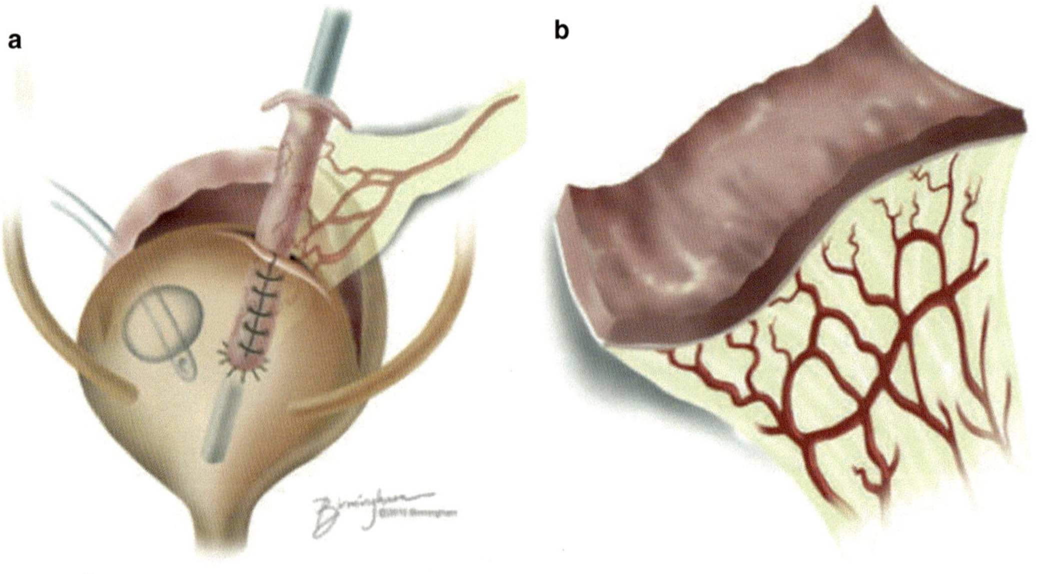

Fig. 9.5 Coronal cystotomy (**a**) and detubularization of ileum on antimesenteric border (**b**) (reproduced with permission from Gundeti et al. [10])

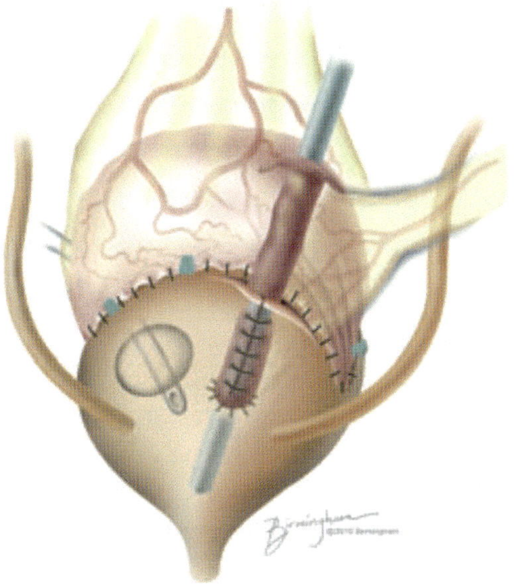

Fig. 9.6 Completed ileocystoplasty and appendicovesicostomy (reproduced with permission from Gundeti et al. [10])

9.3.8 Stoma Maturation, Antegrade Colonic Enema Channel Formation, and Port Closure

If ACE formation is planned, a stay suture is placed to the appendiceal stump or cecal flap and used to pull the stoma up to the abdominal wall at the right lower quadrant trocar site. A skin flap is created using the surgeon's preferred technique (V, VQ, VQZ techniques), and the stoma is matured using a 3–0 PDS II suture. The author prefers the VQZ flap for optimal cosmetic and functional outcome [17]. A similar technique is used to mature the APV channel to the umbilicus or an alternate stoma site.

A final inspection of the abdominal cavity is performed to assess for hemostasis, and the remaining ports are removed and robot undocked. The fascia of the remaining port sites is then closed, followed by the skin.

9.4 Postoperative Care

Patients are monitored in the hospital postoperatively until discharge criteria are met, including adequate pain control, ability to ambulate, ability to tolerate general diet, and patient/family comfort with caring for drainage tubes. Pain control is initiated with intravenous ketorolac for 48 h postoperatively, followed by oral ibuprofen and acetaminophen. Intravenous morphine is given as needed, though we strive to limit narcotic use to prevent the associated ileus. Patients who undergo RALMA alone are started on a clear liquid diet immediately postoperatively, while those undergoing RALIMA are started on clear liquids on postoperative day 1. Diet is then advanced as tolerated. Patients with baseline constipation are resumed on their home bowel regimen. Our approach to postoperative management is summarized in Table 9.2.

The suprapubic catheter is maintained to gravity drainage and 8-Fr feeding tube in APV channel is secured in place with a Tegaderm. Four weeks postoperatively, the APV catheter is removed and patient/family are instructed in clean intermittent catheterization. The suprapubic catheter is left in place as a "safety valve" for one additional week, or longer as needed until CIC is performed without difficulty. A postoperative renal ultrasound is performed to assess the upper urinary tracts.

Table 9.2 Summary of postoperative management and follow-up routine

Postoperative management
Intravenous ketorolac for 48 h
Acetaminophen
Early feeding: regular diet day of surgery for RALMA, postoperative day 1 for RALIMA
Home bowel regimen
Discharge criteria
Tolerating diet
Pain controlled
Baseline ambulation
Family/caregiver comfort with drains and tubes
Drains
8-Fr feeding tube in APV secured to skin for 4 weeks
SP catheter(s) and Foley catheter (if present) to gravity for 4 weeks
At 4-week postoperative visit, APV stent removed and SP catheter capped; commence CIC
SP catheter removed 1 week later if CIC going well
Follow-up
Upper tract evaluation with renal ultrasound 2–3 months postoperatively

Abbreviations: *APV* appendicovesicostomy, *SP* suprapubic, *CIC* clean intermittent catheterization

9.5 Complications

Potential complications following AC are similar between the open and laparoscopic approach, with the notable exception of potential complications from gaining access during a laparoscopic procedure. These potential complications have been well described [18], and are related to potential injury to intraperitoneal and retroperitoneal organs with placement of the laparoscopic trocars. In our practice, we have minimized complications related to access by using an open Hasson technique to place the camera port, and subsequently placing all other ports under direct vision. This is critical in patients at high risk for complications from port placement, such as obese patients and those with kyphoscoliosis or multiple prior abdominal surgeries.

The potential immediate and long-term complications following formation of a catheterizable channel with or without augmentation cystoplasty are similar, regardless of approach. Data on complications of RALMA and RALIMA are limited to small case series from specialized centers, and are therefore difficult to compare to the gold standard open approach. However, initial results are promising.

Complications from the augmentation itself are quite rare, but include leak from intestinal anastomosis, urine leak from augmented bladder, and perforation of augmented bladder. These events have a reported incidence of 2.9–7.8% among children undergoing open augmentation cystoplasty [19, 20]. No such events have been reported in patients undergoing RALMA or RALIMA, though this could be due to the rarity of events and small sample sizes in the existing published series [5, 6, 11]. Though not technically a complication, bladder stone formation is common following augmentation cystoplasty likely due to mucus/debris in the bladder and urinary stasis. Bladder stone formation rates are comparable between open and laparoscopic series, ranging from 17 to 36% [6, 19–21].

Potential complications specific to catheterizable channel formation include stomal stenosis and channel stenosis. Stomal complications such as stenosis or prolapse have been reported to occur in 5–10% of cases in various open series [20, 22–24], compared to a 16.7% stomal complication rate described in the largest RALMA series to date, which includes 20 patients [11]. Channel stenosis was reported in 3.4–6% of cases in the open series [20, 22], and has not yet been encountered with the robotic approach.

The formation of peritoneal adhesions and subsequent small bowel obstruction (SBO) is a concern with any surgery that violates the peritoneal cavity. SBO has been reported as a rare long-term complication following open AC, affecting 3.4–10.3% of patients [19–21]. SBO has not been reported as a complication of RALMA or RALIMA in current series, though it remains a theoretical risk. However, a study in a porcine model has demonstrated that the rate of peritoneal adhesion formation was significantly lower in animals undergoing robotic ileocystoplasty compared to those undergoing an open ileocystoplasty [25]. This could account for the fact that no SBO has been reported thus far in patients undergoing RALIMA.

Based on all available data, it appears that there is no significant difference in complication rate between the open and robotic approach to augmentation cystoplasty.

9.6 Outcomes

With respect to protecting a patient's renal function, the most important outcome measure is increasing the bladder capacity and compliance. Although not randomized, a retrospective case comparison between robotic and open augmentation cystoplasty did demonstrate a significantly larger bladder capacity following the robotic approach. This series compared 15 patients undergoing RALIMA to 13 undergoing open AC, and found a postoperative bladder capacity of 400 mL and 225 mL, respectively. However, the preoperative capacity was higher in the robotic cohort and there was no difference in the percent change in bladder capacity [6]. These data suggest that the robotic and open approaches are at least equivalent with respect to increasing bladder capacity.

An important functional outcome is continence of the catheterizable channel. Large series of patients undergoing open AC report continence rates ranging from 91.1 to 98% [22, 23]. Data for the robotic approach are again limited to small series, but results are encouraging with reported continence rates of 90–94.4% [5, 11].

The need for surgical revision is also an important measure of outcomes, and appears to be equivalent between the two approaches. Surgical revision has been necessary in 16–17% of patients undergoing open AC [23, 24], versus 10–11% of those treated with an initial robotic approach [5, 11].

9.7 Discussion

Minimally invasive, robotic approaches to bladder augmentation remain in their early stages and are currently performed only at specialized centers with extensive robotic expertise. However, the existing data does suggest that the robotic approach is both safe and effective. Given the small sample sizes of existing RALIMA series, ongoing study is needed to ensure that these initial results are replicated.

Decreased length of hospital stay, decreased postoperative pain, and faster return to regular activities are all proposed benefits of the robotic approach. The authors' series on RALIMA did demonstrate a significantly shorter median length of hospital stay (6 vs. 8 days), with no difference in use of narcotic analgesics [6]. However, mean operative time in this series is significantly longer in the robotic cohort than the open (623 vs. 287 min). There is no doubt that the learning curve is steep for this procedure, and it is our hope that operative times will decline with greater surgeon experience. Further study will be useful to assess the perceived benefits of the robotic approach over the open.

Conclusion

In the hands of an experienced robotic pediatric surgeon, RALIMA is a safe and effective minimally invasive approach to managing pediatric patients with neurogenic bladder requiring augmentation cystoplasty.

References

1. Biers SM, Venn SN, Greenwell TJ. The past, present and future of augmentation cystoplasty. BJU Int. 2012;109(9):1280–93.
2. Jordan GH, Winslow BH. Laparoscopically assisted continent catheterizable cutaneous appendicovesicostomy. J Endourol Soc. 1993;7(6):517–20.
3. Pedraza R, Weiser A, Franco I. Laparoscopic appendicovesicostomy (Mitrofanoff procedure) in a child using the da Vinci robotic system. J Urol. 2004;171(4):1652–3.
4. Gundeti MS, Eng MK, Reynolds WS, Zagaja GP. Pediatric robotic-assisted laparoscopic augmentation ileocystoplasty and Mitrofanoff Appendicovesicostomy: complete intracorporeal—initial case report. Urology. 2008;72(5):1144–7.
5. Nguyen HT, Passerotti CC, Penna FJ, Retik AB, Peters CA. Robotic assisted laparoscopic Mitrofanoff Appendicovesicostomy: preliminary experience in a pediatric population. J Urol. 2009;182(4):1528–34.
6. Murthy P, Cohn JA, Selig RB, Gundeti MS. Robot-assisted laparoscopic augmentation ileocystoplasty and Mitrofanoff Appendicovesicostomy in children: updated interim results. Eur Urol. 2015;68(6):1069–75.
7. Adams MC, Joseph DB. Urinary tract reconstruction in children. In: Wein AJ, editor. Campbell-walsh urology. 10th ed. Philadelphia: Elsevier Saunders; 2012.
8. Gundeti MS, Godbole PP, Wilcox DT. Is bowel preparation required before cystoplasty in children? J Urol. 2006;176(4):1574–7.
9. Storm DW, Fulmer BR, Sumfest JM. Laparoscopic robot-assisted Appendicovesicostomy: an initial experience. J Endourol. 2007;21(9):1015–8.
10. Gundeti MS, Acharya SS, Zagaja GP, Shalhav AL. Paediatric robotic-assisted laparoscopic augmentation ileocystoplasty and Mitrofanoff appendicovesicostomy (RALIMA): feasibility of and initial experience with the University of Chicago technique: RALIMA: feasibility and initial experience. BJU Int. 2011;107(6):962–9.
11. Famakinwa OJ, Rosen AM, Gundeti MS. Robot-assisted laparoscopic Mitrofanoff Appendicovesicostomy technique and outcomes of extravesical and intravesical approaches. Eur Urol. 2013;64(5):831–6.
12. Cohen AJ, Pariser JJ, Anderson BB, Pearce SM, Gundeti MS. The robotic Appendicovesicostomy and bladder augmentation. Urol Clin North Am. 2015;42(1):121–30.

13. Wille MA, Zagaja GP, Shalhav AL, Gundeti MS. Continence outcomes in patients undergoing robotic assisted laparoscopic Mitrofanoff Appendicovesicostomy. J Urol. 2011;185(4):1438–43.
14. Bagrodia A, Gargollo P. Robot-assisted bladder neck reconstruction, bladder neck sling, and Appendicovesicostomy in children: description of technique and initial results. J Endourol. 2011;25(8): 1299–305.
15. Chang C, Steinberg Z, Shah A, Gundeti MS. Patient positioning and port placement for robot-assisted surgery. J Endourol. 2014;28(6):631–8.
16. Marchetti PE, Razmaria AA, Zagaja GP, Gundeti MS. Management of the ventriculo-peritoneal shunt in pediatric patients during robot-assisted laparoscopic urologic procedures. J Endourol. 2011;25(2):225–9.
17. Landau EH, Gofrit ON, Cipele H, Hardak B, Duvdevani M, Pode D, et al. Superiority of the VQZ over the tubularized skin flap and the umbilicus for continent abdominal stoma in children. J Urol. 2008;180(4):1761–6.
18. Ost M, Raju G. Complications of laparoscopic and robotic surgery in pediatrics. In: Wetter PA, editor. Prevention and management of laparoendoscopic surgical complications. 2012, 3rd ed. Miami: JLS.
19. Schlomer BJ, Copp HL. Cumulative incidence of outcomes and urologic procedures after augmentation cystoplasty. J Pediatr Urol. 2014;10(6):1043–50.
20. Flood HD, Malhotra SJ, O'Connell HE, Ritchey MJ, Bloom DA, McGuire EJ. Long-term results and complications using augmentation cystoplasty in reconstructive urology. Neurourol Urodyn. 1995;14(4):297–309.
21. Gurung PMS, Attar KH, Abdul-Rahman A, Morris T, Hamid R, Shah PJR. Long-term outcomes of augmentation ileocystoplasty in patients with spinal cord injury: a minimum of 10 years of follow-up: AIC OUTCOMES IN PATIENTS WITH SCI. BJU Int. 2012;109(8):1236–42.
22. Welk BK, Afshar K, Rapoport D, MacNeily AE. Complications of the catheterizable channel following continent urinary diversion: their nature and timing. J Urol. 2008;180(4):1856–60.
23. Harris CF, Cooper CS, Hutcheson JC, Snyder HM. Appendicovesicostomy: the mitrofanoff procedure-a 15-year perspective. J Urol. 2000;163(6):1922–6.
24. Süzer O, Vates TS, Freedman AL, Smith CA, Gonzalez R. Results of the Mitrofanoff procedure in urinary tract reconstruction in children. Br J Urol. 1997;79(2):279–82.
25. Razmaria AA, Marchetti PE, Prasad SM, Shalhav AL, Gundeti MS. Does robot-assisted laparoscopic ileocystoplasty (RALI) reduce peritoneal adhesions compared with open surgery?: adhesion formation after cystoplasty in a porcine model. BJU Int. 2014;113(3):468–75.

10 Robotic Assisted Laparoscopic Complete and Partial Nephrectomy in Children

Shawn C. Smith and Hiep T. Nguyen

10.1 Introduction

The current gold standard for pediatric complete and partial nephrectomy is the open surgical approach. Despite its short surgical times and excellent long-term outcomes, the open surgical approach has historically been associated with increased hospital stays and morbidity. The open approach often requires the patients to be on high doses of narcotics for postoperative pain management. This, in turn, has led to increased postoperative complications of refractory pain and constipation, which could potentially lead to readmission for their treatment. Laparoscopy provides an alternative approach in performing complete and partial nephrectomy. This approach is associated with less pain, shorter hospitalization, and more rapid recovery time compared to its open counterpart. However, laparoscopy is technically more demanding, leading to potentially higher rates of intraoperative complications, surgical time, and costs.

Approved by the Food and Drug Administration in 2000, the da Vinci surgical system provides a means of decreasing the technical demands of laparoscopy. The robotic system provides a three-dimensional, stable visualization of the surgical field, eliminates the counterintuitive movement associated with conventional laparoscopy, and provides fine control of the laparoscopic instruments. However, it is associated with significantly higher equipment/instrumentation costs compared to that of the open and conventional laparoscopic approach. Recognizing its advantages in reducing the technical complexities associated with laparoscopy, proponents of robotic assisted laparoscopic surgery (RALS) utilized this approach for more complex surgeries [1]. The application of robotic technologies to urologic procedures has been rapidly adopted in the management of adults, while in children its use has lagged behind. Currently, it is not known if in children RALS can become the gold standard for total nephrectomy due to its persistently higher cost. In contrast, for partial nephrectomy, which has a higher degree of technical complexity compared to the more straightforward complete nephrectomy, RALS could potentially become the gold standard of care [2].

10.2 Indications

In children, the indications for complete and partial nephrectomy are more commonly related to benign diseases rather than from malignancies. Obstruction (such as ureteropelvic junction or ureterovesicular junction), vesicoureteral reflux, multicystic dysplasia, and recurrent urinary tract infections (specifically from pyelonephritis) may result in a nonfunctioning or poorly functioning renal unit

S.C. Smith (✉) • H.T. Nguyen, M.D.
Banner Children's Specialists, Urology, Cardon Children's Hospital, Mesa, AZ, USA
e-mail: shawn.c.smith@bannerhealth.com; hiep.t.nguyen@bannerhealth.com

G. Mattioli, P. Petralia (eds.), *Pediatric Robotic Surgery*, DOI 10.1007/978-3-319-41863-6_10

that in the long term may lead to hypertension and significant proteinuria [3]. It is generally recommended that kidneys with relative renal function less than 10% as measured on DMSA scan should be removed. In determining whether renal units associated with a duplicated collecting system should be removed or reconstructed, there is not a consensus on a threshold amount of renal function required. More often, a subjective decision is based on the amount of renal parenchyma seen on ultrasound (US) and the differential renal function between the upper and lower pole segments.

The decision as to whether to perform the procedure with an open versus conventional laparoscopic versus RALS approach is dependent on numerous factors such as the patient/parental preference, assessment of the relative risks versus benefits of each surgical approach, surgeon's experience and comfort with the various surgical modalities, availability of instruments and equipment, cost/insurance coverage, time available, and accessibility of trained assistants and operating room personnel. When a minimally invasive surgical approach is chosen, the advantages and disadvantages of conventional laparoscopy and RALS must be considered and compared. The principal advantages of RALS include simplification and precision of exposure and suturing; movements of the robotic arm in real time providing an increased degree of freedom in the movement of the laparoscopic instruments; and a magnified three-dimensional view [4]. Other advantages include computer elimination of tremor, increased range of motion at the distal end of the instruments, and improved surgeon ergonomics. As with the conventional laparoscopic approach, RALS epitomizes the idea of minimally invasive surgery with its miniaturized and precise movements that ultimately result in smaller incisions, less blood loss and pain, shorter hospital stays, and quicker convalescence [5].

10.3 Equipment and Instruments

With the da Vinci system, which evolved from the telepresence machines developed for NASA and the United States Army and is the most commonly used equipment, there are essentially three components: a vision cart that holds a dual-light source and two high-definition cameras, a master console where the operating surgeon sits, and a moveable cart, where three instrument arms and the camera arm are mounted [6]. The camera arm contains dual cameras and the image generated is three-dimensional. The master console consists of (1) an image-processing computer that generates a true three-dimensional image with depth of field; (2) the view port where the surgeon views the image; (3) foot pedals used to control electrocautery, camera focus, and instrument/camera arm clutches; and (4) master control grips that drive the servant robotic arms at the patient's side. The instruments are cable driven and provide seven degrees of freedom, mimicking the natural movements of the surgeon's hands, wrists, and arms. The system displays its three-dimensional image above the hands of the surgeon so that it gives the surgeon the illusion that the tips of the instruments are an extension of the control grips, thus giving the impression of being at the surgical site [7].

In performing complete or partial nephrectomy, a very limited number of instruments are required. Dissection can be performed using a forceps, such as a DeBakey or ProGrasp, and a cautery instrument, such as a monopolar curved scissors or cautery hook. In performing a partial nephrectomy, the use of a Harmonic curved shears is very helpful in removing the nonfunctioning renal unit from the rest of the kidney without excessive bleeding. Since in most cases the vascular supply to the nonfunctional renal unit is diminished, a 5 mm vascular clip applier can be used to ligate the renal vessels. A vascular stapler or suture ligation is rarely required. To remove the specimen, it is useful to place the specimen in a laparoscopic bag so that it can be removed easily and intact through the umbilical port.

10.4 Surgical Approach

Much debate has centered on the best laparoscopic approach, transperitoneal versus retroperitoneal. The advantages and disadvantages of both

Table 10.1 Advantages and disadvantages of transperitoneal and retroperitoneal approach

Approach	Advantages	Disadvantages
Transperitoneal	Familiar anatomy	Theoretical risk of postoperative intraperitoneal adhesions
	More working space, especially in young children	
	Can perform concurrent procedures such as extravesical ureteral reimplantation	
Retroperitoneal	Short distance to the kidney	Limited working space and unfamiliar layout of anatomy
	Less risk of subjecting peritoneum to complications such as urine leak, infection, and tumor seeding	Inability to perform total ureterectomy without adjunct inguinal incision
	Less interference from surrounding organs such as the liver, spleen, and bowel	Risk of peritoneal tear and subsequent conversion to open surgery
	Easier exposure to the renal hilum (due to the kidney falling anteriorly with gravity)	Risk of balloon rupture used to develop the retroperitoneal space, which necessitates meticulous retrieval of fragments
	Ureter and pelvis are posterior for easier dissection	
	Theoretical reduction in postoperative intraperitoneal adhesions and easy conversion to lumbodorsal approach	

Modified from Freilich DA and Nguyen HT. Robotic-Assisted Laparoscopic heminephrectomy in Current Clinical Urology: Pediatric Robotic Urology. Editor Palmer JS. 2009. Chapter 10: page 137–172. Humana Press, NY

approaches are listed in Table 10.1. In most instances, the surgeon's preference and comfort with the surgical approach are the prime determinants of which approach is selected.

10.5 Preparation

All patients require a thorough clinical evaluation and a complete discussion of all surgical options, expected outcomes, and potential complications. Unless there is a history of coagulopathy, preoperative blood values are often not necessary. Further, there is no need for considering blood type and cross, but this should be left to the surgeon's preference, experience, and comfort. A complete bowel preparation is also not necessary under most circumstances. However, decompression of the colon with enemas done the evening prior to surgery is often helpful, especially in smaller children in which the abdominal space is limited. For anxious patients, an appropriate dose of anxiolytic may be prescribed prior to surgery. In cases of a duplicated collecting system, placement of a ureteral stent prior to the RALS procedure to identify the normal ureter in partial nephrectomy is often not necessary since the grossly dilated affected ureter sufficiently enables proper identification [8].

10.6 Patient Positioning

One of the most important aspects of the procedure is appropriate patient positioning to prevent inadvertent injury of the patient during the procedure and to allow the robotic equipment to be in the optimal location for proper functioning. Once the patient has been anesthetized and the endotracheal tube is secured in place, a Foley catheter should be inserted, and the patient should be moved into a lateral decubitus position. It is important to bring the patient toward the edge of the table and rotated off the vertical plane at approximately 45°. This will help to prevent the robotic arms from colliding with the table.

Some surgeons prefer to use a beanbag to support the patient's positioning, while others prefer

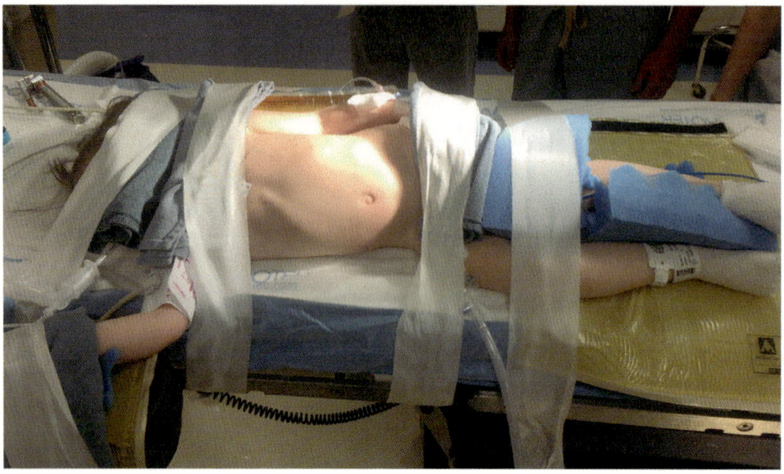

Fig. 10.1 Patient position for the transperitoneal approach. In this instance, a *left* partial nephrectomy was performed. The patient's *left side* was up, approximately 45° off the bed. The *left arm* was placed straight down the patient's side. Safety straps were placed over the head, shoulder, pelvis, and lower extremities to prevent the patient from moving when tilting the table

the use of gel rolls. The beanbag should be placed on the operative table prior to moving the patient from the transport gurney. The upper aspect of the beanbag or gel rolls should reach just below the patient's neck. The bottom arm should then be placed on an arm board and padded with egg crate foams or pressure point gels. The upper arm should then be secured along the side of the body with appropriate foam padding. Placing the upper arm crossed over the upper chest, as in the conventional lateral decubitus position, may impede the robotic equipment from properly coming over the shoulder and having adequate range of movements without hitting the body. The upper leg should be placed straight while the lower leg crossed with both being carefully padded to prevent pressure injury. This configuration of the lower extremities helps to stabilize the lower body while in the lateral decubitus position. Security straps or, preferably, large fabric tape are used to secure the shoulder, pelvis, and lower extremities to prevent movement when the table is tilted; if a beanbag is used, it should be deflated to fix the patient's position, and then inflated when the proper positioning has been achieved (Fig. 10.1).

Especially in younger children, the head accounts for a significant portion of the body weight. Consequently, the head should also be padded and secured to the table with fabric tape to prevent movement during the procedure. Anesthesia and grounding cables should be placed in such a way to remain clear of the patient and to avoid resting on exposed skin. Finally, some surgeons prefer to raise the kidney rest to provide additional flexion to improve the exposure of the kidney. While this may be important in the open surgical approach to help bring the kidney into the surgical field, it is less important in transabdominal laparoscopic approach.

10.7 Port Placement for the Transperitoneal Approach

In most pediatric cases, RALS complete and partial nephrectomy can be performed with a camera port and two instrument ports. An additional 5 mm assistant port may be helpful for retraction and passing sutures and vascular clips. There are currently two sizes of laparoscopes on the market, 8.5 and 12 mm, and two sizes of robotic instruments, 5 and 8 mm. The previously available 5 mm laparoscope has been discontinued because of its inability to allow for three-dimensional binocular vision [9].

It is often assumed that the smaller laparoscope and instruments are preferable in the pediatric cases. However, it is actually more advantageous to use the 12 mm laparoscope and 8 mm instruments in these cases. The 12 mm laparoscope has much brighter lighting components compared to its 8 mm counterpart. The concern that a larger port is needed for the 12 mm laparoscope is ameliorated by the fact that the excised renal unit could be more easily and safely removed through the larger port site. Moreover, there is a greater variety of 8 mm instruments available compared to the 5 mm instruments, most importantly, the availability of those that provide hemostasis such as cauterizing scissors and Harmonic scalpel. In addition, due to the difference in joint configuration of the 8 and 5 mm instruments, the 5 mm instruments require more of the instrument to be in the abdominal cavity, which is a significant issue in smaller children. Based on personal experience, placement of the larger instrument port needed for 8 mm instruments has not been an issue even in small children.

Once the patient has been prepped and draped in the usual sterile fashion, a semilunar incision is made around the umbilicus. The table should be tilted so that the patient is leveled as much as possible (correcting for the 45° lateral decubitus position). This maneuver will aid in obtaining a 90°, straight access into the abdominal cavity. Some surgeons prefer to obtain access into the peritoneal cavity using the open Hasson technique, while others use a needle system to insufflate the abdomen and then place the port using a self-retracting bladed trocar. Once the camera port is in place and pneumoperitoneum is achieved (approximate pressure 12–14 mmHg in adolescents and 10–12 mmHg in younger children), the laparoscope is placed into the peritoneal cavity, and careful inspection of the abdominal cavity is performed to identify any bleeding or inadvertent vascular, bowel, or organ injuries. The instrument and assistant ports are then placed under direct vision. The robotic trocar ports are used to mark circular indentations in the skin at the preferred port sites; the 8 mm ports will be inserted for the robotic arms and a 5 mm port for the assistant. Local anesthesia is applied to the port insertion sites and then skin incisions are made within the circular indentations. The underlying fascia is widened with a blunt mosquito under direct vision; this method of obtaining port access allows for well-fitted ports and eliminates the need for mooring the ports with sutures to prevent dislodgement.

When placing the ports, the size of the patient is taken into consideration. For older children, the upper instrument port (closer to the head) is placed at midline, approximately 8 cm from the camera port (Fig. 10.2). The lower instrument port is placed in the midclavicular line at a 30° angle (rotated away from midline toward the affected kidney), 6 cm away from the camera port. Finally, a 5 mm assistant port can be placed either in between the upper instrument and the camera port or inferior to the camera port in the midline depending on the

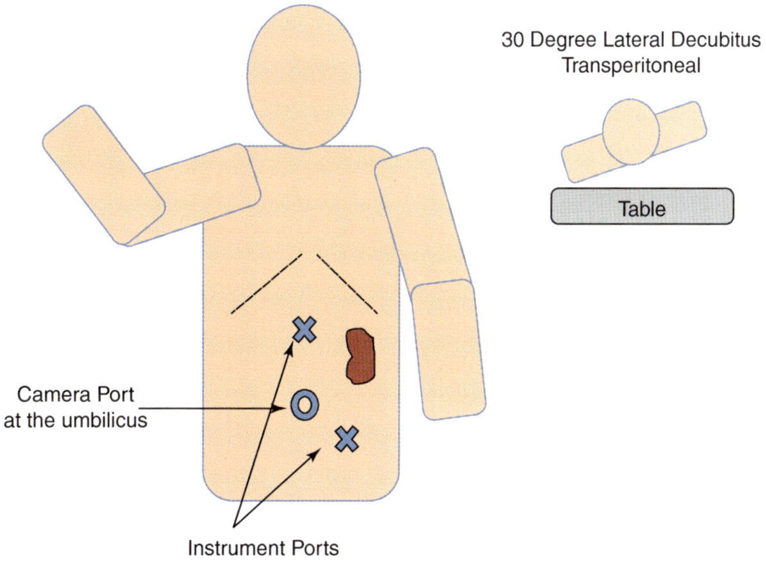

Fig. 10.2 Position of the camera and instrument ports when performing transperitoneal approach with the patient in a 45° lateral decubitus position

size of the patient (Fig. 10.3) [5]. For smaller and younger children, the distance between the camera ports and instruments can be reduced by 2–3 cm. In addition, the lower instrument port may be moved closer to the midline if the width of the abdomen is limited. It should be noted that with the abdomen fully insufflated, there should be ample space to accommodate all the robotic ports even in the smallest children. Once all the ports have been place, the table should be tilted in the opposite direction of the side of the surgery in order for the bowel to fall to a more dependent position in the abdomen, away from the kidney being operated on. The robotic system is then brought over the patient's shoulder, and the ports are clipped onto the robotic arm. It is crucial to line the center robotic arm up with the midportion of the kidney. This can be accomplished by leaving the laparoscope in the abdomen and directly visualizing the kidney while moving the robot into place (Fig. 10.4). This alignment

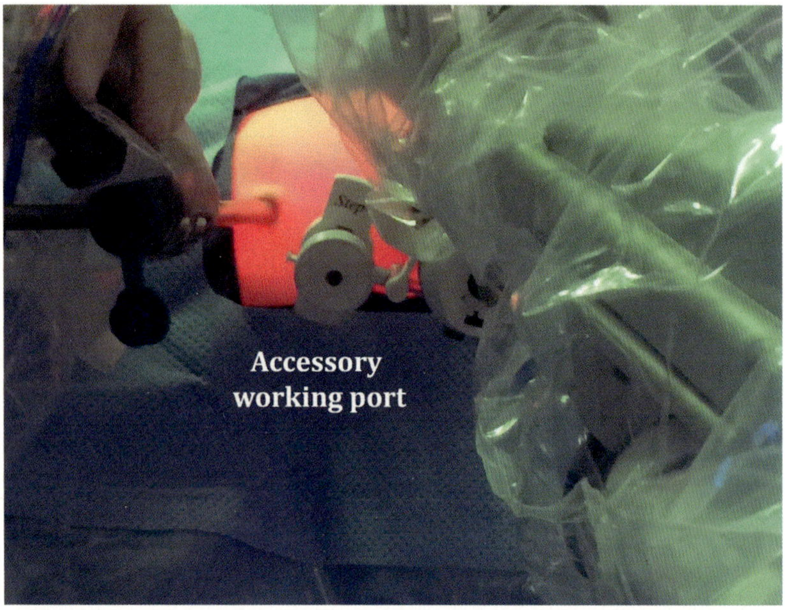

Fig. 10.3 Location of the accessory working port. In this instance, it is placed between the midline instrument port and the camera port

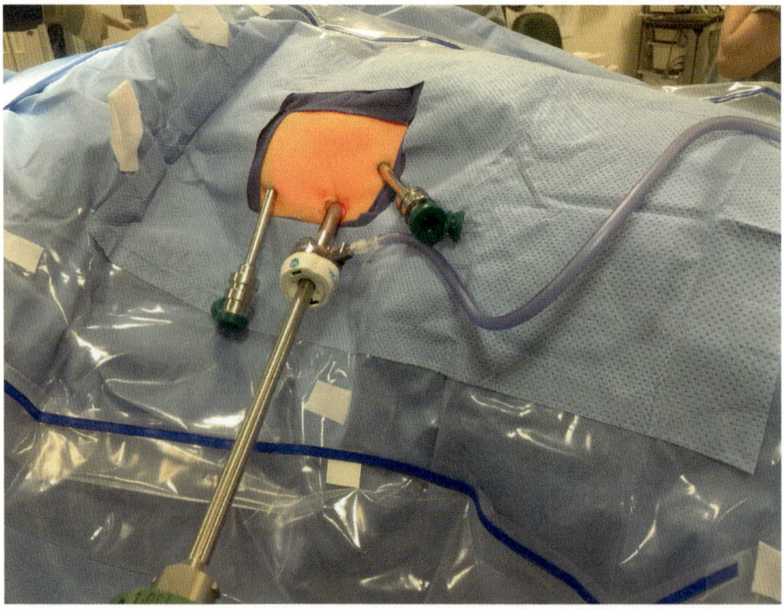

Fig. 10.4 To properly align the robotic system, the camera is *left* in place to visualize the kidney when the robotic system is moved into place. This allows the center robotic arm to be aligned up with the kidney

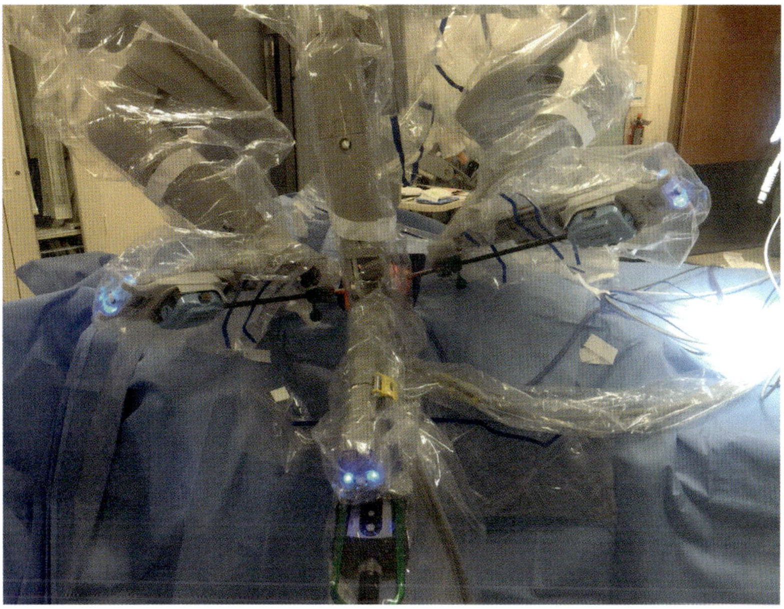

Fig. 10.5 Proper setup of the robotic system with maximal working space between the instrument and camera arms to prevent collision

allows the robotic arms to be in optimal location for proper functioning (Fig. 10.5). Especially in younger children, it is important to lift the ports and robotic arms upward and outward from the abdominal wall to maximize the space available inside the abdominal cavity for the instruments to maneuver (Fig. 10.6).

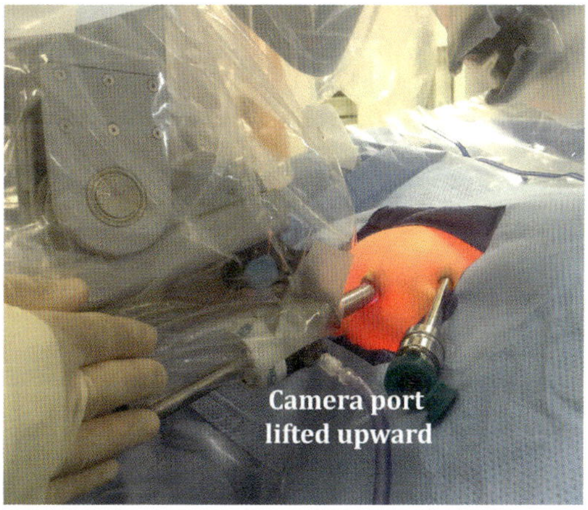

Fig. 10.6 All ports should be lifted up and away from the abdominal wall to maximize intra-abdominal working space

10.8 Positioning and Port Placement for Lateral and Prone Retroperitoneal Approach

For the lateral retroperitoneal (RP) approach, the patient is positioned on the operating table laterally with flexion to facilitate trocar placement between the last rib and iliac crest (Fig. 10.7). The camera port is placed 3 cm below the 12th rib. The Gerota fascia is approached with a muscle-splitting technique via blunt dissection along the lumbodorsal fascia. An anchoring suture is placed to secure the port, allowing it to pull back and tent the skin in order to increase the retroperitoneal working space. The working space is developed either with gas insufflation, balloon dilator, or blunt finger dissection. The first instrument port is placed posteriorly in the costovertebral angle and the second along the anterior axillary line 10 mm superior to the iliac crest.

For the prone RP approach, the patient is placed in the prone position (Fig. 10.8). The camera port is inserted laterally along the posterior clavicular line, just above the iliac crest. The first instrument port is placed at the costovertebral angle at the edge of the paraspinous muscles and the 12th rib, and the second port is placed medial to the paraspinous muscles, just above the iliac crest.

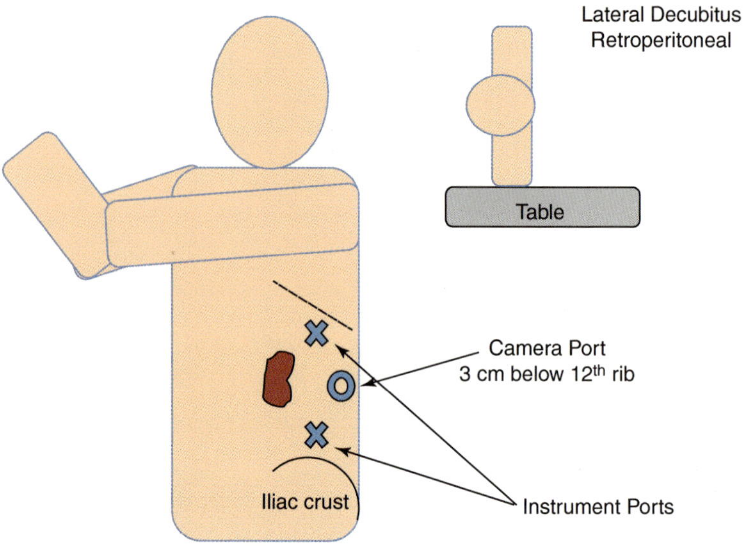

Fig. 10.7 Position of the camera and instrument ports when performing retroperitoneal approach with the patient in a lateral decubitus position

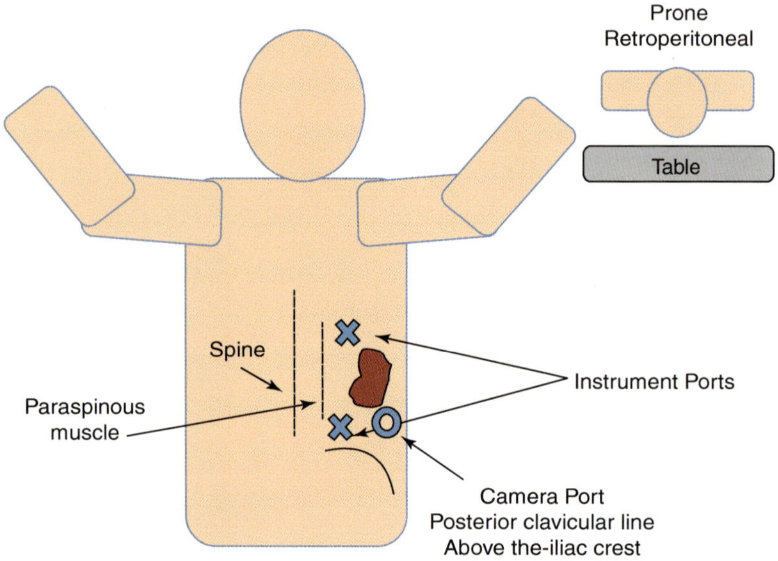

Fig. 10.8 Position of the camera and instrument ports when performing retroperitoneal approach with the patient in a prone position

10.9 General Technique for Transperitoneal Approach

In performing the complete or partial nephrectomy, it is important to maximally tilt the table away from the side of the affected kidney. This allows the bowel to fall into a more dependent position on the downside of the abdomen, thus increasing the available abdominal space for unrestricted movement of the robotic instruments. It is important to first take down the splenic (for left-sided surgery) or the hepatic flexure (for right-sided surgery), and then carry the dissection along the white line of Toldt to the pelvic brim in order to efficiently mobilize the large bowel away from the kidney. Some surgeons prefer to avoid this step and operate through a mesenteric window. Since the hilum is often difficult to directly visualize due to the surrounding fat tissue, it is often easier to identify the ureter near the pelvic brim and, using the ureter as a landmark, to advance the dissection superiorly toward the renal hilum. Of note, it is helpful to avoid initially dissecting laterally to the kidney and releasing the kidney from the lateral abdominal wall. Instead, this should be done last, in order to prevent the kidney from flopping over the hilum and obscuring it.

Dividing the ureter and using it as a handle will provide traction and facilitate the dissection around the hilum as well as the identification of the renal artery and vein. When performing a partial nephrectomy, it is important to trace the ureters to their corresponding renal units. For a nonfunctioning upper pole system, the upper pole ureter should be dissected free from the surrounding tissues and then divided. The ureteral stump is then passed below the lower pole renal hilum and then re-grabbed from above. It can then be used to facilitate the dissection of the upper pole hilum. After ligating its vasculature, the upper pole parenchyma can be removed with a Harmonic curved shear. Using this instrument will help to reduce bleeding. Careful attention should be paid to avoiding the collecting system of the lower pole. If the collecting system is violated, suture closure with absorbable sutures such as Chromic or Vicryl can be performed, which can be expediently done using the robotic system.

Cauterizing the bed that remains following the excision of the upper pole will help to destroy any residual functioning renal tissue. In addition, perinephric fat should be placed into this area. These maneuvers, in addition to the application of a sealing agent such as fibrin glue (from personal experience), can help to reduce the chance of developing a urinoma in this area postoperatively. After carrying out the complete or partial nephrectomy, the hilum should be observed at a low abdominal pressure (approximately 5 mmHg) to make sure that there is no venous bleeding. In dealing with the remaining distal ureteral stump, if the pathology is from an obstructive process then the remnant ureter should be left open; if the pathology is from vesicoureteral reflux then the remnant ureter should be ligated.

10.10 Removal of Specimen

Once the nonfunctioning renal unit is removed from the functional portion of the kidney, or, in the case of total nephrectomy, the kidney is isolated from the renal hilum and hemostasis is obtained, the robotic telescope is removed from the 12 mm port and a smaller laparoscope is introduced through one of the 8 mm ports. The pneumoperitoneum tubing is then attached to one of the smaller ports. Under direct visualization, the laparoscopic specimen bag is placed through the 12 mm port and into the surgical field (Fig. 10.9). The specimen is maneuvered into the

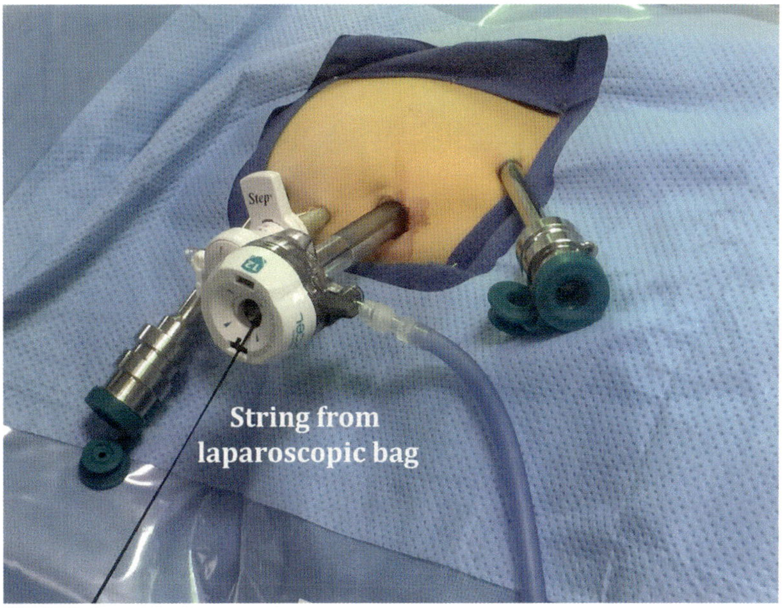

Fig. 10.9 The laparoscopic specimen bag was placed through the 12 mm camera port. The string is *left* outside in order to retrieve the bag

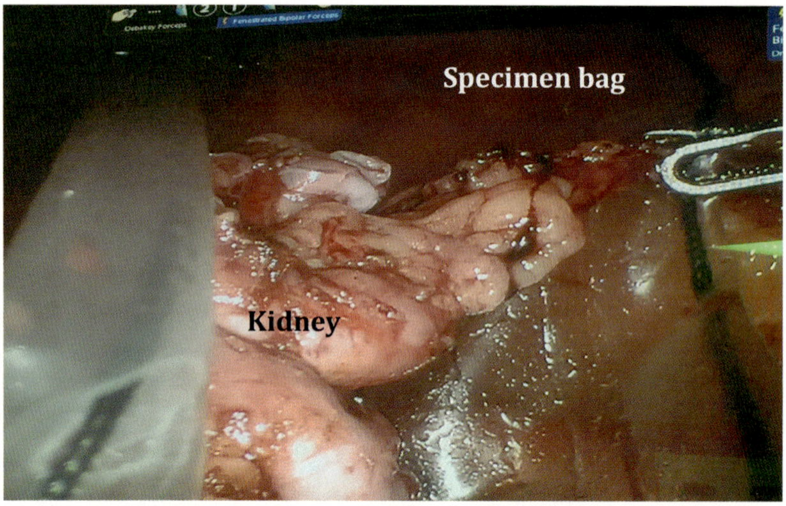

Fig. 10.10 The specimen is maneuvered into the specimen bag

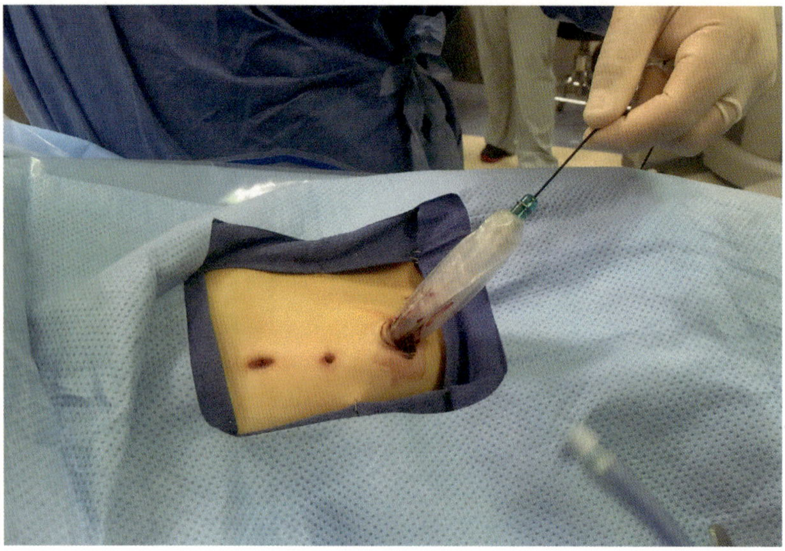

Fig. 10.11 The laparoscopic specimen bag is removed through the umbilical incision after removing the camera port

specimen bag with the forceps (Fig. 10.10). The laparoscopic bag is closed and removed through the 12 mm port site (Fig. 10.11).

The surgical field should be surveyed one last time to ensure that no damage has been caused to surrounding viscera and proper hemostasis has been obtained. Irrigation may be used to check for small areas of bleeding and for better visualization of sutures and staples that were applied. Once the field has been assessed and there are no other concerns to address, the robotic arm is disengaged from the 12 mm port site and the robot is pushed away from the field. The smaller laparoscope is returned and the remaining trocars are removed under direct visualization to ensure that there is no other bleeding from the port sites. When all ports have been safely removed, the field is prepared for closure of the port sites and completing the procedure.

10.11 General Technique for Retroperitoneal Approach

Since there are no overlying bowel or organs, the kidney and ureter are easily identified in this approach. The renal hilum can be identified anterior to the renal pelvis. The ureter should be transected to help manipulate the kidney. After ligation of the hilum and isolation of the nonfunctioning segment of kidney, the specimen can be removed through the larger 12 mm camera port. A Penrose drain in the surgical bed is recommend since there is limited fluid absorptive ability of the retroperitoneum as compared to the transperitoneal approach.

10.12 Postoperative Care

In most cases, a regular diet can be resumed, usually within 4 hours, despite the transperitoneal approach. In the management of pain, narcotics should be avoided in order to decrease the risk of an ileus. Instead, nonsteroidal anti-inflammatory drugs such as ketorolac, acetaminophen, and ibuprofen should be encouraged. Removing the Foley catheter early (either later in the evening following the completion of the procedure or the next morning) will help to decrease bladder spasms and encourage early ambulation. Obtaining a follow-up CBC the next day is left to the discretion of the surgeon, but is not mandatory. The patients are discharged on post-op day one when tolerating a diet, afebrile with no signs of wound infection, and are able to void. In some cases, such as simple nephrectomy, same-day discharge may be considered. A follow-up ultrasound is performed at 1 month postoperatively to assess for complications such as a hematoma or urinoma and evaluation of the remnant renal units.

10.13 Complications

There are few complications specific to performing RALS. Technical problems such as non-overridable fault and instrument failure may require conversion to conventional laparoscopy or open surgery. When performing any type of laparoscopic intraperitoneal procedure, there is a low risk of serious complications such as bowel perforation, trocar or needle trauma to major blood vessels, thermal injury from coagulation elements, splenic or liver injuries, and pneumothorax. Specific to partial nephrectomy, hematoma or urinoma and their potential for infection may occur postoperatively. In the majority of the cases, these complications are self-limiting and do not require intervention. However, urinoma may require an extensive amount of time before resolving. Inadvertent injury of the remnant renal unit may occur but this complication is uncommon.

10.14 Current Literature

It has been well demonstrated that RALS procedure in general is safe in children [10–12] and has greater efficiency and safety over standard laparoscopic approach [13]. A review of the most up-to-date published literature on RALS complete and partial nephrectomy reveals that there are a limited number of studies in the pediatric population compared to the more extensive body of literature in adults. Currently, there are no studies available to support the notion that RALS is a superior modality to laparoscopic or open surgical procedures in children. However, RALS and conventional laparoscopic approach are associated with shorter hospital stay with RALS (decreased by approximately 1 day), less blood loss, and decreased use of narcotics for postoperative pain control. On the other hand, these approaches are associated with an initial increase in operative time, which decreases with experience, and a significant increase in operative cost (especially with RALS).

When comparing conventional laparoscopy with RALS, the role of RALS has been more clearly established in reconstructive procedures such as pyeloplasty and ureteral reimplantation, while its role in extirpative surgery such as nephrectomy remains unclear. However, the use of RALS may serve as a learning procedure in preparation for performing more complicated reconstructive cases. Inarguably, performing a laparoscopic partial nephrectomy is technically more demanding than performing a complete nephrectomy. Consequently, the application of RALS in accomplishing this procedure has been more widely adopted and hence more reported in the literature.

In review of the over 30 articles with information on pediatric partial nephrectomy, some common observations can be identified. Comparing transperitoneal (TP) versus retroperitoneal (RP) approach, most surgeons preferred TP to RP approach due to more working space and the ability to excise the ureter completely [9]. TP was the best approach when a total ureterectomy was needed or when the child was less than a year old [14] or in small children because it provided greater working space and hence less risk of damage to the functional renal unit when performing a partial nephrectomy [15]. Some surgeons have noted that the RP approach was limited in space to properly visualize the hilum and distal ureter in infants [16]. RP approach may be best utilized for complete nephrectomy in children greater than 2 years of age [17].

In a study of 48 children who underwent RAL partial nephrectomy, Castellan et al. observed three complications out of 32 patients with the TP approach and three out of 16 with the RP approach; 80% of complications involved children less than 1 year of age [14]. In the TP approach, these complications included pneumothorax secondary to diaphragm perforation, postoperative hypertension requiring pharmacological treatment, and recurrent UTI requiring excision of a remnant ureteral stump left after RALS partial nephrectomy. In the RP approach, there was a peritoneal tear, which necessitated conversion to TP, conversion to open surgery due to scarring of the affected pole and anterior pole vasculature, postoperative urine leak, and postoperative urinoma. In another study of 22 children who underwent RP upper (18) versus lower (4) pole heminephrectomy, Wallis observed associated complications including converting to open due to peritoneal tears, the inability to develop adequate pneumoperitoneal space with which to work, postoperative urine leakage, aspiration of seroma, and fever [15]. The author suggested that the RP approach is preferable to the TP approach because it more closely resembles the open surgical technique. However, the TP approach may be more appropriate in smaller children because it offers more working space and potentially decreased risk of damage to the residual moiety.

In a randomized study of 19 children, Borzi examined posterior RP versus lateral RP approach in performing RALS partial nephrectomy [18]. The authors found that in children 5 years of age and older, the posterior RP was less favorable when compared to lateral RP since posterior RP approach did not provide for a more complete ureteral excision. However, the posterior RP provides superior vascular control.

There are many disadvantages associated with RALS. The use of the daVinci robot system is limited by its cost for many institutions. While most fellowship trained pediatric urologists are comfortable in the utilization of the robotic assisted technique, the modality remains a daunting task for more seasoned pediatric urologists to undertake. Additionally, when compared to RALS, the argument can be made that the open technique takes less time, has fewer complications, and can have the patient discharged from the hospital in little more than an extra day of recovery. However, with time, experience, increased comfort, and improved technique in using the robotic system, patient outcomes can be improved. RALS partial nephrectomy is superior to traditional open surgery in regard to cosmesis, postoperative length of hospitalization, and narcotic utilization [8]. Ultimately, many factors will have significant impacts on the future of RALS, namely, cost of the robotic system and the comfort level of the hands and eyes performing the surgery behind the console and not at the operative field. However, additional clinical experience is required to determine the long-term efficacy of this method. As there are many surgical techniques available that do not offer a conclusive endorsement, the best modality is that which the specialist is most comfortable.

Conclusion

Although it is not yet possible to demonstrate the superiority of one single surgical modality over another, RALS has been shown to be feasible, well tolerated, and advantageous in reconstructive urological procedures [19]. With increased experience, the surgeon utilizing the robotic approach will significantly decrease the operative time for RALS; this will, in turn, decrease the overall cost involved in using the robot. Furthermore, with the added benefits of precision of exposure and suturing in a magnified three-dimensional view and improved cosmesis, RALS may become the modality of choice for pediatric partial and, potentially, complete nephrectomy.

References

1. Traxel EJ, Minevich EA, Noh PH. Early uses of laparoscopy in pediatric urology included management of non-palpable testes (A review: the application of minimally invasive surgery to pediatric urology: upper urinary tract procedures). Urology. 2010;76:122–33.
2. Stifelman MD, Caruso RP, Nieder AM, Taneja SS. Robot-assisted laparoscopic partial nephrectomy. J Soc Laparoendoscopic Surgeons. 2005;9(1):83–6.
3. Hammad FT, Upadhyay V. Indications for nephrectomy in children: what has changed? J Pediatr Urol. 2006;2(5):430–5.
4. Casale P, Kojima Y. Robotic-assisted laparoscopic surgery in pediatric urology: an update. Scand J Surg. 2009;98(2):110–9.
5. Chang C, Steinberg Z, Shah A, Gundeti M. Patient positioning and port placement for robot-assisted surgery. J Endourol. 2014;28(6):631–8.
6. Satava RM. Surgical robotics: the early chronicles: a personal historical perspective. Surg Laparosc Endosc Percutan Tech. 2002;12(1):6–16.
7. Lanfranco AR, Castellanos AE, Desai JP, Meyers WC. Robotic surgery: a current perspective. Ann Surg. 2004;239(1):14–21.
8. Freilich DA, Nguyen HT. Robotic-assisted laparoscopic heminephrectomy in current clinical urology. In: Palmer JS, editor. Pediatric robotic urology. New York: Humana Press; 2009. p. 137–72. (Chapter 10).
9. Piaggo L, Franc-Guimond J, Figueroa TE, Barthold JS, Gonzalez R. Comparison of laparoscopic and open partial nephrectomy for duplication anomalies in children. J Urol. 2006;175(6):2269–73.
10. Volfson IA, Munver R, Esposito M, Dakwar G, Hanna M, Stock JA. Robot-assisted urologic surgery: safety and feasibility in the pediatric population. J Endourol. 2007;21(11):1315–8.
11. Meehan JJ, Sandler A. Pediatric robotic surgery: a single-institutional review of the first 100 consecutive cases. Surg Endosc. 2008;22(1):177–82.
12. Sinha CK, Haddad M. Robot-assisted surgery in children: current status. J Robot Surg. 2008;1(4):243–6.
13. Yee DS, Klein RB, Shanberg AM. Case report: robotic-assisted laparoscopic reconstruction of a ureteropelvic junction disruption. J Endourol. 2006; 20(5):326–9.
14. Castellan M, Gosalbez R, Carmack AJ, Prieto JC, Perez-Brayfield M, Labbie A. Transperitoneal and retroperitoneal laparoscopic heminephrectomy—what approach for which patient? J Urol. 2006;176(6 Pt 1):2636–9. discussion 9
15. Wallis MC, Khoury AE, Lorenzo AJ, Pippi-Salle JL, Bagli DJ, Farhat WA. Outcome analysis for retroperitoneal laparoscopic heminephrectomy in children. J Urol. 2006;175(6):2277–80. discussion 80-2
16. Sydorak RM, Shaul DB. Laparoscopic partial nephrectomy, nephroureterectomy and heminephroureterectomy in the pediatric population. J Urol. 2000;163(5):1531–5.
17. Miranda ML, Oliveira-Filho AG, Carvalho PT, Ungersbock E, Olimpio H, Bustorff-Silva JM. Laparoscopic upper-pole nephroureterectomy in infants. Int Braz J Urol. 2007;33(1):87–91.
18. Borzi PA. A comparison of the lateral and posterior retroperitoneoscopic approach for complete and partial nephroureterectomy in children. BJU Int. 2001;87(6):517–20.
19. Trevisani L, Nguyen HT. Current controversies in pediatric urologic robotic surgery. Curr Opin Urol. 2013;23(1):72–7.

11 Gynecological Procedures

Gloria Pelizzo

11.1 Introduction

The most substantial improvements in minimally invasive gynecologic surgery have been documented in the adult population [1–8]. The advent of robotic surgery, with its improved approach to narrow cavities such as the pelvis, has modified outcomes in gynecological interventions [9–22]. The robotic instrument which rotates with precise movements and superior articulation was introduced into clinical practice and has maximized ergonomics for the surgeon. Robotic surgery has an edge over open surgery with its smaller incisions, reduced blood loss and pain, shorter hospital stays, and quicker convalescence. Furthermore, the three-dimensional visualization provides high definition in complicated procedures when extensive dissection and proper anatomy reestablishment are required [18, 21].

Most operations performed with the da Vinci can also be performed by laparoscopy, which is a simpler and less expensive method. Robotic surgery however, especially in the gynecologic field, simplifies the laparoscopic approach [22, 23].

Up to now, outcomes in robotic gynecology have been encouraging and the da Vinci System has become fully applicable even in pediatric gynecological surgery [24]. In children, in nonemergency conditions, robotic surgery may be considered not only an "enabling technology" but also a "facilitating technology." As a facilitating technology the robotic approach in pediatric and adolescent surgery ameliorates the operative learning curve allowing a greater diffusion of the laparoscopic procedure, which has already proven beneficial for patients.

The da Vinci Si Surgical System® was designed for educational purposes. The learning experience using the double-console da Vinci Si Surgical System® is considered an excellent opportunity for the surgeon in training and provides the same view as the operating surgeon, in high-definition 3D [25–28]. For all these reasons even robotic gynecologic surgery is becoming a clinical reality and is gaining increased acceptance even in the pediatric field.

11.2 Robot-Assisted Gynecological Procedures in the Pediatric Age

The indications for robotic gynecologic surgery are similar to conventional laparoscopy. Because of the increased setup time, robotic gynecologic procedures are primarily for treatment, as opposed to diagnostic laparoscopy [22, 23].

Robotic assisted gynecologic surgery has been implemented in all adult fields of gynecology, including reproductive endocrinology,

G. Pelizzo
Pediatric Surgery Unit, Children's Hospital, Istituto Mediterraneo di Eccellenza Pediatrica, Palermo, Italy
e-mail: gloriapelizzo@gmail.com

G. Mattioli, P. Petralia (eds.), *Pediatric Robotic Surgery*, DOI 10.1007/978-3-319-41863-6_11

infertility, urogynecology, and gynecologic oncology. Hysterectomy, myomectomy, sacrocolpopexy, endometriosis, and pelvic reconstructive surgery are the most common procedures in the adult age [9–22].

Successful application of minimally invasive surgery in pediatric gynecology has been introduced in recent years and a variety of gynecological surgeries, almost 50% of performed robotic procedures (as well as in adult patients), involve the adnexal structures [24], such as oophorectomy, ovarian cystectomy, ovarian drilling, salpingectomy, and adhesiolysis. Among these, the salpingo-oophorectomy and paratubal cystectomy for idiopathic cysts are the most frequent indications, while abdominal pain due to subtorsion mechanisms secondary to teratomas in older children is the second most common indication for robotic surgery. All pathological ovarian treatments with a robotic approach have been reported as safe and feasible.

A minimally invasive approach including robotic surgery in young infants has been reported with a conversion rate of 4% and no major complications [29]. The main surgical indications in infants remain limited to large functional cysts, and therapeutic intervention consists of decapsulation and incision.

As reported in Table 11.1, the most common procedures performed in pediatric gynecological procedures are the following:

1. The management of benign and malignant adnexal masses (ovarian and nonovarian masses): A high-definition 3D panorama allows maximal fertility preservation potential in the pediatric and adolescent population, which is important in oncologic conditions or other medical diseases that lead to continuation of life beyond the reproductive years [30–34].
2. The surgical treatment of congenital reproductive tract anomalies (isolated mullerian anomalies, disorders of sexual differentiation, anorectal malformation).

Table 11.1 Surgical concerns in (1) adnexal masses and (2) congenital reproductive tract anomalies

Indications for surgery	Surgical concerns
(1) *Adnexal masses*	
Benign ovarian (follicular cyst, mature teratoma, ovarian torsion, serous and mucinous cystadenoma, theca-lutein cyst)	
Malignant ovarian (borderline tumors, epithelial carcinoma, epithelial carcinoma, ovarian germ cell tumor, ovarian sarcoma, sex cord, or stromal tumor)	Need for excision or enucleation
Benign nonovarian (endometrioma, hydrosalpinx, leiomyoma, tubo-ovarian abscess)	
(2) *Congenital reproductive tract anomalies*	
Isolated mullerian anomaly	
• Uterovaginal aplasia	Need for vaginal reconstruction. If uterine remnants are present and result in pain, they may need to be removed
• Cervicovaginal agenesis	Need for vaginal reconstruction. May be necessary to remove uterine remnants
• Lower vaginal atresia	Need vaginal pull-through procedure
Disorders of sexual differentiation	Personalize surgical management
Anorectal malformation	Personalize surgical management

11.3 Patient Positioning

Proper patient positioning on the operating table is essential to allow optimal surgical exposure and to prevent neuromuscular injuries [35]. Positioning is even more critical in robotic surgery because it must provide access to the surgical field and also accommodate the robotic camera system and working arms.

The patient is placed in a semilithotomy position (utmost precaution must be made to ensure that the patient's knees are not in the path of the robotic arm, so as to prevent collisions). The hands are padded and placed at the patient's side with palms up to prevent ulnar nerve damage. Both arms are tucked to the side and are kept in place by arm boards. A safety strap or tape can be used to secure the patient to the table [35, 36]. A piece of foam must be placed on the patient's face to protect the endotracheal tube from inadvertent damage or dislodgement during movement of the robotic endoscope [35]. Foley catheters are inserted in all patients.

A Trendelenburg position (roughly inclined 25–30°) is routinely maintained during robotic gynecologic surgery also in the pediatric age, since once the robot is docked with arms engaged to the instruments, adjusting the table is not feasible without undocking the robot. This has led to a tendency to use the steepest Trendelenburg degree possible to maximize the surgical field and avoid having to readjust the table if increased inclination is required [35, 36].

Performing robotic gynecologic surgery in steep Trendelenburg is associated with rare but serious perioperative complications in the adult age [35]. Position-related injuries include musculoskeletal, neurologic, and vascular. The position-related lower extremity neurologic injuries are estimated to be 1.5% following laparoscopic surgery in the lithotomy position. Other studies have shown that the incidence of brachial plexus injuries following gynecologic surgery is 0.16% [37]. In pediatrics, there are very limited data evaluating the incidence of musculoskeletal and vascular injuries as these events are extremely rare [35]. Although the incidence of similar injuries is unknown in the pediatric age, measures to prevent them are mandatory.

11.4 Camera, Ports, and Instruments

Despite differences in body size, the use of conventional instruments, although designed for adult patients, also provides safe laparoscopic procedures in children and young girls [38, 39]. For standard interventions use conventional 5-mm instruments (8, 5 mm scope size) or 8-mm instruments (12 mm scope size) [36, 40, 41].

Surgery is possible in abdominopelvic procedures using only two operative instruments. The arm n.1 (usually right sided) handles the Endo Wrist monopolar cautery hook and the 5-mm EndoWrist Harmonic Ace (Ethicon Endo-Surgery, Cincinnati, Ohio); left-sided instruments (arm n. 2) include the 5-mm Schertel Grasper, the 5-mm EndoWrist Maryland dissector, and the 5-mm EndoWrist needle drivers. Trocars are inserted with patients in the supine position.

The primary consideration with pediatric procedures is the planning of the trocar placement. In infants and younger children the proper placement of port sites will increase intracorporal instrument length, maximize dexterity, and circumvent external robot arm collisions. Port configuration, and angulation between the trocars and the camera, should allow full rotation of movements and the inversion of working instruments should be very wide (between 135 and 180°). The maximum dexterity of the 5-mm robotic instrument is obtained only when the trocars are positioned more caudally and laterally with respect to the camera position. Five-mm instruments need full 3 cm rotation to obtain at widest working space exceeding the distance of 3 cm from bones, Fig. 11.1 [41].

The limited size of the patient and the narrow surgical field in small children and in small patients necessitate that the operative trocars be inserted before carrying out the telescope docking procedure. The robot is positioned at the foot of the operating bed in older children and adolescents, while in young girls the robot may also be placed at the inferior side of the operating table.

Children and adolescents are usually placed in the Trendelenburg position which is less inclined than in traditional robotic gynecologic surgery [35, 36].

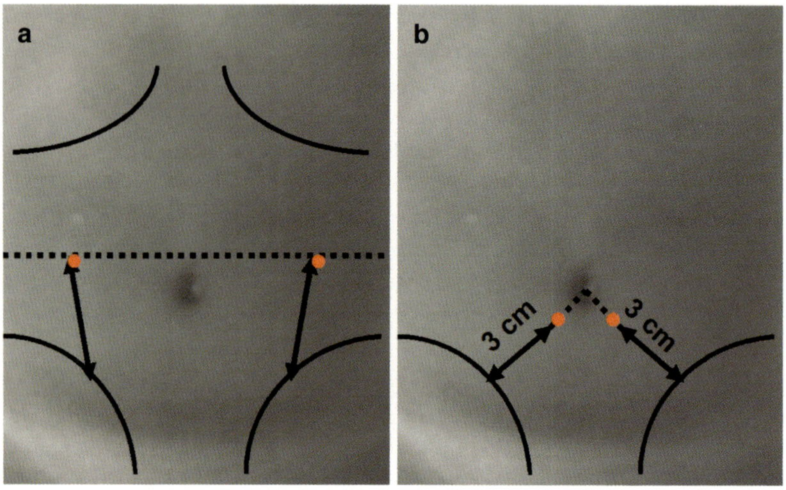

Fig. 11.1 Standard port placement protocol: Panel (**a**): port placement in small children (<8 years); Panel (**b**) port placement in children (>8 years) and adolescents

In this position, insufflation pressure can be lower than usually applied in laparoscopic procedures (8–10 mmHg and a maximum flow at 1.5 L/min). In small patients, inverted instrument orientation may be used. This position allows the suspension of the abdominal wall when instruments are turned away from the abdominal wall, resulting in a lower insufflation pressure [24, 41].

The surgical process includes robot docking time, console operating time, and total operating time.

The docking time includes maneuvering of robotic arms, insertion of robotic instruments into cannulas, and surgeon positioning at the console, while the console time includes the time devoted to the surgical procedure.

11.5 Room Setup

The operating room should be large enough to accommodate all of the robotic components so there is a clear view of the patient from the surgeon's console, tension-free cable connections between the equipment, and clear pathways for operating room personnel to move freely around the room. The positioning of the robotic dual console, robot, scrub station, and anesthesia machines should be optimized to ensure the most effective arrangement for seamless workflow [36]. A schematic of the room setup for gynecological procedures in children and adolescents is illustrated in Figs. 11.2 and 11.3.

The surgeon performs the procedure from the da Vinci Si Surgical System® console, while the surgical assistant standing at the patient's right or left side is ready to prepare special introduction sites depending on the nature of the pathology.

Robotic surgeries may be conducted using the dual console which has the great advantage of being utilized as an integral part of training for current residents, fellows, and visiting surgeons. The double console may be located in the same surgical room or elsewhere. Dual-console robotic surgery is being utilized as a training tool even in pediatric surgery. The learning curve which is achieved during these training procedures is becoming shorter and reached early by fellows [25–28]; thus, the robotic surgical approach in children should rapidly become safer and more effective.

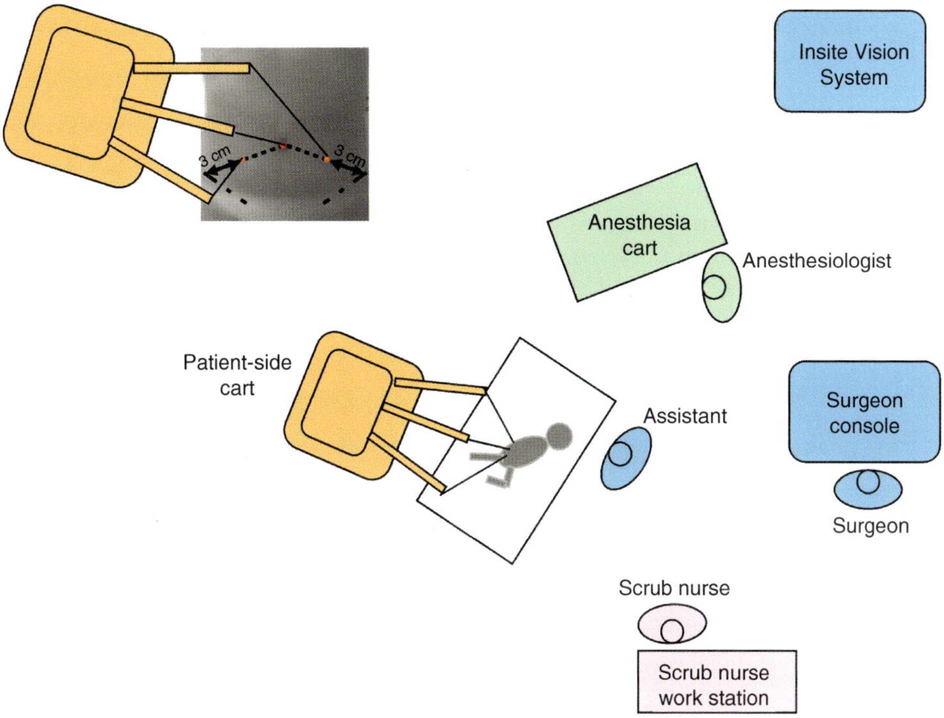

Fig. 11.2 Schematic room setup for gynecological procedures in small children (<8 years)

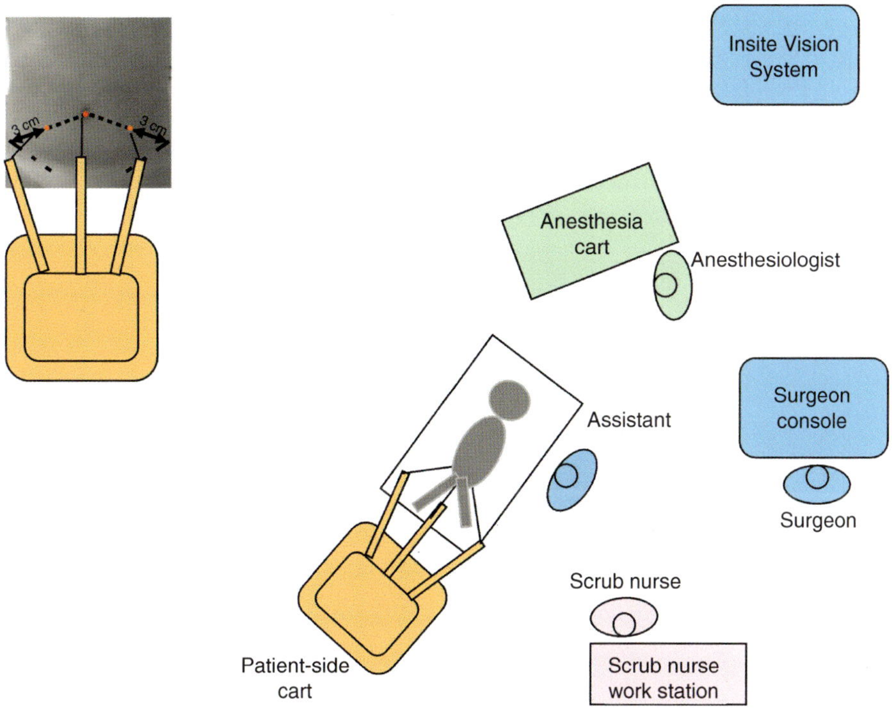

Fig. 11.3 Schematic room setup for gynecological procedures in children (>8 years) and adolescents

11.6 Other Considerations

Robotic-gynecologic assisted surgery offers the best field of view in the rectovesical and recto-uterine pouch in case of congenital malformations and contributes to fertility preservation in case of pediatric ovarian benign tumors [32, 34]; its advantage over laparoscopic view, already reported in adults, is confirmed even in the pediatric age [42, 43].

Although several studies have demonstrated similar surgical outcomes, consisting in decreased surgical morbidity and recovery time comparing robotic to laparoscopic surgery [18, 21–23], it is still premature to conclude that pediatric robotic assisted gynecologic surgery provides better clinical outcomes than traditional laparoscopic surgery. Randomized, prospective, comparative studies will help characterize the advantages and disadvantages of this technology as a routine procedure in pediatric patients.

All reports indicate that it is a promising tool in surgical education [25–28]. Resident training and participation in robotic assisted surgeries will promote shorter adaption to the use of robotic equipment to achieve a safe management even in pediatrics. In fact the dual-console system seems to improve the incorporation of fellow education and resident training in pediatric surgery [44, 45]. Surgeons who have had training in robotics are also expected to better adapt and improve their performance in laparoscopic surgery with the aim of increasing the number of children who will benefit from mini invasive technology.

References

1. Law KS, Abbott JA, Lyons SD. Energy sources for gynecologic laparoscopic surgery: a review of the literature. Obstet Gynecol Surv. 2014;69:763–76.
2. Bhagavath B, Benjamin A. Minimally invasive gynecologic surgery for benign conditions: progress and challenges. Obstet Gynecol Surv. 2015;70:656–66.
3. Rabinovich A. Minimally invasive surgery for endometrial cancer. Curr Opin Obstet Gynecol. 2015;27:302–7.
4. Arimoto T, Kawana K, Adachi K, et al. Minimization of curative surgery for treatment of early cervical cancer: a review. Jpn J Clin Oncol. 2015;45:611–6.
5. Palomba S, Fornaciari E, Falbo A, et al. Safety and efficacy of the minilaparotomy for myomectomy: a systematic review and meta-analysis of randomized and non-randomized controlled trials. Reprod Biomed Online. 2015;30:462–81.
6. Carbonnel M, Revaux A, Frydman R, et al. Single-port approach to benign gynecologic pathology. A review. Minerva Ginecol. 2015;67:239–47.
7. Sisodia RM, Del Carmen MG, Boruta DM. Role of minimally invasive surgery in the management of adnexal masses. Clin Obstet Gynecol. 2015;58:66–75.
8. Bush SH, Apte SM. Robotic-assisted surgery in gynecological oncology. Cancer Control. 2015;22:307–13.
9. van den Haak L, Alleblas C, Nieboer TE, et al. Efficacy and safety of uterine manipulators in laparoscopic surgery: a review. Arch Gynecol Obstet. 2015;292:1003–11.
10. Shazly SA, Murad MH, Dowdy SC, et al. Robotic radical hysterectomy in early stage cervical cancer: a systematic review and meta-analysis. Gynecol Oncol. 2015;138:457–71.
11. Mäenpää M, Nieminen K, Tomás E, et al. Implementing robotic surgery to gynecologic oncology: the first 300 operations performed at a tertiary hospital. Acta Obstet Gynecol Scand. 2015;94:482–8.
12. Zanotti KM, Abdelbadee AY. Robotic management of endometriosis: where do we stand? Minerva Ginecol. 2015;67:257–72.
13. Liu H, Lu D, Shi G, et al. WITHDRAWN: robotic surgery for benign gynaecological disease. Cochrane Database Syst Rev. 2014;12:CD008978.
14. Liu H, Lawrie TA, Lu D, et al. Robot-assisted surgery in gynaecology. Cochrane Database Syst Rev. 2014;12:CD011422.
15. White WM, Pickens RB, Elder RF, et al. Robotic-assisted sacrocolpopexy for pelvic organ prolapse. Urol Clin North Am. 2014;41:549–57.
16. Paraiso MF. Robotic-assisted laparoscopic surgery for hysterectomy and pelvic organ prolapse repair. Fertil Steril. 2014;102:933–8.
17. Sinno AK, Fader AN. Robotic-assisted surgery in gynecologic oncology. Fertil Steril. 2014;102:922–32.
18. Ng AT, Tam PC. Current status of robot-assisted surgery. Hong Kong Med J. 2014;20:241–50.
19. Smorgick N, As-Sanie S. The benefits and challenges of robotic-assisted hysterectomy. Curr Opin Obstet Gynecol. 2014;26:290–4.
20. Tarr ME, Paraiso MF. Minimally invasive approach to pelvic organ prolapse: a review. Minerva Ginecol. 2014;66:49–67.
21. Ayala-Yáñez R, Olaya-Guzmán EJ, Haghenbeck-Altamirano J. Robotics in gynecology: why is this technology worth pursuing? Clin Med Insights Reprod Health. 2013;7:71–7.
22. Gala RB, Margulies R, Steinberg A, et al. Systematic review of robotic surgery in gynecology: robotic techniques compared with laparoscopy and laparotomy. J Minim Invasive Gynecol. 2014;21:353–61.
23. Fanfani F, Restaino S, Ercoli A, et al. Robotic or laparoscopic gynecology. What should we use? Minerva Ginecol. 2016;68(4):423–30.

24. Nakib G, Calcaterra V, Scorletti F, et al. Robotic assisted surgery in pediatric gynecology: promising innovation in mini invasive surgical procedures. J Pediatr Adolesc Gynecol. 2013;26:e5–7.
25. Nezhat C, Lakhi N. Learning experiences in robotic-assisted laparoscopic surgery. Best Pract Res Clin Obstet Gynaecol. 2016;35:20–9. pii: S1521-6934(15)00221-7
26. Catchpole K, Perkins C, Bresee C, et al. Safety, efficiency and learning curves in robotic surgery: a human factors analysis. Surg Endosc. 2016;30(9): 3749–61.
27. El Hachem L, Momeni M, Friedman K, et al. Safety, feasibility and learning curve of robotic single-site surgery in gynecology. Int J Med Robot. 2016;12(3):509–16. doi:10.1002/rcs.1675.
28. Sheth SS, Fader AN, Tergas AI, et al. Virtual reality robotic surgical simulation: an analysis of gynecology trainees. J Surg Educ. 2014;71:125–32.
29. Sinha CK, Haddad M. Robot-assisted surgery in children: current status. J Robot Surg. 2008;1:243–6.
30. Long CJ, Ginsberg JP, Kolon TF. Fertility preservation in children and adolescents with cancer. Urology. 2016;91:190–6. pii: S0090–4295(15)01176–0
31. Estes SJ. Fertility preservation in children and adolescents. Endocrinol Metab Clin N Am. 2015;44:799–820.
32. Lipskind ST, Gargiulo AR. Computer-assisted laparoscopy in fertility preservation and reproductive surgery. J Minim Invasive Gynecol. 2013;20:435–45.
33. Pathiraja P, Tozzi R. Advances in gynaecological oncology surgery. Best Pract Res Clin Obstet Gynaecol. 2013;27:415–20.
34. Gargiulo AR. Fertility preservation and the role of robotics. Clin Obstet Gynecol. 2011;54:431–48.
35. Ulm MA, Fleming ND, Rallapali V, et al. Position-related injury is uncommon in robotic gynecologic surgery. Gynecol Oncol. 2014;135:534–8.
36. Chang C, Steinberg Z, Shah A, et al. Patient positioning and port placement for robot-assisted surgery. J Endourol. 2014;28:631–8.
37. Barnett JC, Hurd WW, Rogers RM Jr, et al. Laparoscopic positioning and nerve injuries. J Minim Invasive Surg. 2007;14:664–72.
38. Jackson HT, Kane TD. Advances in minimally invasive surgery in pediatric patients. Adv Pediatr Infect Dis. 2014;61:149–95.
39. Blatnik JA, Ponsky TA. Advances in minimally invasive surgery in pediatrics. Curr Gastroenterol Rep. 2010;12:211–4.
40. Tomaszewski JJ, Casella DP, Turner RM II, et al. Pediatric laparoscopic and robot-assisted laparoscopic surgery: technical considerations. J Endourol. 2012;26:602–13.
41. Pelizzo G, Nakib G, Romano P, et al. Five millimetre-instruments in paediatric roboticsurgery: advantages and shortcomings. Minim Invasive Ther Allied Technol. 2015;24:148–53.
42. Anderson KM, Ruckle HC, Baldwin DD. Robotic-assisted surgery and the evolution of the radical prostatectomy. Minerva Urol Nefrol. 2012;64:97–122.
43. Bianco FJ. Robotic radical prostatectomy: present and future. Arch Esp Urol. 2011;64:839–46.
44. Smith AL, Krivak TC, Scott EM, et al. Dual-console robotic surgery compared to laparoscopic surgery with respect to surgical outcomes in a gynecologic oncology fellowship program. Gynecol Oncol. 2012;126:432–6.
45. Wedmid A, Llukani E, Lee DI. Future perspectives in robotic surgery. BJU Int. 2011;108:1028–36.

12 Robotic Bladder Outlet Procedures

Patricio C. Gargollo, Gianantonio Manzoni,
and Bernardo Rocco

12.1 Introduction

Minimally invasive techniques are rapidly being developed and integrated into standard open urologic surgery. Over the last 10 years, the urologic literature is replete with novel techniques and adaptations to conventional laparoscopy, including but not limited to laparo-endoscopic single-site surgery, natural orifice transluminal endoscopic surgery, and robot-assisted laparoscopic surgery (RALS). Pediatric urology is no exception to this trend, and the benefits of minimally invasive surgery may be accentuated in children given the relatively more confined working spaces and also a heightened awareness of cosmetic results for the pediatric population. Increasingly, complex pediatric urologic procedures are being performed with robot assistance. The feasibility of nephrectomy, pyeloplasty, ureteral reimplantation, and bladder surgery has been clearly established. A few case reports and a small series have been published describing robot-assisted Mitrofanoff appendicovesicostomy (APV) with or without augmentation ileocystoplasty or creation of an anterograde continent enema colon tube [1–3].

12.2 Urinary Incontinence and Bladder Outlet Surgery

Urinary incontinence secondary to an incompetent urethral sphincter mechanism is an entity commonly encountered in pediatric urology with multiple etiologies. Regardless of the primary cause (exstrophy/epispadias, cloacal anomalies or neurogenic bladder secondary to spinal cord injury or dysraphisms) urine leakage in the absence of a detrusor contraction is the definition of an incompetent urinary sphincter mechanism [4]. It is in this patient population that a bladder outlet procedure, with possible concomitant procedures depending on the patient, is indicated to achieve urinary continence. Whether or not a concomitant bladder augmentation procedure should be performed is a highly contested topic and beyond the scope of this chapter and thus will not be covered here.

The essential mechanism behind all surgical procedures for urinary incontinence secondary to an incompetent sphincter is to somehow tighten the bladder outlet. This can be accomplished through placement of a sling or an artificial urinary sphincter or through a bladder neck reconstruction (BNR). In some cases a bladder neck closure can

P.C. Gargollo (✉)
Department of Pediatric Urology, Texas Children's Hospital, Baylor College of Medicine, Houston, TX, USA
e-mail: pcgargol@texaschildrens.org

G. Manzoni
Pediatric Urology Unit, Fondazione IRCCS à Granda, Ospedale Maggiore Policlinico, Milan, Italy

B. Rocco
Department of Urology, University of Milan Fondazione IRCCS à Granda, Ospedale Maggiore Policlinico, Milan, Italy

G. Mattioli, P. Petralia (eds.), *Pediatric Robotic Surgery*, DOI 10.1007/978-3-319-41863-6_12

also be performed. At one of the author's institutions (PG), management of neurogenic bladder with persistent urinary incontinence despite clean intermittent catheterization (CIC) and anticholinergic therapy includes a Leadbetter/Mitchell bladder neck reconstruction (BNR) with or without a bladder neck sling (BNS) and, when needed, the creation of a Mitrofanoff APV (or Monti channel when the appendix is inadequate).

The unique anatomical view of the bladder neck and posterior urethral region which is achieved with the 3D robotic exposure has potential further applications. A very preliminary and initial experience in partial cysto-prostatectomy for rhabdomyosarcoma is also discussed in this chapter.

12.2.1 Robotic Assisted Bladder Neck Reconstruction

Establishing urinary continence in pediatric patients with sphincteric incompetence usually involves a combination of medical therapy, clean intermittent catheterization (CIC), and sometimes surgical intervention. This condition is most often encountered in children with spina bifida, and is diagnosed by persistent incontinence despite CIC and anticholinergics in patients with detrusor areflexia and DLPP <50 cm H_2O on urodynamic testing. Cystography demonstrates a smooth-walled bladder and, typically, an open bladder neck. The most commonly used procedure to gain continence in these patients is bladder neck sling (BNS). However, our data indicate that a Leadbetter/Mitchell bladder neck reconstruction to reduce the caliber of the outlet, plus sling (LMS), has higher continence rates than a sling alone [5]. Consequently, we perform this procedure and APV (or Monti channel when the appendix is inadequate) to achieve urinary continence in this patient population using robotic assistance. Whether or not an augmentation ileocystoplasty should be concomitantly performed is beyond the scope of this article but the below techniques can be implemented and easily modified to accommodate an augmentation when indicated.

It is clear from our data (see below) that the robotic approach offers the same continence for a LMS with the added advantages of small "band-aid" incisions, less postoperative pain, and shorter hospitalization. We have previously reported our initial results [3] and provide our technique and outcomes.

12.3 Description of Technique

Below is the step-by-step description of the technique for a robotic assisted bladder neck sling with bladder neck reconstruction (Leadbetter/Mitchell) and an appendicovesicostomy. Given the excellent exposure to the pelvis and the bladder this technique can be modified to accommodate any type of bladder neck repair (Salle, Kropp, Young-Dees, etc).

12.3.1 Patient Positioning

The child is placed supine on a padded beanbag patient positioner (Fig. 12.1). Alternatively the

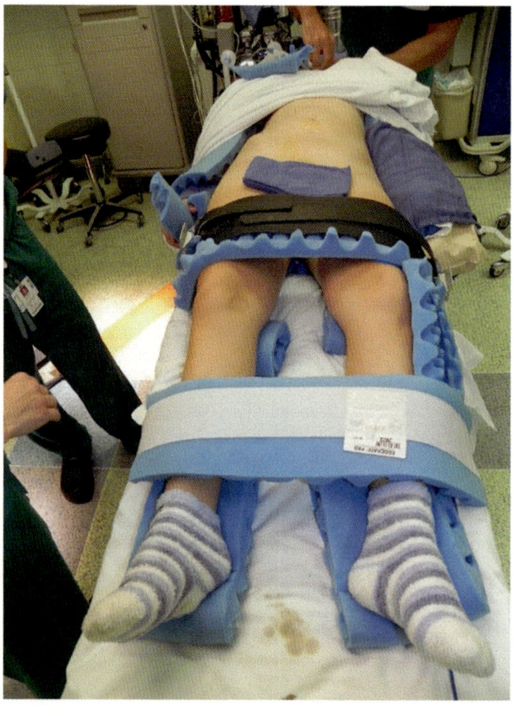

Fig. 12.1 Patient positioning. It is imperative to meticulously pad every possible pressure point. Alternatively the patient can be placed in lithotomy although we do not recommend it given the potential for lower extremity nerve injury during long cases

legs can be placed in lithotomy stirrups. It is imperative to pad all pressure points including the heels (Fig. 12.2). The patient is secured to the bed using wide tape. The shorter end of the base of the OR table should be oriented towards the patient's feet to allow as much space as possible for the base of the robot (Fig. 12.3). Along these lines the patient should be moved down on the operating table as much as possible. The patient is prepped and draped. The head of the operating table is lowered (Trendelenburg position) for the bladder neck portion of the surgery. A Foley catheter is inserted transurethrally and the balloon inflated to later help identify the bladder neck. This is done sterile on the field. Prior to positioning it is recommended (especially early in the surgeon's experience) to cystoscopically place externalized ureteral catheters to aid in ureteral orifice identification during the bladder neck reconstruction. They are secured to the Foley and prepped onto the field.

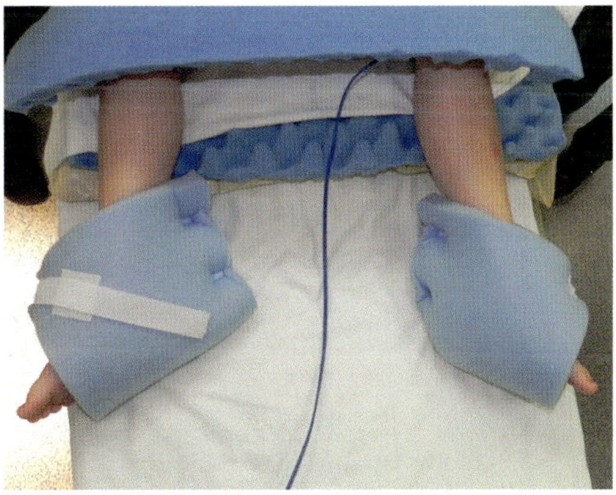

Fig. 12.2 Padding at the ankles and heels

12.3.2 Skin Incision and Port Placement

If a final umbilical stoma is chosen an inverted "V"-shaped incision is made in the umbilicus with the apex of the "V" at the base of the umbilicus. The umbilical stalk is grasped with a Kocher clamp and access is obtained with a veress needle technique. A 5 mm VersaStep™ trocar is placed and a 5 mm laparoscopic camera is used to place the remaining ports. Port placement is as shown in Fig. 12.4. The robotic ports are secured to the patient's skin as shown in Fig. 12.5 using two ½ in. Steri-Strips™ which are wrapped around the trocar and a small Tegaderm™ adhesive dressing is used these to secure them to the skin. A 2–0 Vicryl suture on a UR6 needle is then used to secure the above dressing to the skin and deep subcutaneous tissues. These sutures are then wrapped around the 8.5 mm trocars. In case of a

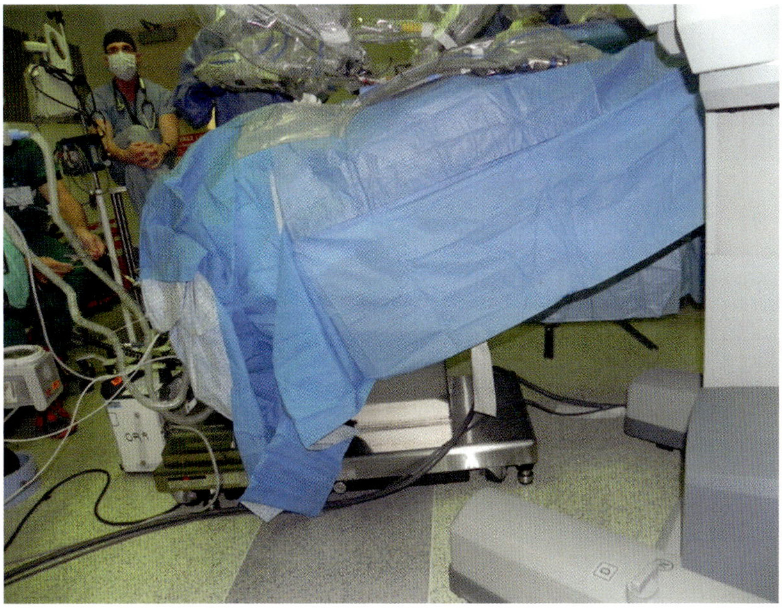

Fig. 12.3 Docking. The shorter end of the base of the OR table should be oriented towards the patient's feet to allow as much space as possible for the base of the robot

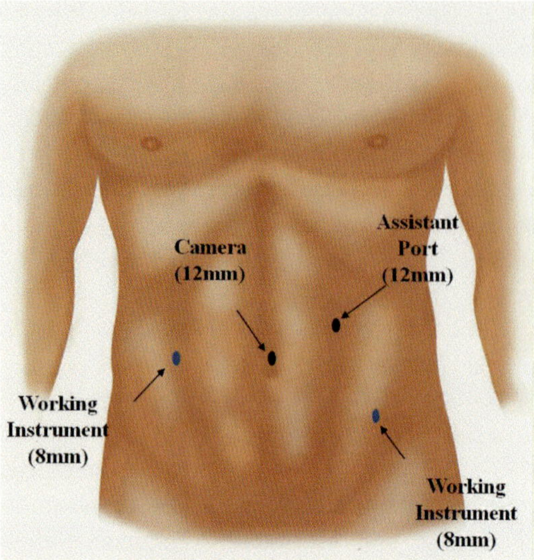

Fig. 12.4 Port placement. We use a 12 mm camera and two 8.5 working ports. If any bowel work is going to be performed or if a sling is going to be used we use a 12 mm assist in the left upper quadrant. If just an appendicovesicostomy is going to be performed a 5 mm assist port can be used

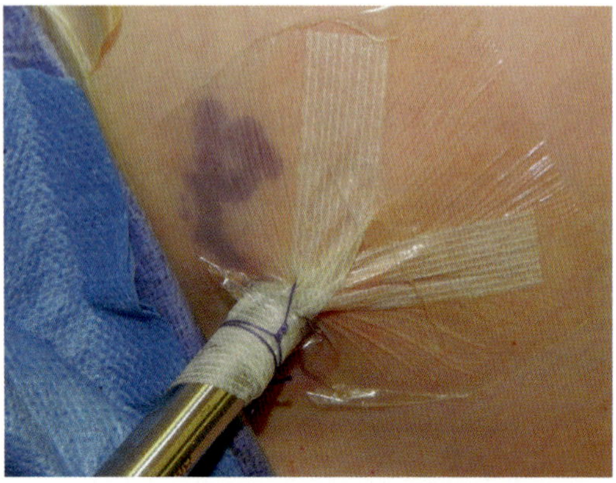

Fig. 12.5 The robotic ports are secured to the patient's skin as shown using two ½ in. Steri-Strips™ which are wrapped around the trocar and a small Tegaderm™ adhesive dressing is used these to secure them to the skin. A 2–0 Vicryl suture on a UR6 needle is then used to secure the above dressing to the skin and deep subcutaneous tissues. These sutures are then wrapped around the 8.5 mm trocars

right iliac fossa final stoma the skin incision is made accordingly in the VQZ technique as described by Ransley [6] at the end of the robotic procedure (Fig. 12.6).

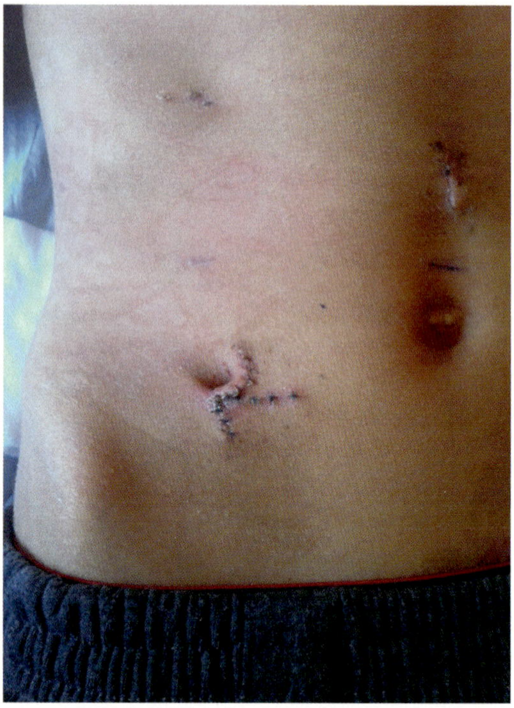

Fig. 12.6 Alternate placement for catheterizable conduit in this instance shown as a VQZ flap in the right lower quadrant

12.3.3 Dissection of the Appendix

Before the robot is docked the entire right and mid-transverse colon are mobilized laparoscopically to allow for the appendix to be dissected as inferiorly in the pelvis as possible. The appendix is harvested with a 12 mm laparoscopic endo-gia stapler. A cecal extension of the stable line can be used at this point and is particularly helpful in obese patients or in patients with a short appendix.

12.3.4 Robotic Docking

The da Vinci robot is docked either directly in the midline from inferior (if the patient is in lithotomy) or slightly from the patient's right side and inferior (Fig. 12.7). The second position allows the surgeon a bit more flexibility to work above the pelvis and to the right of the patient in cases where the appendix needs to be further mobi-

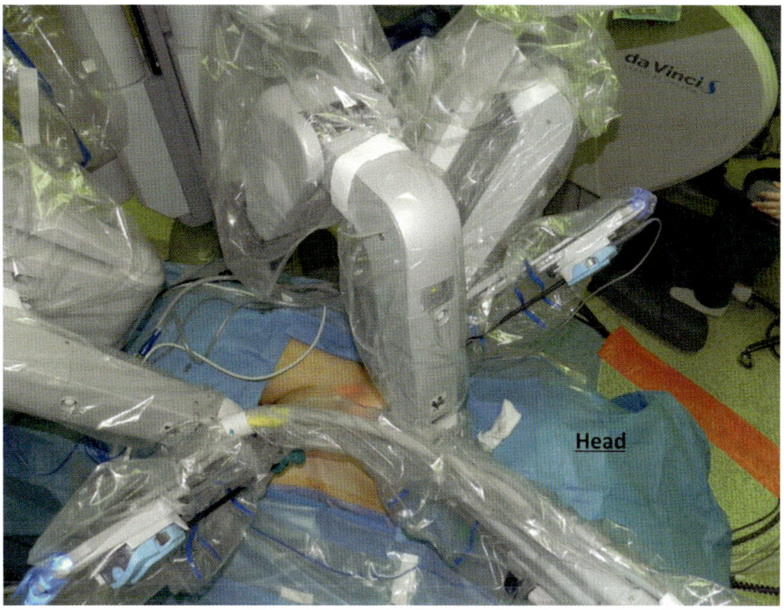

Fig. 12.7 The da Vinci robot is docked either directly in the midline from inferior (if the patient is in lithotomy) or slightly from the patient's right side and inferior

lized. In the second method the base of the robot should straddle the right corner of the operating table (Fig. 12.3). Ports are secured to the robotic arms. A 12 mm camera at the 30 degree up position is used.

Bladder Neck Reconstruction and Sling Placement:

Camera: 30 degree up.

Working Instruments:

Right Arm: Monopolar cautery scissors.

Left Arm: Robotic deBakey or bipolar Maryland.

The plane between the vagina and posterior bladder in females or the rectum and posterior bladder in males is developed. The peritoneum between these structures is opened using a wide horizontal incision. The assistant grasps the inferior lip of this incision and retracts towards themselves (back and down). This plane is dissected as distal as possible. Movement of the Foley and visualization of the balloon can help identify where the end of the bladder neck is. Care must be taken to identify and preserve the vas deferens bilaterally in males. Care must also be taken not to carry the dissection too laterally as this risks potential injury to the ureters. Once this dissection is complete a second incision is made above the bladder to release the peritoneum, the urachus, and the lateral bladder attachments. This dissection is carried all the way to the lateral pelvic floor at which point the endopelvic fascia is incised bilaterally and the puboprostatic ligaments (in males) are released. In adolescent males a dorsal vein suture (2–0 or 3–0 Vicryl) is placed for hemostasis.

12.3.5 Extracorporeal Preparation of the Sling

The sling material preferred is a Suspend-Tutoplast Processed Fascia Lata sling (2 cm × 7 cm) (Coloplast). The sling is prepared according to the manufacturer's instructions. Two 12-Fr central line introducers cut at 3 cm are then sewn to each end of the sling. Three air knots are made to create three loops in between the introducer and the sling. This facilitates retraction by the bedside assistant in the subsequent sections.

Retrovesical Placement of the Sling.

Camera: 30 degree down.

Working Instruments:

Right Arm: bipolar Maryland.

Left Arm: Monopolar cautery scissors or deBakey forceps.

The sling is passed intracorporeally through the assist port, if 12 mm, if not through one of the 8.5 mm robotic working ports. The attached introducers are placed behind the bladder. One at a time, each introducer is grasped with the Maryland and the space of Retzius is entered bilaterally (Fig. 12.8a and b). Alternatively this plane can be developed with the bipolar Maryland and once the plane is developed the introducers can be passed anteriorly. At this point both sides of the sling are passed (Fig. 12.8c).

Leadbetter/Mitchell Bladder Neck Revision:

Camera: 30 degree down.

Working Instruments:

Right Arm: Monopolar cautery scissors.

Left Arm: deBakey forceps.

The assistant grasps the loops of suture placed on each end of the sling and retracts cephalad and down. The urethra is incised from 3 to 9 o'clock using the monopolar scissor. The incision is deepened until the urethral catheter and the ureteral stents (if placed) are exposed. The transverse incision is grasped with the left hand and retracted cephalad. The urethra and bladder neck are "unroofed" by carrying the 3 and 9 o'clock incisions in parallel fashion ending just below the trigone (Fig. 12.8d) The ureteral orifices can be identified by the previously placed ureteral catheters or by having the anesthesiologist give the patient intravenous indigo carmine. Continuous traction on the midline of the urethra cephalad helps keep the incisions in the same plane, exposing a strip of dorsal urethra as seen in these photos.

For the tubularization of the bladder neck:

Camera: 30 degree down.

Working Instruments:

Right Arm: DaVinci black diamond microforceps.

Left Arm: DaVinci black diamond microforceps.

A 5-Fr feeding tube is placed into the distal urethra and then the urethra is retubularized using two layers continuous, submucosal 4–0 Vicryl and then 3–0 Vicryl stitches from distally to proximally (Fig. 12.8e). It is important to suture close to the edge of the urethral strip—especially through the bladder neck—to ensure that the lumen remains uniform in caliber. The feeding tube is left in place and secured to the foreskin or labia minora with a 4–0 silk suture.

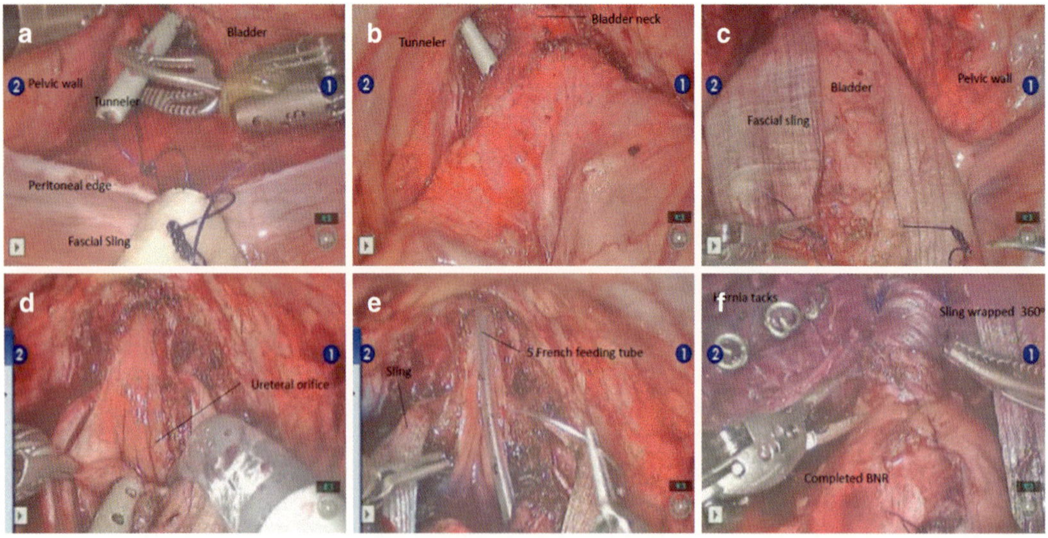

Fig. 12.8 Steps in the bladder neck reconstruction: The tunnelers are then passed ventrally from the posterior bladder dissection into the developed space of Retzius (**a**), (**b**). Once the sling is passed from posterior to anterior (**c**) the urethra is unroofed up through the bladder neck to the level of the interureteric ridge (**d**). At this point, the Foley catheter is exchanged for a 5F feeding tube, and the urethra is retubularized in two layers with a running simple suture of 4–0 Vicryl followed by 3–0 Vicryl (**e**). After the Leadbetter/Mitchell repair is completed the sling is tightly wrapped 360° and attached to the pubic bone using six screws from a hernia tacker (**f**)

Sling Placement:

Right Arm: bipolar Maryland.

Left Arm: deBakey forceps.

The central line introducers attached to the sling are detached from the sling and removed. The Maryland on the right arm is passed behind the sling and behind the bladder and the sling end on the patient's right is passed to the Maryland with the left arm (deBakey forceps). The sling is thus wrapped 360 degrees. The sling is cinched tight.

Right Arm: DaVinci black diamond microforceps.

Left Arm: DaVinci black diamond microforceps.

The sling is secured to itself using two interrupted 5–0 prolene sutures. The ends of the sling are lifted up to the pubic bone. The assistant passes a hernia Tacker™ Fixation Device (Covidien) and tacks the sling to the pubis using two or three titanium spiral screws (Fig. 12.7f).

Bladder Hitch:

Camera: 30 degree down.

Working Instruments:

Right Arm: deBakey forceps.

Left Arm: deBakey forceps.

The bladder is hitched to the anterior abdominal wall using three interrupted 3–0 PDS sutures passed through the abdominal wall or secured intracorporeally. The purpose of this is to bring the bladder as close to the umbilicus and as cephalad as possible and thus minimize the tension on the appendicovesical anastomosis. If the hitch stitches are passed through the abdominal wall it is helpful to pass them through a 14 G angiocath. The hitch stitches are not tied down until the end of the case after the robot is undocked. They are secured at the skin surface using hemostats.

Appendicovesicostomy:

Working Instruments:

Right Arm: deBakey forceps followed by monopolar scissors.

Left Arm: deBakey forceps.

The staple line is removed and the tip of the appendix is cut. A 10-Fr feeding tube cut at 10 cm is passed from proximal to distal and the tube is suture ligated to the cecal end of the appendix with a 3–0 PD suture cut to 10 cm. This allows the tube to be manipulated instead of the appendix. A 4 cm detrusor tunnel is fashioned on the posterior aspect of the bladder.

Appendicovesical Anastomosis.

Right Arm: DaVinci black diamond microforceps.

Left Arm: DaVinci black diamond microforceps.

A mucosal opening is made on the inferior apex of the detrusor tunnel. The distal end of the appendix is anastomosed using two running simple sutures of 5–0 Vicryl on TF needles one up each side.

Detrusor closure.

Right Arm: deBakey forceps or large needle driver.

Left Arm: deBakey forceps.

The detrusor tunnel is closed over the appendix using a running simple 3–0 V-lock suture with a laparaty at the looped end of the suture. Every other throw incorporates adventitia on the appendix.

12.3.6 Maturing Stoma

The robot is undocked. The 5 mm laparoscopic camera is turned back on. A Maryland or bowel grasper is passed through the umbilical trocar, the tube sutured to the appendix is grasped, and the appendix is delivered through the umbilical stoma. The appendix is secured to the fascia using a single 4–0 PDS. The appendix is spatulated and the stoma is matured circumferentially to the skin using interrupted 5–0 Vicryl sutures. The 10-Fr feeding tube is exchanged for a 12- or 14-Fr mentor catheter. The mentor catheter is secured to the skin using a 3–0 nylon suture.

12.3.7 Port Closure

All ports are removed and the fascia closed with 2–0 Vicryl on UR6 needles. Skin is closed with 5–0 monocryl. Dermabond skin adhesive is used. Dressings are optional. All tubes are secured to the skin and attached to drainage bags.

12.4 Results

We have now performed 38 robotic assisted LMS and APV at one of the author's institutions (PG) and have a mean follow-up of 21 months (range 5–33). One of these patients had previously undergone an appendectomy and therefore had a robotic Monti channel created. The male:female ratio is 16:22 and 90% of these patients had myelomeningocele and neurogenic bladder. Mean patient age was 10 years (range 5–16) and mean BMI was 22.3 (16–31). The mean preoperative bladder capacity was 206 mL (162–308). None of our patients had prior or simultaneous augmentation. Mean operative time was 5.8 h (3.6–12.25) with the longer operative times being significantly higher in the first 10 versus the last 28 cases ($p = 0.0001$). In four cases conversion to open surgery was necessary, due to extensive intra-abdominal adhesions in two and an appendix that was not sufficient for APV and so required Monti in two. Mean hospital length of stay was 52 h (34–86).

Of the patients 31/38 (82%) are completely dry during the day on CIC every 3 h. Of the seven that are wet four are noncompliant with CIC. One is wet from his urethra and Monti channel and two developed decreased bladder compliance that was unresponsive to increased anticholinergics and Botox injection and so underwent ileocystoplasty. Additional complications include four cases of de novo reflux (grade 2 and 3), and two patients who developed bladder stones. Figure 12.9 shows the postoperative appearance at 6 months.

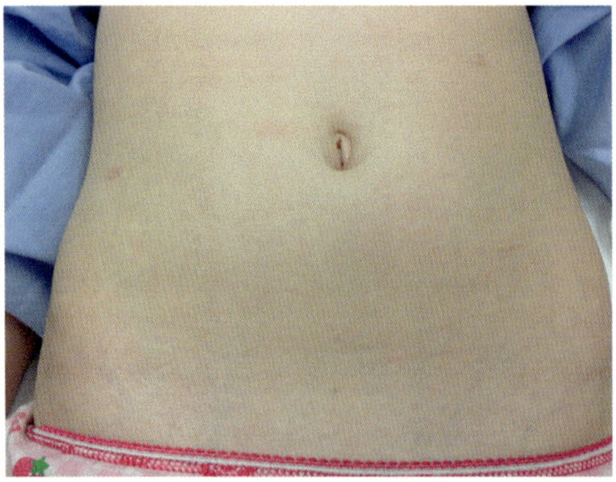

Fig. 12.9 Postoperative appearance at 6 months post-op

12.4.1 Robotic Assisted Partial Cysto-Prostatectomy

The multiple advantages of robotic technology have allowed for a vast expansion in the surgical armamentarium for both the pediatric and adult urologist. As described above access to the bladder neck is feasible and may provide benefits over traditional open access to this anatomic location. Recently there have been two descriptions of robotic assisted prostatectomy or partial cystectomy and prostatectomy for residual masses after chemotherapy and radiation for prostate and bladder rhabdomyosarcoma [7, 8]. In one of these reports Minoli et al. describe a case of a 2-year-old male with bladder and prostate involvement who initially presented with bilateral hydroureteronephrosis and renal failure. After percutaneous decompression the patient underwent chemotherapy and targeted radiation. Posttreatment imaging revealed a residual mass involving the bladder and prostate (Fig. 12.10). A transvesical cysto-prostatectomy without ureteral

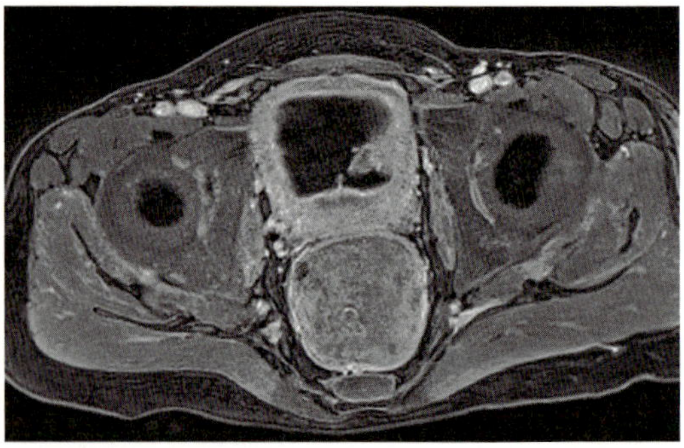

Fig. 12.10 Magnetic resonance imaging showing a sagittal view of pelvis revealing residual left-sided mass after chemotherapy and radiation treatment

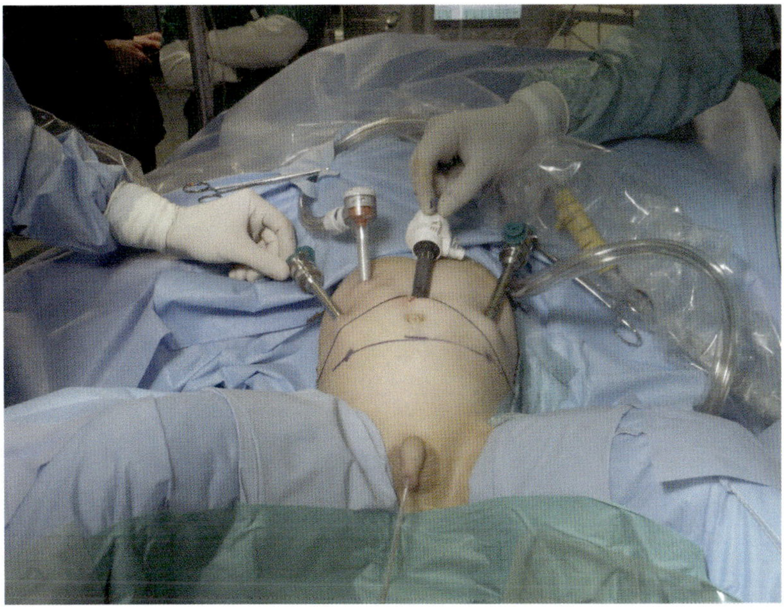

Fig. 12.11 Robotic setup for transvesical partial cystectomy and prostatectomy for rhabdomyosarcoma. 12 mm camera port, 8.5 mm working ports, and 5 mm assist port

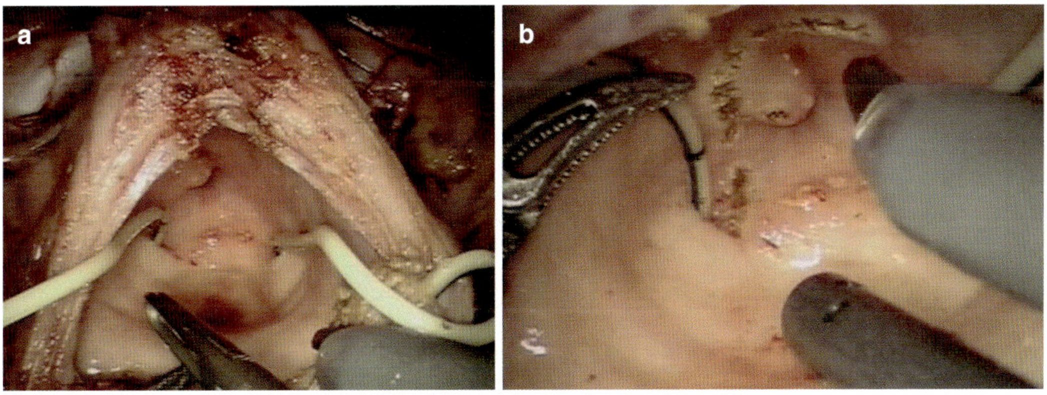

Fig. 12.12 Transvesical view of trigone with ureteral stents in place (**a**). Demarcation of tumor margin with monopolar cautery scissors prior to resection (**b**)

reimplantation was performed (Figs. 12.11 and 12.12). Ureteral stents were left indwelling for 2 months. Histology revealed no residual tumor cells. Postoperative imaging and follow-up at 18 months revealed urinary continence, spontaneous voiding, and low-grade vesicoureteral reflux (Figs. 12.13 and 12.14). These reports again emphasize the feasibility of robotic assisted technology for access to pelvic structures in both benign and malignant disease.

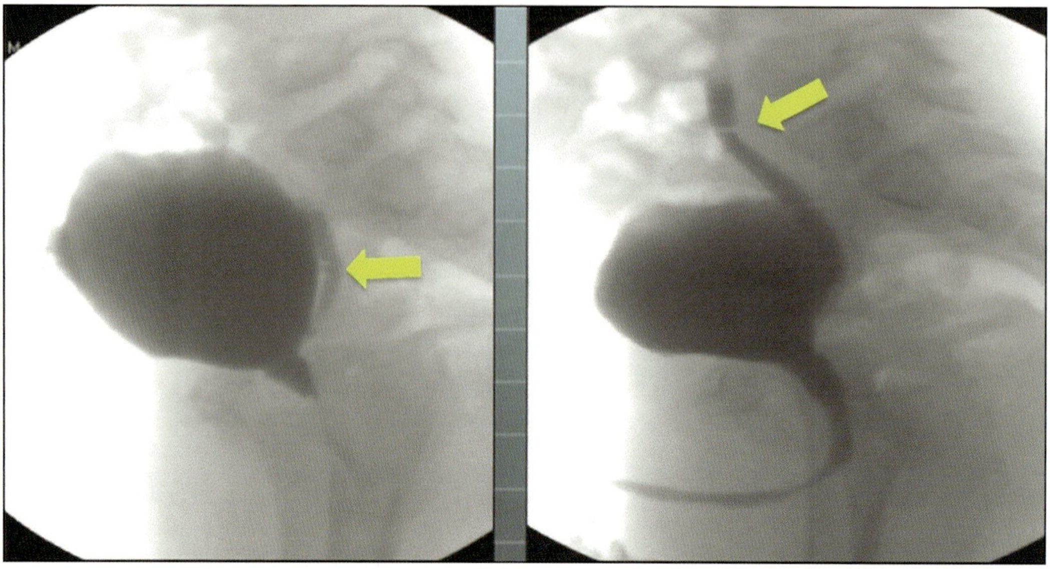

Fig. 12.13 Postoperative voiding cystourethrogram showing a competent bladder neck and low-graded left vesicoureteral reflux

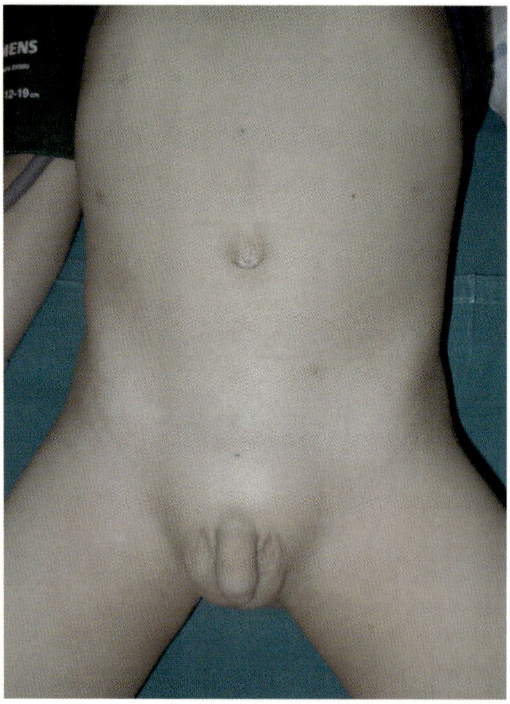

Fig. 12.14 Post-op appearance of the abdomen 18 months after surgery

12.5 Tips and Tricks

Robotic assisted bladder neck reconstruction with creation of a continent catheterizable conduit should be considered an "advanced" robotic procedure and we strongly recommend that surgeons become very familiar and facile with robotic assisted pyeloplasty and ureteral reimplant prior to attempting these cases. The following tips and tricks have helped reduce operative time significantly:

- We strongly advise that all the ports be secured to the patient's skin using a device similar to that shown in Fig. 12.5. Accidental removal of the ports during instrument and robotic arm manipulation can add a significant amount of time to the procedure.
- Mobilization of the entire right and mid-transverse colon should be done using free-hand laparoscopy prior to docking the robot. Once the robot is docked it is not possible for the console surgeon to "look" cephalad and thus mobilization of the large bowel (if needed to decrease tension of the appendix to bladder anastomosis) is not possible.

- The ideal initial patient should be prepubertal and a female where there is no concern for the vas deferens during the dissection for the sling. We also strongly recommend that the first patient not have a VP shunt or at least have minimal VP shunt revisions at the abdominal level. VP shunts (especially if they have been revised) cause significant intra-abdominal adhesions which can make the procedure longer and can contribute to a higher conversion rate (Gargollo et al., manuscript in preparation).
- Management of the VP shunt is controversial. Some authors advocate placing it in a sterile laparoscopic specimen bag [9]. Until recently we had had no VP shunt infections without any specific treatment for the shunt. We recently had a CSF pseudocyst form which required shunt externalization.
- We do not routinely perform a bowel prep for these patients although some have advocated it to reduce the overall fecal load especially in the neurogenic bowel patients.
- Using a dorsal venous ligating suture before bladder neck reduction significantly increases visibility.
- All detrusor tunnels were created on the posterior bladder wall because decreased stone formation, urinary tract infection, and increased mucus removal are cited with posterior placement [10]. Maneuvers for improving the operation will surely continue to come to light. The benefits of robot-assisted surgery were evident in the majority of our patients. Three of four patients were discharged on postoperative day 2. Unilateral low-grade reflux did develop in two patients; it has responded to increased anticholinergic dose.

Conclusion

In addition to potential for decreased postoperative pain, rapid convalescence, and improved cosmesis, RALS surgery has immense potential with respect to the type of surgery that can be performed in the deep pelvis in children—one of the main reasons this technology has taken a strong foothold in urologic and gynecologic surgery. Because we can achieve the equivalent continence results with the added benefits of smaller incisions, less intraoperative blood loss, less postoperative pain, and shorter hospital stays using robotic assistance as compared to open surgery, we rarely perform open bladder neck reconstruction for children with bladder outlet incompetency at our respective institutions. Early in the surgical experience the surgeon should expect significantly longer operative times when using robotic assistance. However, over time, operative times become significantly shorter and more similar to the duration expected for traditional open surgery for these procedures. While we perform the Leadbetter/Mitchell technique for our bladder neck repairs based on analysis of our outcomes in open surgery, other bladder neck repair techniques could also be adapted to be done robotically. Regardless, when learning such procedures we recommend the initial patients be thin and prepubertal without prior abdominal surgery, and especially without a ventriculoperitoneal shunt.

- Our series is the largest to date reporting complex robotic assisted lower urinary tract reconstruction for urinary continence. Our data supports that these procedures are safe and feasible and achieve equivalent continence outcomes to open repairs while providing the additional benefits of shorter hospitalizations and decreased pain. A prospective analysis comparing these methods to open methods is ongoing.

References

1. Gundeti MS, et al. Robotic-assisted laparoscopic reconstructive surgery in the lower urinary tract. Curr Urol Rep. 2013;14(4):333–41.
2. Gundeti MS, et al. Paediatric robotic-assisted laparoscopic augmentation ileocystoplasty and Mitrofanoff appendicovesicostomy (RALIMA): feasibility of and initial experience with the University of Chicago technique. BJU Int. 2011;107(6):962–9.

3. Bagrodia A, Gargollo P. Robot-assisted bladder neck reconstruction, bladder neck sling, and appendicovesicostomy in children: description of technique and initial results. J Endourol. 2011; 25(8):1299–305.
4. Abrams P, et al. The standardisation of terminology of lower urinary tract function: report from the standardisation sub-committee of the international continence Society. Neurourol Urodyn. 2002;21(2):167–78.
5. Snodgrass WT, Gargollo PC. Urologic care of the neurogenic bladder in children. Urol Clin North Am. 2010;37(2):207–14.
6. Itesako T, et al. Clinical experience of the VQZ plasty for catheterizable urinary stomas. J Pediatr Urol. 2011;7(4):433–7.
7. Minoli D, et al. Robotic assisted partial cystoprostatectomy for embryonal rhabdomyosarcoma. In: 26th congress of the European society of pediatric urology. Prague, Czechoslovakia; 2015.
8. Venegas AM, et al. Robotic prostatectomy in a child of 7 years: a case report. In: 26th congress of the European society of pediatric urology. Prague, Czechoslovakia; 2015.
9. Marchetti P, et al. Management of the ventriculoperitoneal shunt in pediatric patients during robot-assisted laparoscopic urologic procedures. J Endourol. 2011;25(2):225–9.
10. Berkowitz J, et al. Mitrofanoff continent catheterizable conduits: top down or bottom up? J Pediatr Urol. 2009;5(2):122–5.

Robotic Treatment of Utricular Cysts

13

Mario Lima, Tommaso Gargano, Michela Maffi, Giovanni Ruggeri, and Michele Libri

13.1 Introduction

Müllerian duct remnants (MDR) derive from incomplete regression of female structures, presumably as a consequence of delayed or insufficient production or effect of anti-Müllerian hormone (AMH) [1–3]. Dilatation of the Müllerian duct remnants can lead to an enlarged prostatic utricle or a Müllerian duct cyst which is known to be present in 4% of newborns and 1% of adults [4]. The prevalence of symptomatic remnants is still unknown. In 11–14% of cases an enlarged prostatic utricle is associated to distal hypospadias or disorders of sexual differentiation (DSD) and to a perineal hypospadias in 50% of cases [5, 6].

M. Lima (✉)
Department of Pediatric Surgery, Bologna University, Bologna 40138, Italy

Department of Pediatric Surgery, Bologna University, Via Massarenti 11, Bologna 40138, Italy
e-mail: mario.lima@unibo.it

T. Gargano • M. Maffi • G. Ruggeri • M. Libri
Department of Pediatric Surgery, Bologna University, Bologna 40138, Italy

MDR can be asymptomatic but also present with urinary tract infections (UTI), stones in the pouch, dysuria, back pressure changes, and pseudoincontinence due to entrapment of urine [5]. Moreover, risk of malignant degeneration has been reported [2, 7].

Diagnosis is often easy. Ultrasounds (US) reveal a retrovesical hypoechoic cystic lesion and voiding cystourethrogram (VCUG) detects communication between the urethra and the cyst (Fig. 13.1). MRI can also be used as a second-level investigation to confirm dimensions of the lesion and the relations with the other pelvic structures (Fig. 13.2).

Treatment of MDR can be challenging in order to preserve fertility and prevent pelvic nerves' injuries. Historically several open approaches have been attempted: (a) perineal; (b) retropubic or suprapubic extravesical; (c) transvesical transtrigonal; (d) transperitoneal; (e) posterior sagittal transanorectal; (f) anterior sagittal transanorectal (ASTRA); and (g) posterior perirectal or pararectal [8].

In 1994, McDougall first reported a successful laparoscopic removal of MDR in adult with preservation of continence and potency

G. Mattioli, P. Petralia (eds.), *Pediatric Robotic Surgery*, DOI 10.1007/978-3-319-41863-6_13

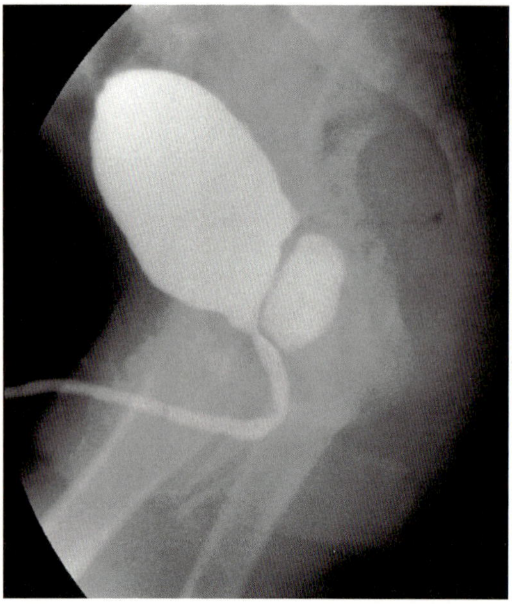

Fig. 13.1 VCUG showing a Müllerian remnant in a 6-year-old patient

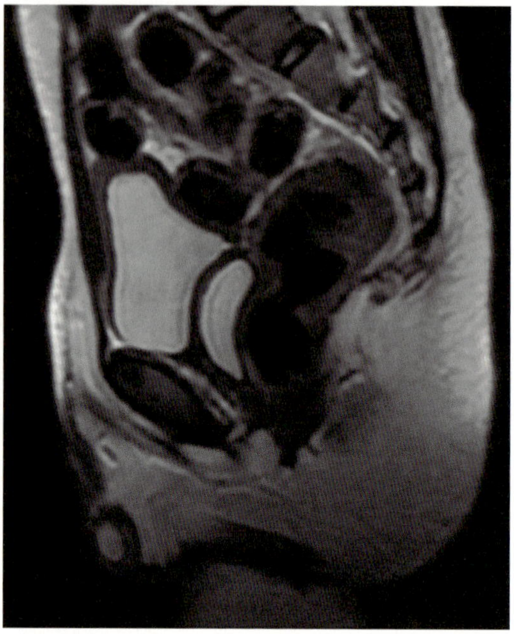

Fig. 13.2 MRI of the previous case confirming the presence of a cystic retrovesical lesion

[9]. Since then, laparoscopic removal has been considered the treatment of choice. Robot-assisted resection of MDR has been rarely described and only few reports and small case series are present in literature [2, 4, 5, 10, 11].

13.2 Preoperative Preparation

A complete endocrinologic and genetic assessment is mandatory to guide the management in case of associated DSD. We suggest to define karyotype and hormone panel including AMH, estradiol, follicle-stimulating hormone, luteinizing hormone, and testosterone.

If these lesions are associated to UTI, antibiotic prophylaxis should be provided during the preoperative period.

13.3 Preoperative Setup

The patient lays in mild Trendelenburg position with legs apart. The patient cart is positioned on the right of the patient in the case of the da Vinci Xi® surgical system or at patient's feet in case of previous models without boom movements. Before the procedure, a cystoscopy and placement of urethral catheter and ureteric catheter in the remnant are performed (Fig. 13.3). Three 8 mm trocars are positioned along the transum-

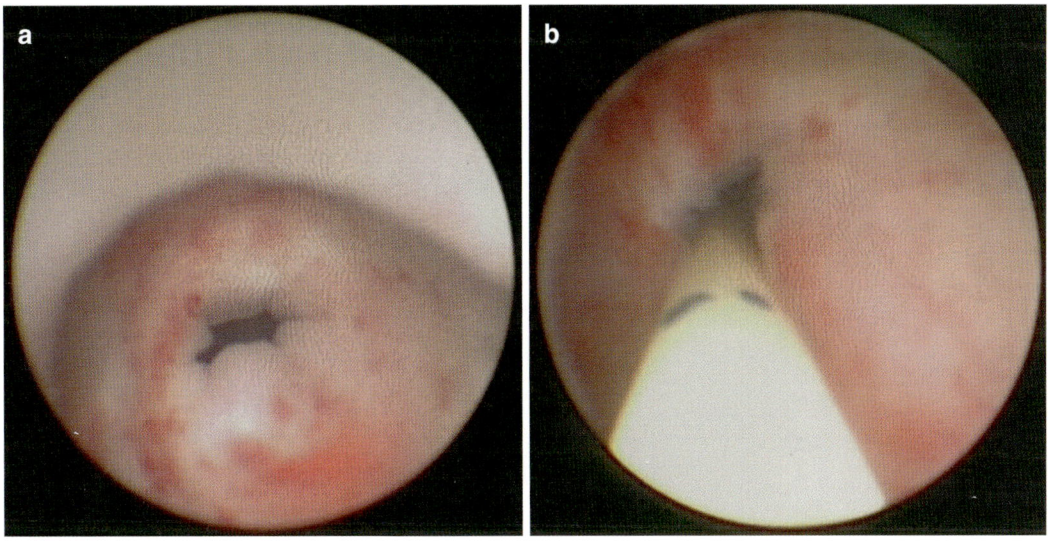

Fig. 13.3 Cystoscopic visualization of Müllerian remnant opening (**a**) and placement of a ureteral catheter in MDR lumen (**b**)

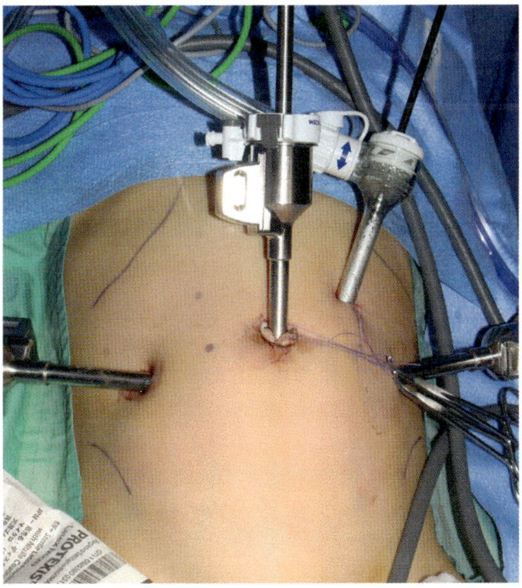

Fig. 13.4 Three 8 mm trocars for the robotic arms are placed along the transumbilical line. An additional 5 mm trocar is placed some centimeters above the transumbilical line between the umbilical trocar and the left one

bilical line at a minimum distance of 6 cm from each other. An additional 5 mm assistant port is placed some centimeters above the transumbilical line (Fig. 13.4).

13.4 Procedure

A single stitch can be placed on the posterior bladder wall to suspend pelvic structures. The stitch is inserted through the abdominal wall and held externally with mosquito forceps.

The pelvic peritoneum is opened and a blind dissection is performed till the remnant can be grasped. A gentle traction on this structure allows to continue dissection using monopolar hook or scissors and grasper. The traction can be done with a laparoscopic forceps through the accessory trocar, so the first surgeon can use both robotic arms. The remnant is dissected carefully as much as possible paying attention to avoid injuries to the bladder neck, urethra, rectum, ureters, vas deferens, prostate, and seminal vesicles. A selective unilateral vasectomy can be performed if the vas deferens drains ectopically into the remnant as it would not be functioning. When the dissection is complete, the neck of the remnant can be closed by suturing or placing preformed loops. Then the MDR is resected just above its junction with urethra and removed through one of the accesses (Fig. 13.5). At the end of the procedure the transurethral catheter is left in place.

13.5 Postoperative Care

The patient resumes free full oral intake on the same day of surgery. Postoperative pain and discomfort can be controlled by paracetamol and nonsteroidal analgesics. The transurethral catheter is left in place for 3 or 4 days and the patient can be discharged after a normal micturition.

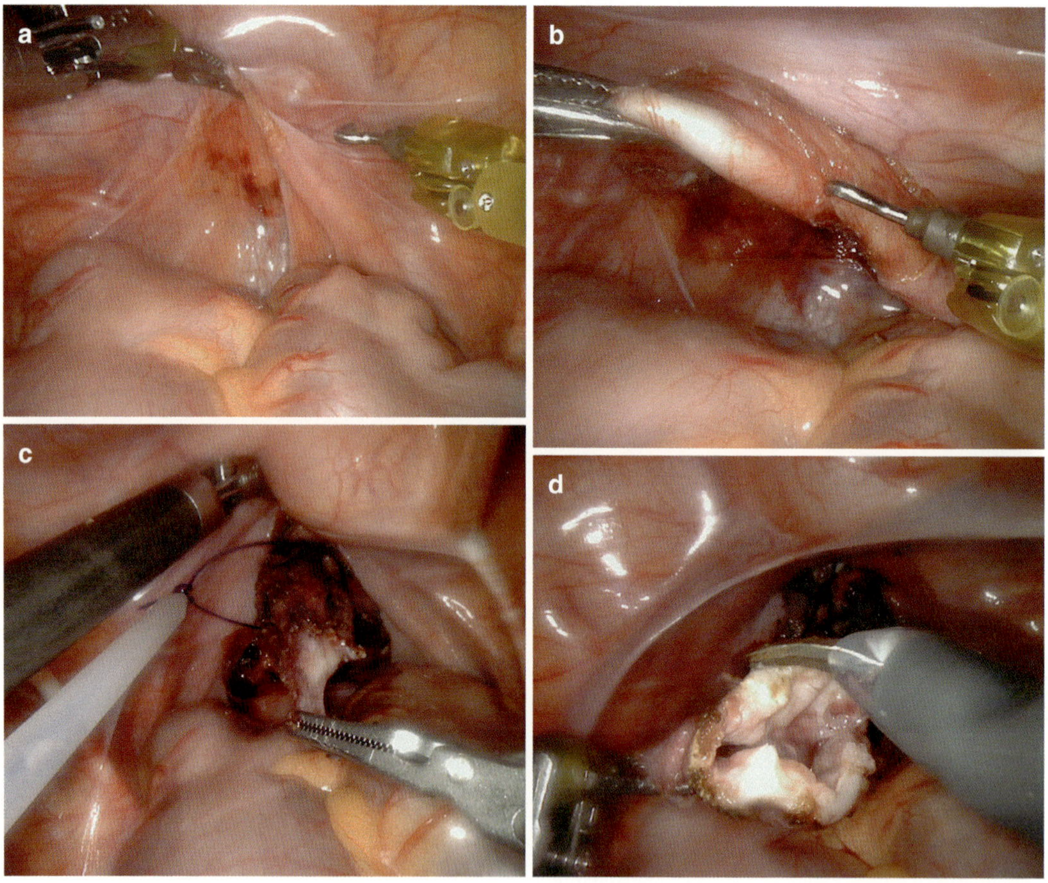

Fig. 13.5 The pelvic peritoneum is opened with monopolar hook (**a**); the MDR is identified (using the ureteral catherer placed cystoscopically as a guide) and grasped to allow dissection (**b**); an endoloop is placed at remnant neck as near as possible to its junction with the urethra (**c**); the remnant is resected and removed (**d**)

13.6 Complications

If the stitch on the residual neck is too close to the urethra, the patient will develop a urethral stricture, while if a substantial portion of the residue is left, there will be persistence of symptoms. Besides these technical mistakes, the risk of damage to nearby structures must always be considered. The vas deferens requires particular attention because they are in close contact with the MDR in their distal part. However, rather than risking irreversible damage to the delicate pelvic structures, it is preferable to leave a few millimeters of the remnant and schedule a close monitoring both clinical and instrumental [8].

13.7 Discussion

The management of symptomatic MDR has been a challenge for a long time. Laparoscopic treatment, since its introduction in 1990s, provided a safer approach associated with less postoperative pain, lower morbidity, shorter hospital stay, and reduced convalescence [4]. In our experience minimally invasive approach allowed MDR removal without complications nor residual morbidity [1]. Robot-assisted surgery represents a natural improvement of conventional laparoscopic surgery which provides the advantages of 3D vision, easy control of instruments, and possibility to reach lower pelvic structures.

References

1. Lima M, Aquino A, Dòmini M, Ruggeri G, Libri M, Cimador M, Pelusi G. Laparoscopic removal of müllerian duct remnants in boys. J Urol. 2004;171(1):364–8.
2. Smith-Harrison LI, Patel MS, Smith RP, Schenkman NS. Persistent Müllerian duct structures presenting as hematuria in an adult: case report of robotic surgical removal and review of the literature. Urol Ann. 2015;7(4):544–6.
3. Josso N, Belville C, di Clemente N, Picard JY. AMH and AMH receptor defects in persistent Müllerian duct syndrome. Hum Reprod Update. 2005;11:351–6.
4. Hong YK, Onal B, Diamond DA, Retik AB, Cendron M, Nguyen HT. Robot-assisted laparoscopic excision of symptomatic retrovesical cysts in boys and young adults. J Urol. 2011;186(6):2372–8.
5. Goruppi I, Avolio L, Romano P, Raffaele A, Pelizzo G. Robotic-assisted surgery for excision of an enlarged prostatic utricle. Int J Surg Case Rep. 2015;10:94–6.
6. Meisheri IV, Motiwale SS, Sawant VV. Surgical management of enlarged prostatic utricle. Pediatr Surg Int. 2000;16:199–203.
7. Farikullah J, Ehtisham S, Nappo S, Patel L, Hennayake S. Persistent Müllerian duct syndrome: lessons learned from managing a series of eight patients over a 10-year period and review of literature regarding malignant risk from the Müllerian remnants. BJU Int. 2012;110(11 Pt C):E1084–9.
8. Lima M, Aquino A, Domìni M. Laparoscopic treatment of utricolar cysts. In: Bax KMA, Geogeson KE, Rothenberg SS, Valla JS, Yeung CK, editors. Endoscopic surgery in infants and children. Berlin: Springer; 2008. p. 737–41. (Chapter 99).
9. McDougall EM, Clayman RV, Bowles WT. Laparoscopic excision of müllerian duct remnant. J Urol. 1994;152(2 Pt 1):482–4.
10. Najmaldin A, Antao B. Early experience of tele-robotic surgery in children. Int J Med Robot. 2007;3:199–202.
11. JA W, Hsieh MH. Robot-assisted laparoscopic hysterectomy, gonadal biopsy, and orchiopexies in an infant with persistent Mullerian duct syndrome. Urology. 2014;83:915–7.

Retroperitoneal Robotic Procedures

14

L. Henning Olsen

14.1 Introduction

The retroperitoneal access with laparoscopic instruments in children was first described by Yeung et al. [1]. The author has taken this approach with slight modifications ever since in the robotic access to the retroperitoneum for renal procedures [2] with comparable success rates for pyeloplasty [3] and heminephrectomy [4]. However, this approach has not gained wide acceptance due to technical challenges [5, 6]. The retroperitoneal route is the preferred approach in open surgery. The slightly longer learning curve is outbalanced by the potential benefits as the lower risk of damage of intra-abdominal organs. In pyeloplasty, leakage to the retroperitoneum from the anastomosis is self-limiting, like minor oozing from the resection surface in heminephrectomies. Only few studies have compared the two approaches with no clear preference for one or the other approach [7, 8]. Larger randomized trials are not available.

L.H. Olsen, M.D.,D.M.Sc.,F.E.A.P.U.,F.E.B.U.
Paediatric Urology, Department of Urology,
Aarhus University and Aarhus University Hospital,
Aarhus 8200 N, Denmark
e-mail: henning.olsen@clin.au.dk

14.2 Indications

Essentially the same indications, like pyeloplasty as the main issue, apply for the use of the retroperitoneal route. However, the small space and the limited flexibility of the robotic arms make the management of a pelvic kidney, horseshoe kidney, and retrocaval ureteral stenosis difficult if not impossible. In addition, one should not embark on a redo procedure in the retroperitoneum, fibrosis and the lack anatomical landmarks will make it hazardous. The lower weight limit for the retroperitoneal access is around 10–12 kg. Smaller infants, if ever, should be approached with a transperitoneal access or open due to the bulky robotic instruments.

14.3 Patient Positioning

With the patient in an 80–90 degree flank position, a gel roll is placed under the contralateral iliac crest. This stretches the costo-iliac distance. No further bending, as used in adults, is needed. On the contrary, bending of the table would decrease the anterior-posterior diameter of the retroperitoneal space and eventually led to port and instrument collisions. The upper leg is stretched while the lower leg is flexed (Fig. 14.1). Care is taken to avoid contact between the legs to avoid pressure lesions.

G. Mattioli, P. Petralia (eds.), *Pediatric Robotic Surgery*, DOI 10.1007/978-3-319-41863-6_14

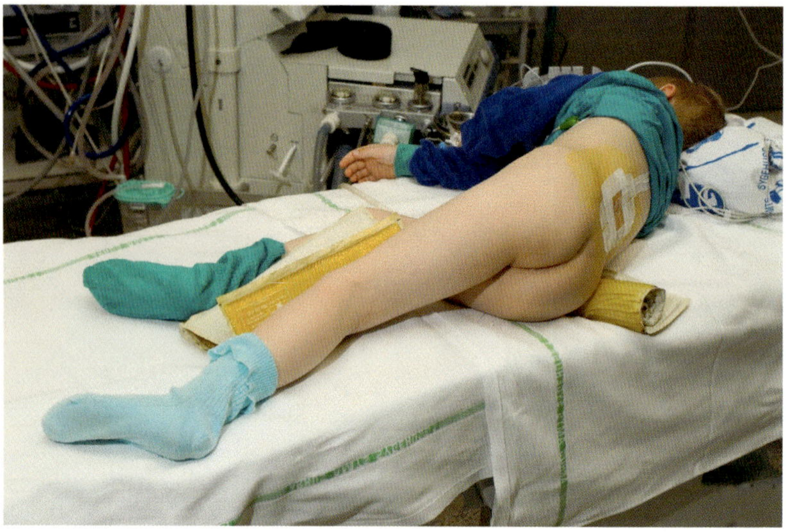

Fig. 14.1 Patient positioning for the retroperitoneal access. The upper leg is stretched, lower leg is flexed. A small gel roll supports the contralateral iliac crest. The table is not bent

14.4 Retroperitoneal Access

The most important issue in the retroperitoneal access is the correct port placement. The first step is a 10–12 mm splitting incision approximately 1.5 cm cranial to the iliac spine (Fig. 14.2). The three muscular layers are split step by step using small Langenbeck retractors until one reaches the lumbo-dorsal fascia. The fascia is subsequently incised. With an index finger introduced in the surgical wound, the lower kidney pole and the inner surface of the costal margin should be easily palpated. The initial finger dissection of the retroperitoneal space should be done in a cranioposterior direction to avoid tearing of the peritoneum. Once an appropriate space has been developed, a dissecting balloon is introduced. While a commercial balloon dilator is available for adolescence and adults, a simple homemade balloon is used in children. The inner proportion of the commercial balloon dilator is far too large to fit into the retroperitoneal space of infants and children. The homemade balloon consists of a finger of a size 8 surgical glove ligated to the tip of a 10–12 Fr catheter. The dilating balloon is inflated with 200–300 mL of air depending on the size of the patient. The dilation should be maintained for approximately 3–5 min to obtain hemostasis. In the meantime, 3-0 sutures are

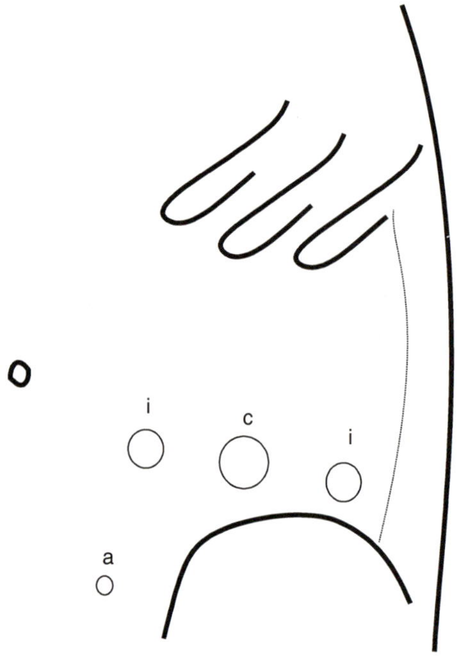

Fig. 14.2 Port placement with the robotic-assisted retroperitoneal approach. Camera port (c), instrument ports (i), optional port for assistance (a)

placed in the external fascia and the skin and left for later knotting around the camera port to avoid CO_2 leakage.

14.5 Port Placement

Once the balloon has been deflated and removed, the medial and lateral robotic ports are introduced in the retroperitoneal space under finger guidance (Fig. 14.2). We prefer the finger guidance instead of visual guidance because of a more precise placement and the fact that the abdominal wall can be compressed around the port. This is important since the limited space makes it crucial not to insert the ports too far into the retroperitoneum, especially in smaller children and infants. In fact, the ports are seldom introduced so far that the pivot point of the ports is placed at the fascial layer as recommended by the producer of the robot. In addition we prefer to use the dilating VersaStep™ system in combination with the da Vinci System™ blunt trocar, which makes placement easier and probably safer. An additional 5 mm assistant port can be placed in the iliac fossa helps to provide suction, needles or hemostatic devices during the procedure. A 10 mm balloon port for the telescope is eventually placed in the primary incision and the previously mentioned sutures around the port are knotted. The surgical cart is docked from the patient's head.

14.6 Aspects of Retroperitoneal Procedures

As soon as the ports are in place CO_2 is insufflated at a maximum pressure of 8–10 mmHg and the telescope and the instruments are introduced. The initial view will be Gerota's fascia, which should be incised widely in a cranio-caudal manner close to the lateral musculature using a bipolar deBakey and monopolar scissors. Attention should be drawn to the fat below the lower end of the incision, which may contain some significant veins. It is important to keep meticulous hemostasis at this point of the procedure maintaining a clear vision and thereby orientation in a space with few anatomical landmarks. However, the psoas muscle on the lateral aspect and the kidney on the medial aspect can be clearly identified. Once Gerota's fascia has been opened including the underlying tissue the kidney will fall medially exposing its dorsal aspect including the vessels and the collecting system. In pyeloplasties it is crucial to dissect the lower kidney pole completely to avoid overlooking lower pole vessels. From this point the retroperitoneal procedures do not differ significantly from the transperitoneal approach as described elsewhere in this book. Furthermore, access to the artery is straightforward and much easier than in the transperitoneal approach. The limitation of this approach with the robot is the difficulty to access the lower ureter. In cases of heminephrectomies, where one wants to dissect the typically upper pole ureter far down to the bladder, pulling out the freed ureter through the assistant port in the iliac fossa makes it easy to divide the ureter very close to the bladder.

Conclusion

The initial steps of the retroperitoneal approach with the robot require some training. Once familiar with the approach the procedures are straightforward and, at least theoretically, with a lower inherent risk of damage to intra-abdominal organs. An approach most surgeons will prefer in open surgery for renal/ureteric disorders.

References

1. Yeung CK, Tam YH, Sihoe JD, Lee KH, Liu KW. Retroperitoneoscopic dismembered pyeloplasty for pelvi-ureteric junction obstruction in infants and children. BJU Int. 2001;87(6):509–13. PM:11298045
2. Olsen LH, Jorgensen TM. Computer assisted pyeloplasty in children: the retroperitoneal approach. J Urol. 2004;171(6 Pt 2):2629–31.
3. Olsen LH, Rawashdeh YF, Jorgensen TM. Pediatric robot assisted retroperitoneoscopic pyeloplasty: a 5-year experience. J Urol. 2007;178(5):2137–41.

4. Olsen LH, Jorgensen TM. Robotically assisted retroperitoneoscopic heminephrectomy in children: initial clinical results. J Pediatr Urol. 2005;1(2):101–4. http://www.sciencedirect.com/science/article/B7GX6-4FJXNBT-3/2/2d7d9e5fdf88408fcc6b7b9738ece73f
5. Anderberg M, Kockum CC, Arnbjornsson E. Paediatric computer-assisted retroperitoneoscopic nephrectomy compared with open surgery. Pediatr Surg Int. 2011;27(7):761–7.
6. Casale P. Robotic pediatric urology. Curr Urol Rep. 2009;10(2):115–8.
7. Abuanz S, Game X, Roche JB, Guillotreau J, Mouzin M, Sallusto F, Chaabane W, Malavaud B, Rischmann P. Laparoscopic pyeloplasty: comparison between retroperitoneoscopic and transperitoneal approach. Urology. 2010;76(4):877–81.
8. Canon SJ, Jayanthi VR, Lowe GJ. Which is better--retroperitoneoscopic or laparoscopic dismembered pyeloplasty in children? J Urol. 2007;178(4 Pt 2):1791–5.

Part 3

Gastrointestinal Surgery

Robot Assisted Surgery for Choledochal Cyst

15

Naved K. Alizai, Michael J. Dawrant, and Azad S. Najmaldin

15.1 Introduction

For the child with a choledochal cyst the treatment of choice is cyst excision with hepaticoenterostomy [1]. Traditionally this has been performed as an open procedure with hepaticojejunostomy. In 1995, the first report of this condition being treated by minimally invasive laparoscopic surgery was published [2]. Initially the uptake of this procedure was slow, because it is a technically demanding procedure. However the last 7 years have seen a marked upsurge in the application of laparoscopic treatment of choledochal cyst with the publication of some large [3–5] and some staggeringly large series [6–8] from centres in South-East Asia, where the condition is more prevalent. The minimally invasive approach has clearly become their standard approach. We adopted this technique in 2007. However, as a department with an interest in robotic surgery and providing supra-regional paediatric liver care, in 2009, we made the transition from conventional laparoscopic to robot assisted excision of choledochal cyst and Roux-en-Y hepaticojejunostomy. This new technique has become our standard approach for treating patients with choledochal cysts [9, 10].

15.2 Operative Technique

As part of the patient's preoperative work up we advocate a detailed MRCP (Fig. 15.1a, b) to map the ducts and any possible strictures.

Given the limited working space in infants and small children, we prefer the use of three arms of the standard da Vinci surgical system (Intuitive Surgical, Sunnyvale, CA): using one optic and two working arms. The patient is positioned supine with a slight head up tilt (reverse Trendelenburg), with a nasogastric tube and a urinary bladder catheter. Prophylactic intravenous antibiotics (Co-Amoxiclav) are given to cover the perioperative period. The theatre setup is similar for all robotic assisted hepatobiliary procedures. The operating table may have to be moved and turned around to suit the theatre environment and optimise safe surgical and anaesthetic access. The patient-side cart is placed above the right shoulder and the vision cart further down to the right hand side of the patient. The assistant sits comfortably at the patient's left-hand side. The scrub nurse and their instrument trolley are also positioned on the left, close to the foot of the table.

Our technique with port placement has developed with time. Initially we used to place a

N.K. Alizai (✉) • M.J. Dawrant • A.S. Najmaldin
Children's Liver Unit, Leeds Children's Hospital, Leeds General Infirmary, Great George Street, Leeds LS1 3EX, UK
e-mail: naved.alizai@nhs.net

A.S. Najmaldin
Department of Paediatric Surgery, Leeds Children's Hospital, Leeds General Infirmary, Great George Street, Leeds LS1 3EX, UK

G. Mattioli, P. Petralia (eds.), *Pediatric Robotic Surgery*, DOI 10.1007/978-3-319-41863-6_15

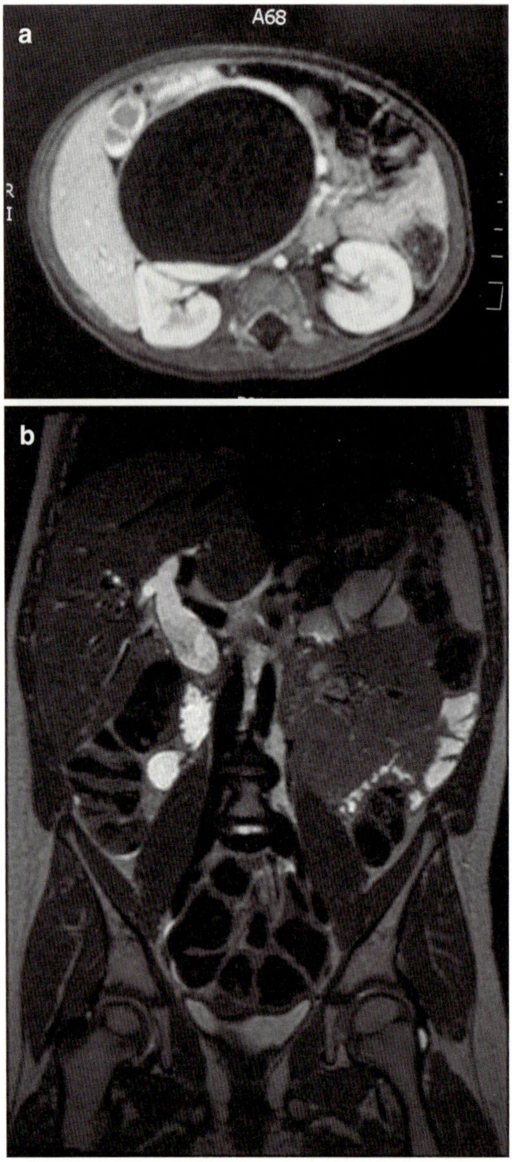

Fig. 15.1 A typical Type 1c (**a**) and Type 1f (**b**) cyst

12 mm port through an infra-umbilical curved incision using a standard open technique [11]. However, since we create the Roux loop extracorporeally, this wound would need to be extended at a later stage of the operation. We now start by making a suitable sized infra-umbilical curved incision for this later step of the operation, right from the beginning and place an Alexis® laparoscopic system wound protector/retractor (Applied Medical, Rancho Santa Margarita, CA, USA). The camera can be placed through the lid of this system whilst maintaining a pneumoperitoneum. The lid is removed and then reapplied as required for the removal and replacement of the bowel from the abdomen for the formation of the Roux loop. Previously we would remove the telescope port once the robotic excision of the choledochal cyst is completed and the umbilical incision would be extended, in order to fashion the Roux loop externally. Once the intestine is reduced into the peritoneal cavity, the incision is partially closed to re-accommodate the telescope port, a pneumoperitoneum is re-established, and the final robotic manipulation and hepaticojejunostomy anastomosis can be completed (Fig. 15.2). The exact sites of the working ports depend on the size of the patient and the cyst. In general two robotic working ports (5–8 mm) are placed under direct vision, just lateral to the midclavicular lines with the right port being at or just below the umbilicus and the left slightly higher (Fig. 15.3). In the majority of hepatobiliary procedures, the authors advocate the use of a 30° 12 mm telescope and the 8 mm robotic instruments. The 0° telescope is less versatile than 30° and the 12 mm scope provides better visualisation than the 8.5 mm scope. The 8 mm instruments are more versatile and have a wider range of movements than the 5 mm instruments. An accessory laparoscopic port (3.5–5 mm) is placed in a far left lateral position for the bedside assistant. This enables assistance to the robot for the insertion of sutures and additional instruments to retract tissues, provide suction and irrigate or cut sutures, as required. In choosing the best position for the accessory port and avoiding collisions, the direction and position of the patient's left-sided robotic arm and its range of movement needs to be considered. A Nathanson's retractor is inserted through a stab incision in the right upper quadrant to retract the liver gently. If the cyst is large (Fig. 15.3) it may be necessary to aspirate the cyst percutaneously, after the insertion of the camera port, in order to be able to create intra-abdominal space to place the working ports and execute the procedure successfully.

The dissection is performed with a pair of insulated curved monopolar scissors in the surgeon's

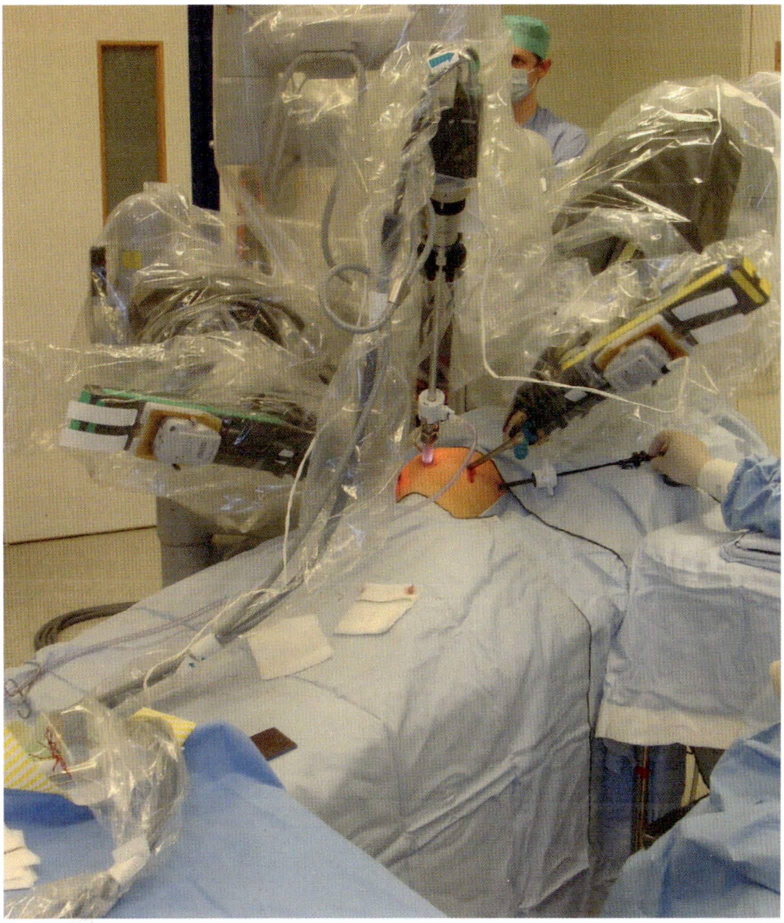

Fig. 15.2 Ports in position and assistant sitting comfortably on patient's left

right hand (alternatively a bipolar or plasmakinetic grasping forceps can be used), helped by an atraumatic grasping forceps (Cadiere) in the left hand. The surgical dissection is commenced by opening the hepaticoduodenal ligament over the choledochal cyst and then dissecting around it, keeping close to the cyst wall and away from the portal vein and hepatic artery. The dissection is continued down to the distal aspect of the choledochal cyst as it tapers into the pancreas, whilst the assistant retracts the duodenum downwards using a blunt accessory laparoscopic instrument. This may be the easiest point to get around the back of the choledochal cyst, staying away from the portal vein. Care must be taken not to damage the pancreas or the pancreatic duct. In a typical cystic form of choledochal cyst it is not unusual to find that the distal end of the common bile duct is very narrow with an 'elephant's tail' appearance. This end can be cut deep in the pancreatic head, without the need to ligate the distal end [12]. In some cystic types and all fusiform cysts the distal end is transfixed (Fig. 15.4) or ligated once or twice, using an absorbable braided suture (alternatively one or two clips are used to secure the distal end) before dividing.

The choledochal cyst is then mobilised off the portal vein (Fig. 15.5), towards the hepatic ducts. Once the cyst is completely mobilised, only then the gall bladder is dissected off its bed. The common hepatic duct is divided just below the confluence of the hepatic ducts. The hepatic ducts are then inspected and flushed if required. It is safer to divide the duct low and then trim, to avoid cutting too high and ending up separating the left and right hepatic ducts. Once the lumen is clearly seen and anatomy is understood (Fig. 15.6), the cut end of the hepatic duct is extended towards

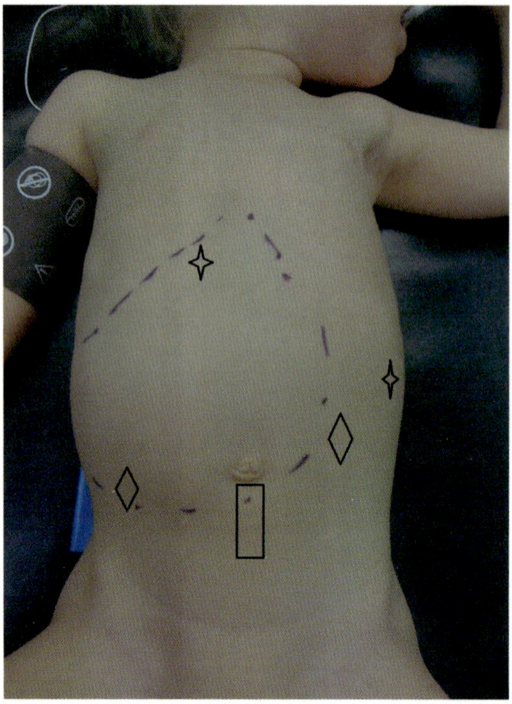

Fig. 15.3 Cyst and expected port positions marked after the patient is anaesthetised. This cyst required aspiration of the cyst following the insertion of the telescope, to create space for other ports and instruments. The port site on the right side of the epigastrium is for Nathanson retractor; left lateral side for 5 mm assistant port; *Infra-umbilical rectangular mark* for camera port and the *square boxes* for the right and left hand working ports

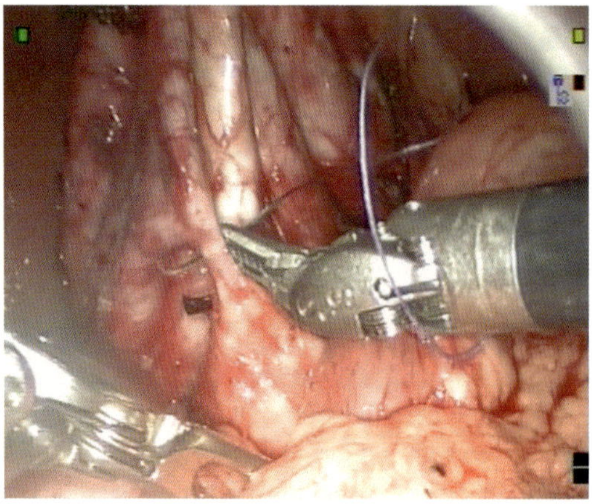

Fig. 15.4 Transfixation of the lower end in a type 1C type choledochal cyst

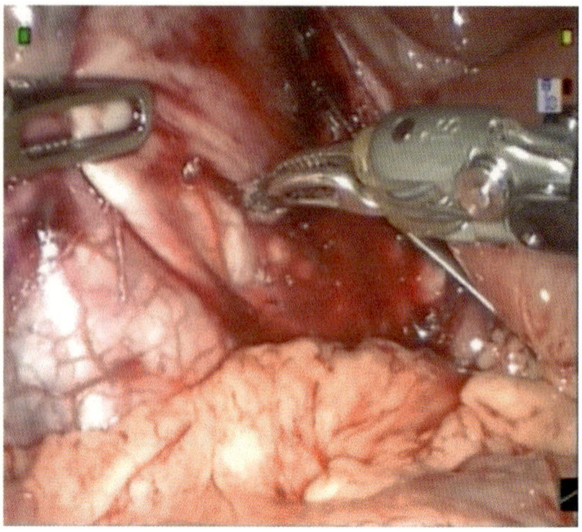

Fig. 15.5 Dissection of the posterior part of the cyst, lifting it off the portal vein

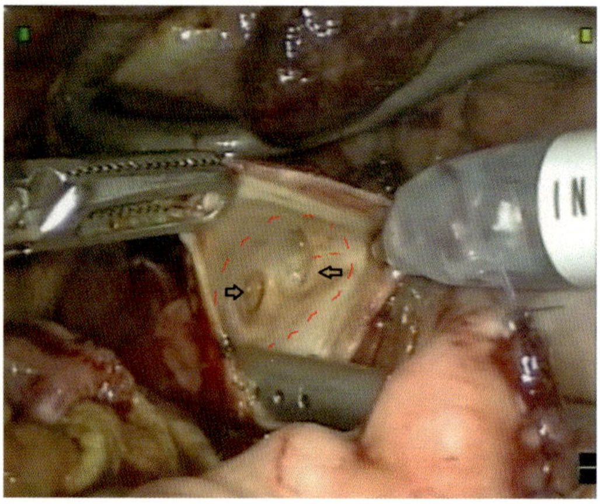

Fig. 15.6 The cyst is opened, flushed and hepatic duct openings visualised (*arrows*). The *red line* denotes the final level of trimming and fish-mouthing into the left hepatic duct

the left hepatic duct to increase the size of the hepaticojejunostomy [13]. If the left and right hepatic ducts do get separated, they can either be anastomosed separately or joined together, before performing a single hepaticojejunostomy anastomosis. Low inserting sectoral hepatic duct branches should be carefully looked for, as they can be easily missed on the preoperative MRCP. Care should be taken not to handle the wall of the hepatic duct aggressively or dissect too far up onto the bifurcation of the hepatic ducts as over-dissection can impair the blood supply and increase the risk of postoperative anastomotic leak and/or stricture formation.

The next step is to create the Roux loop. The assistant is asked to lift the large bowel with an atraumatic (Johan) grasper through the accessory port, while the operating surgeon identifies the duodeno-jejunal flexure. The bowel is carefully orientated and fed into the assistant's grasper. The assistant must make every effort not to disengage, twist the grasper, or generally disorientate the bowel whilst the robot is undocked, the sub-umbilical opening is prepared and the jejunal loop delivered externally. If an Alexis® retractor is being used then the assistant can push the jejunal loop that is within the jaws of their grasper out through the retractor. A 30 cm Roux loop is fashioned externally (Fig. 15.7) and then returned into the abdominal cavity. A small window is made in the transverse meso-colon to take the Roux loop retrocolic to the transected hepatic duct. The retrocolic positioning of the roux loop can be accomplished extracorporeally in infants and small children but is performed intracorporeally in older children. The lid of the Alexis® retractor is replaced, pneumoperitoneum re-established, telescope inserted and the robot redocked (alternatively the extended wound is narrowed slightly to refit the 12 mm robotic telescope port). For the intracorporeal tunnelling, the left hand Cadiere robotic instrument is placed behind the transverse colon with the tip facing the camera and the assistant then lifts up the transverse colon towards the abdominal wall using an accessory atraumatic grasper (Johan) while the surgeon creates a window in the meso-colon using the robotic monopolar scissors (or a bipolar/plasmakinetic forceps). Once an adequate sized opening is made, the Roux loop is pulled through and placed in close proximity of the previously prepared and transected hepatic duct using the atraumatic left-hand robotic instrument. The surgeon must now double check that there is no torsion or tension of the mesentery, no constriction of the bowel in the mesocolic window and that the Roux loop is sitting comfortably at the porta hepatis. An antimesenteric enterotomy is made using monopolar diathermy scissors, a few millimetres away from the end of the Roux loop, to match the size of the prepared hepatic duct. A tension-free anastomosis is now created (Fig. 15.8) using interrupted 5/0 or

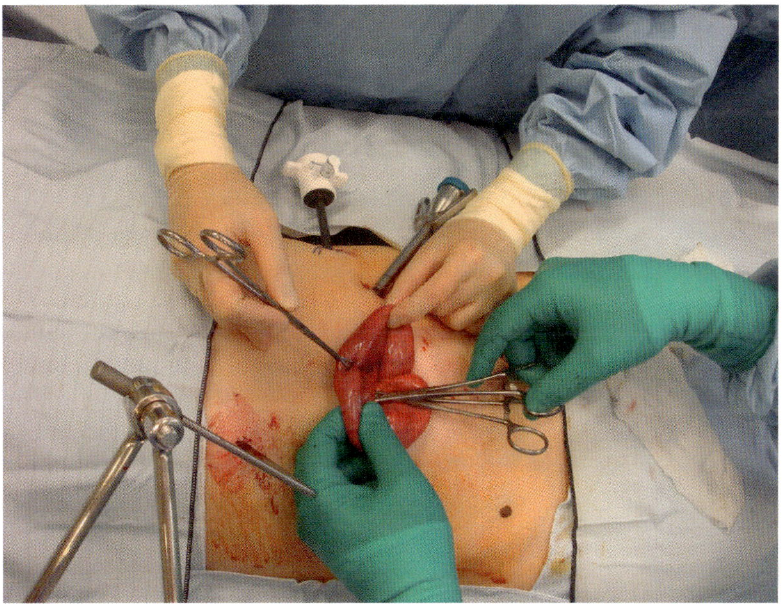

Fig. 15.7 Extracorporeal Roux en Y formation

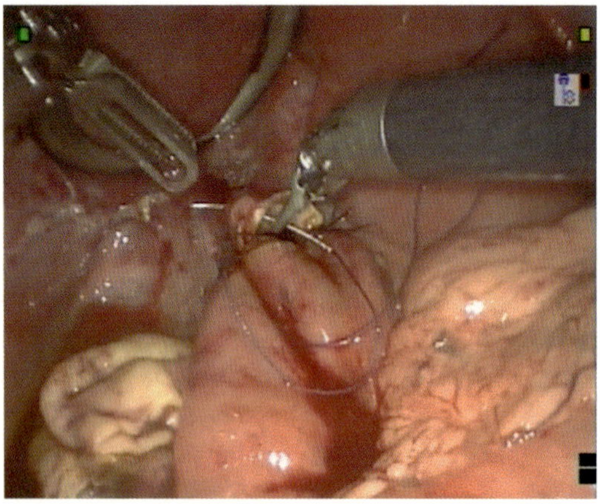

Fig. 15.8 Hepaticojejunostomy, using interrupted absorbable sutures

4/0 absorbable sutures starting at the 6 o′clock position on the posterior wall.

The peritoneal cavity is aspirated thoroughly and irrigated with warm saline if thought necessary. A suction drain is placed through the Nathanson retractor stab incision and positioned near the anastomosis. The specimen is removed and port sites closed in layers.

Intravenous prophylactic antibiotic is continued for 48 hours and oral feed commenced on day three. Typically, the drain is removed on day four and patient sent home anytime between day four and day six.

15.3 Discussion

Although choledochal cysts have traditionally been treated as an open procedure, the recent increase in publications suggests that minimally invasive surgery is becoming the new standard approach, particularly in large volume centres [6–8]. In line with this, since the first reported case of robotic assisted choledochal cystectomy in 2006 [14] there has been a gradual rise in the number of centres reporting cases. There have been 90 cases published in the literature so far [9, 10, 14–27]. These have mostly been performed in children with only nine cases reported in adults [15, 22, 24, 25, 27]. The Roux-en-Y loop tends to be fashioned intracorporeally in adults and extracorporeally in most paediatric cases.

To date the authors have performed 58 robotic assisted choledochal cyst procedures in children. The mean age is 5.6 years (range 0.3–16 years) and the mean console operating time is 302 min (range 202–394). This includes our learning curve. The conversion rate was 15.5%: all for anatomical or technical reasons—none for surgical complications. The complication rate is 3.4%: one bile leak and stricture and one intestinal adhesion obstruction 4 years after surgery. A particular advantage of robotic assistance is the easier and more precise nature of the hepaticojejunostomy anastomosis, when compared to our experience with conventional laparoscopic surgery. It has been reported that in large volume centres the learning curve for laparoscopic choledochal cystectomy and hepaticojejunostomy, in terms of operative time and rate of complications, is over 30 cases [6, 28]. It is not known what this would be in smaller volume centres. It has been shown that robotic assisted surgery can act as an enabler, facilitating surgeons to take on and learn more complex minimally invasive procedures [17, 29]. This option is likely to be more important in centres with a moderate case volumes of choledochal cysts.

Some centres have recently questioned the benefits of hepaticojejunostomy as the method of choice for bile duct drainage following choledochal cystectomy, suggesting that hepaticoduodenostomy would be better, as it lends itself to the minimally invasive approach and allows postoperative endoscopic access to the anastomosis if required [30]. There is only one adult case of choledochal cystectomy and hepaticoduodenostomy, and this was only because the patient had altered gastrointestinal anatomy following previous bariatric surgery [25]. It would take some careful and accurate long-term follow-up to prove that hepaticoduodenostomy is actually a better or comparable approach to warrant a change. Medium term follow-up studies for patients who underwent hepaticoduodenostomy have suggested they are at a higher risk of abdominal pain compared to hepaticojejunostomy, where the concern is the risk of Roux loop complications [31]. Our aim with developing our robotic assisted procedure has been to safely replicate the equivalent of the open procedure that we had previously performed.

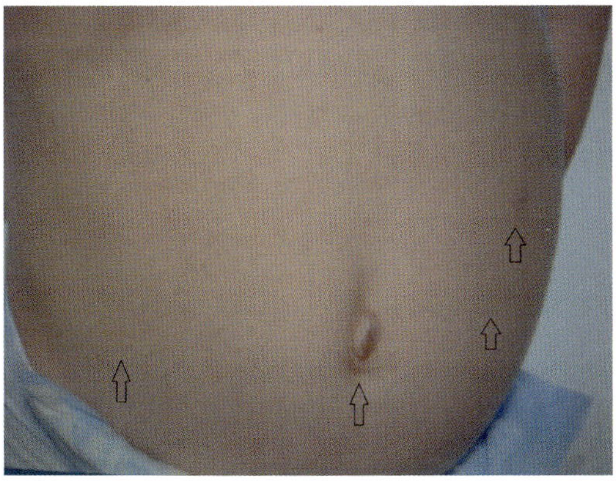

Fig. 15.9 Cosmetic appearance. The port sites are marked with *arrows*, and retractor site is visible at the top right. Note the low position of the working ports, which, in small children, allows more working space for the instruments internally

As with all new techniques, the total operating time for robot assisted resection of choledochal cysts and hepaticojejunostomy can be long. Like other authors, we have found the new approach to be safe and effective in children. It allows early recovery, has a low rate of complications and marked ergonomic advantages for the surgeon. The parents and older children are pleased with the cosmetic results (Fig. 15.9).

References

1. Miyano T, Yamataka A, Kato Y, Segawa O, Lane G, Takamizawa S, Kohno S, Fujiwara T. Hepaticoenterostomy after excision of choledochal cyst in children: a 30 year experience with 180 cases. J Pediatr Surg. 1996;31:1417–21.
2. Farello GA, Cerofolini A, Rebonato M, Bergamaschi G, Ferrari C, Chiappetta A. Congenital choledochal cyst: video-guided laparoscopic treatment. Surg Laparosc Endosc. 1995;5:354–8.
3. Lee KH, Tam YH, Yeung CK, Chan KW, Sihoe JDY, Cheung ST, Mou JWC. Laparoscopic excision of choledochal cysts in children: an intermediate-term report. Pediatr Surg Int. 2009;25:355–60.
4. Tang ST, Yang Y, Wang Y, Mao YZ, Li SW, Tong QS, Cao GQ, Zhao ZX. Laparoscopic choledochal cyst excision, hepaticojejunostomy, and extracorporeal Roux-en-Y anastomosis: a technical skill and intermediate-term report in 62 cases. Surg Endosc. 2011;25:416–22.
5. Wang B, Feng Q, Mao JX, Liu L, Wong KKY. Early experience with laparoscopic excision of choledochal cyst in 41 children. J Pediatr Surg. 2012;47:2175–8.
6. Diao M, Li L, Cheng W. Laparoscopic versus open Roux-en-Y hepatojejunostomy for children with choledochal cysts: intermediate-term follow-up results. Surg Endosc. 2011;25:1567–73.
7. Liem NT, Pham HD, Dung LA, Son TN, Vu HM. Early and intermediate outcomes of laparoscopic surgery for choledochal cysts with 400 patients. J Laparoendosc Adv Surg Tech A. 2012;22:599–603.
8. Qiao G, Li L, Li S, Tang S, Wang B, Xi H, Gao Z, Sun Q. Laparoscopic cyst excision and Roux-Y hepaticojejunostomy for children with choledochal cysts in China: a multicentre study. Surg Endosc. 2015;29:140–4.
9. Dawrant MJ, Najmaldin AS, Alizai NK. Robot-assisted resection of choledochal cysts and hepaticojejunostomy in children less than 10 kg. J Pediatr Surg. 2010;45:2364–8.
10. Alizai NK, Dawrant MJ, Najmaldin AS. Robot-assisted resection of choledochal cysts and hepaticojejunostomy in children. Pediatr Surg Int. 2014;30:291–4.
11. Humphrey GM, Najmaldin A. Modification of the Hasson technique in paediatric laparoscopy. Br J Surg. 1994;81:1319.
12. Diao M, Li L, Cheng W. Is it necessary to ligate distal common bile duct stumps after excising choledochal cysts? Pediatr Surg Int. 2011;27:829–32.
13. Stringer MD. Wide hilar hepatico-jejunostomy: the optimum method of reconstruction after choledochal cyst excision. Pediatr Surg Int. 2007;23:529–32.
14. Woo R, Le D, Albanese CT, Kim SS. Robot-assisted laparoscopic resection of a type I choledochal cyst in a child. J Laparoendosc Adv Surg Tech A. 2006;16:179–83.
15. Kang CM, Chi HS, Kim JY, Choi GH, Kim KS, Choi JS, Lee WJ, Kim BR. A case of robot-assisted excision of choledochal cyst, hepaticojejunostomy, and extracorporeal roux-en-y anastomosis using the da Vinci surgical system. Surg Laparosc Endosc Percutan Tech. 2007;17:538–41.
16. Klein MD, Langenburg SE, Lelli JL, Kabeer M, Lorincz A, Knight CG. Pediatric robotic surgery: lessons learned from a clinical experience. J Laparoendosc Adv Surg Tech A. 2007;17:265–71.
17. Meehan JJ, Elliott S, Sandler A. The robotic approach to complex hepatobiliary anomalies in children: preliminary report. J Pediatr Surg. 2007;42:2110–4.
18. Geiger JD. Robotic excision of choledochal cyst. In: Holcomb GW, Georgeson KE, Rothenberg SS, editors. Atlas of pediatric laparoscopy and thoracoscopy. Philadelphia: Saunders Elsevier; 2008. p. 211–5.
19. Akaraviputh T, Trakarnsanga A, Suksamanapun N. Robot-assisted complete excision of choledochal cyst type 1, hepaticojejunostomy and extracorporeal Roux-en-y anastomosis: a case report and review literature. World J Surg Oncol. 2010;8:87.
20. Alqahtani A, Albassam A, Zamakhshary M, Shoukri M, Altokhais T, Aljazairi A, Alzahim A, Mallik M,

Alshehri A. Robot-assisted pediatric surgery: how far can we go? World J Surg. 2010;34:975–8.
21. Chang EY, Hong YJ, Chang HK, Oh JT, Han SJ. Lessons and tips from the experience of pediatric robotic choledochal cyst resection. J Laparoendosc Adv Surg Tech A. 2012;22:609–14.
22. Chong CCN, Lee KF, Wong J, Fong AKW, Wong JSW, Cheung SYS, Lai PBS. Robotic excision of adult choledochal cyst with total intra-corporeal reconstruction. Surg Pract. 2012;16:86–7.
23. de Lambert G, Fourcade L, Centi J, Fredon F, Braik K, Szwarc C, Longis B, Lardy H. How to successfully implement a robotic pediatric surgery program: lessons learned after 96 procedures. Surg Endosc. 2013;27:2137–44.
24. Carpenter SG, Grimsby G, De Masters T, Katariya N, Hewitt WR, Moss AA, Reddy KS, Castle EP, Mulligan DC. Robotic resection of choledochocele in an adult with intracorporeal hepaticojejunostomy and roux-en-Y anastomosis: encouraging progress for robotic surgical treatment of biliary disease. J Robotic Surg. 2014;8:77–80.
25. Chang J, Walsh RM, El-Hayek K. Hybrid laparoscopic-robotic management of a type Iva choledochal cyst in the setting of prior roux-en-Y gastric bypass: video case report and review of the literature. Surg Endosc. 2015;29:1648–54.
26. Kim NY, Chang EY, Hong YJ, Park S, Kim HY, Bai SJ, Han SJ. Retrospective assessment of the validity of robotic surgery in comparison to open surgery for pediatric choledochal cyst. Yonsei Med J. 2015;56:737–43.
27. Naitoh T, Morikawa T, Tanaka N, Aoki T, Ohtsuka H, Okada T, Sakata N, Ohnuma S, Nakagawa K, Hayashi H, Musha H, Yoshida H, Motoi F, Katayose Y, Unno M. Early experience of robotic surgery for type I congenital dilatation of the bile duct. J Robotic Surg. 2015;9:143–8.
28. Wen Z, Liang H, Liang J, Liang Q, Xia H. Evaluation of the learning curve of laparoscopic choledochal cyst excision and Roux-en-Y hepaticojejunostomy in children: CUSUM analysis of a single surgeon's experience. Surg Endosc. 2016; doi:10.1007/s00464-016-5032-5.
29. Meehan JJ, Sandler A. Pediatric robotic surgery: a single-institutional review of the first 100 consecutive cases. Surg Endosc. 2008;22:177–82.
30. Santore MT, Behar BJ, Blinman TA, Doolin EJ, Hedrick HL, Mattei P, Nance ML, Adzick NS, Flake AW. Hepaticoduodenostomy vs hepaticojejunostomy for reconstruction after resection of choledochal cyst. J Pediatr Surg. 2011;46:209–13.
31. Narayanan SK, Chen Y, Narasimhan KL, Cohen RC. Hepaticoduodenostomy versus hepaticojejunostomy after resection of choledochal cyst: a systematic review and meta-analysis. J Pediatr Surg. 2013;48:2336–42.

16 Gastric Fundoplication

John Meehan

Most minimally invasive surgical equipment are designed for adults. Pediatric surgeons need to find ways of making the adult equipment fit in the world of pediatric surgery. The da Vinci is no exception and was never designed with children in mind. Since the start of the robotic era, very little has been done to redesign or improve the technology for kids. For example, Intuitive Surgical's 5 mm instrument line debuted at the end of 2004. We are now well over a decade later and nothing has been done to expand the 5 mm robotic instrument product line. The selection of instrument choices remains extremely limited with less than ten usable 5 mm robotic instruments and no hint of smaller instruments on the horizon. Moreover, pediatric surgeons are forced to find unique ways to make this technology work in children. Despite these challenges, we can utilize a few simple adaptations to enhance our ability to safely perform robotic surgery in children.

The first step in determining whether a pediatric procedure is possible with the da Vinci is to analyze the steps of the procedure in relation to the potential working region. Procedures which concentrate in a focused location have the highest probability of success. Procedures which may need to sweep from one quadrant of a cavity to an opposite quadrant may need further consideration. Utilizing a hybrid approach incorporating laparoscopy may be appropriate for some procedures. Careful planning includes optimizing patient positioning, port placement, and port depth. Planning the case should include detailed discussions with all team members to avoid difficulties later in the procedure.

16.1 Positioning

With a height of about 2 m, the current robot appears enormous hovering over a small child. Access to the patient is limited. The robotic arms must have adequate clearance in regard to not only the patient but also the OR table and in relation to the other robotic arms. In order to avoid instrument arm to OR table collisions, we recommend elevating the smaller patients using foam padding (Fig. 16.1). This allows the robot arms a greater range of motion external to the patient as the arms of the robot are less likely to collide with the OR table. Raising the patient off the main OR table with a compressible pad also affords better access to the patient for the bedside assistant and anesthesiologist. We routinely place children 10 kg or less on two foam eggcrate-style pads and one foam pad for children between 10 and 20 kg in size. Larger children are usually fine without additional elevation. An important additional consideration is assuring adequate clearance of the external robot arms over the patient.

J. Meehan
Division of Pediatric Surgery, Seattle Children's Hospital, Seattle, WA 98105, USA
e-mail: John.Meehan@seattlechildrens.org

G. Mattioli, P. Petralia (eds.), *Pediatric Robotic Surgery*, DOI 10.1007/978-3-319-41863-6_16

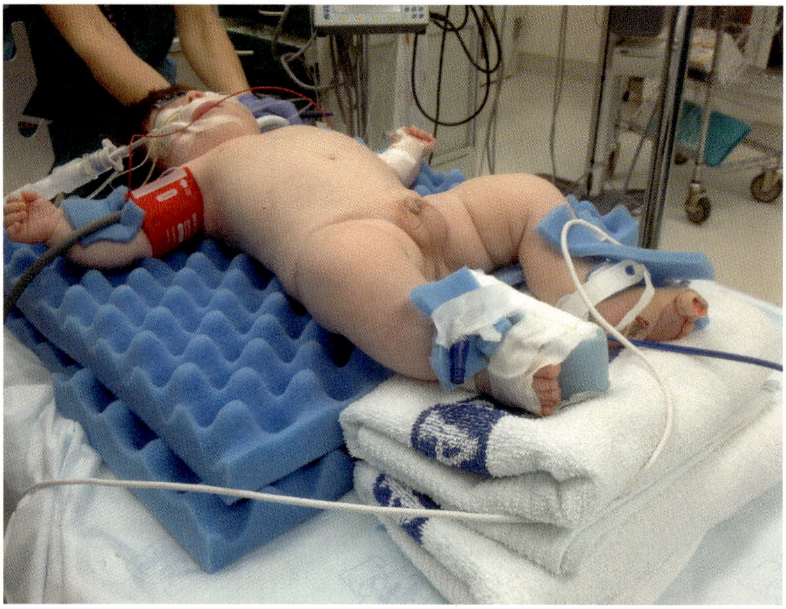

Fig. 16.1 Patient position

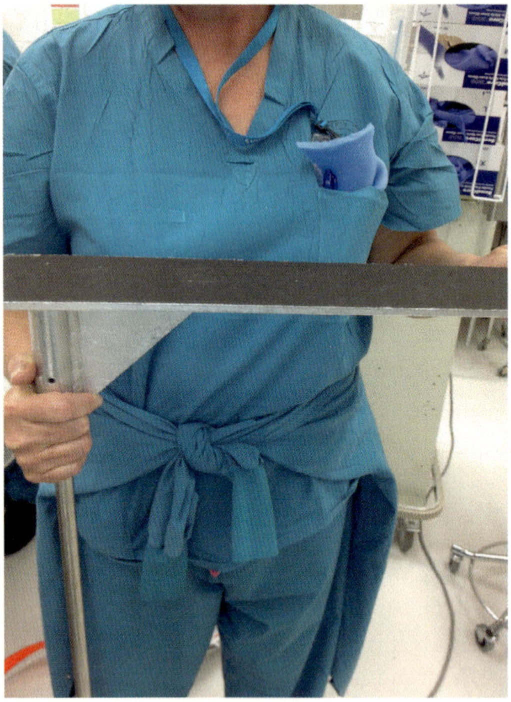

Fig. 16.2 Security barrier placement

Serious injury could occur if the robotic arms torque down onto a patient unchecked. We prefer placing a solid barrier securely mounted to the OR table to help protect the patient. An example is shown in Fig. 16.2.

16.2 Port Location

Port placement in robotic procedures may not be the same as port placement in standard MIS procedures. In standard MIS, ergonomic issues influence how far apart the surgeon may place the trocars. Sites that are too lateral will cause shoulder and neck discomfort for the operating surgeon and can make an otherwise easy case somewhat tedious and physically taxing. However, these ergonomic concerns are eliminated in robotic surgery. But there needs to be a balance. Ports placed too close together create a new problem, namely robotic arm collisions. Conversely, robot arm external collisions can be reduced by making the robot ports further apart. But this benefit is only good up to a certain point; if the ports are too far apart, they may create too shallow of an angle and the external arm could make contact with the patient or the OR table. We will get more in depth with port locations when describing the fundoplication. For now, suffice it to say that the angles between the robotic arms are more important than the distance they are apart.

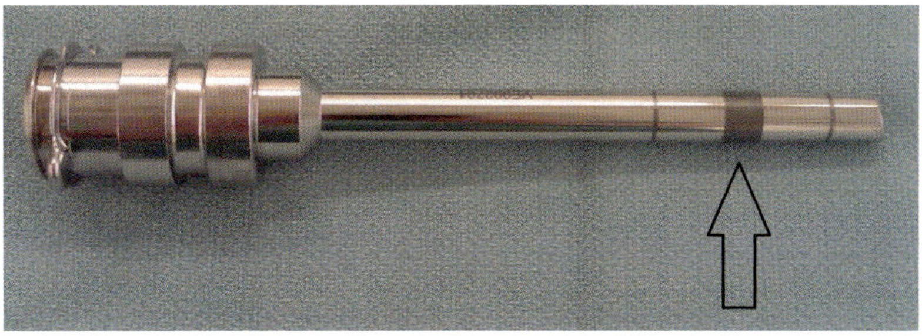

Fig. 16.3 Da Vinci robotic trocar with the *thick black line*

16.3 Port Depth

Usable intra-abdominal or intrathoracic working space is limited by the minimum requirements that are needed for robotic instrument articulation. While this is almost never a problem in adult surgery, the distance between the tip of the instrument and the end of the port can be an enormous issue in the abdomen of a small child. The remote center of the robotic trocar is the point in 3-dimensional space in which the robot arm will pivot around. This location is represented on the da Vinci robotic trocar with a thick black line (Fig. 16.3). The distance from remote center to end of port is a set length at a distance of 2.90 cm. The manufacturer recommends that the robotic port is inserted inside the patient such that the remote center is placed just at the inside edge of the body cavity. Therefore, 2.90 cm of trocar length should be inside the patient. Next, consider the instrument. The shortest 5 mm da Vinci instrument is the needle driver. Measuring the needle driver from the tip of the instrument to the most proximal articulating joint is a distance of 2.71 cm. Adding this distance to the articulating length yields a minimum distance of 5.61 cm. In other words, the target organ must be a minimum of 5.61 cm away from the abdominal or chest wall. Other robotic instruments are even longer. In small children, the amount of usable working space beyond this minimum distance can disappear quickly.

We make an adjustment which allows for additional room in selected patients. Although the remote center marking on the da Vinci trocar was originally intended to be visible just inside a patient, we can adjust the port so it is just outside the patient instead. By routinely retracting the port back such that the remote center is positioned just outside the patient, we can effectively increase our workable domain and potentially improve instrument maneuverability. We have found that this simple adjustment can have tremendous impact on our ability to perform a procedure particularly in smaller children.

16.4 Scope

The optics of the 3-D da Vinci system is a huge advantage in robotic surgery. The 12 mm 3-D da Vinci scope is essentially two 5 mm scopes down the shaft of a single 12 mm tube. The optics are excellent but the diameter is quite large and is too big for some children. In 2005, Intuitive released a 5 mm 2-D scope for use with the da Vinci Standard robot. This 5 mm scope opened the door to neonatal robotic surgery though it was only a 2-D system. The 5 mm camera paved the way for a wave of neonatal cases and allowed robotic neonatal surgery to flourish for a few years [1]. Numerous neonatal congenital anomalies were repaired robotically for the first time in both the abdomen and the chest. These procedures included a duodenal atresia repair in child as young as 1 day of age and a CDH repair in a 2.2-kg 6-day-old baby [2, 3]. Pulmonary lobectomies for congenital pulmonary adenomatoid malformation (CPAM) and pulmonary sequestration were also now possible although there were limitations [4]. At the time, we thought that neonatal robotic surgery was off to a flying start. But it didn't last. The 5 mm scope was discontinued even before the Si had been released. Since then, no attempts have been made to get back towards a 5 mm optical platform. Conveniently, the

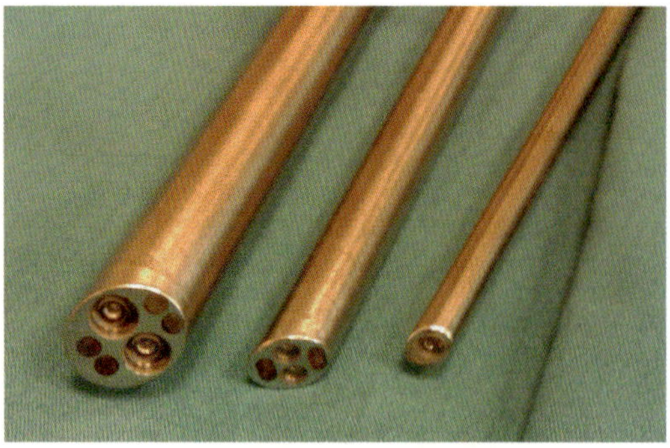

Fig. 16.4 Robotic optics: 12, 8.5, and 5 mm

8.5 mm 3-D scope was released at about this same time. Although the diameter may be a bit too large for the intercostal space in some neonates, it has been a tremendous help for children. The 8.5 mm scope is still in use today and is a key element for the single-site cholecystectomies performed using flexible nonarticulating robotic instruments (Fig. 16.4).

16.5 The Fourth Arm

The da Vinci system has a fourth arm for an additional port if desired. Unfortunately, the robot's large size coupled with the limited space around children limits the usefulness of the fourth arm in pediatric patients. We may consider using the fourth arm in a choledochal cyst, but otherwise rarely find use for it. Our recommendation is to avoid using the fourth arm until you are well acclimated to the robot as the addition of this arm in such a confined space magnifies the complexities of the case significantly.

16.6 Fundoplication

Now that we have addressed the basics, we can move on to discuss the most basic procedure, the robotic fundoplication. The fundoplication is an ideal training procedure to learn pediatric robotic surgery. Along with the cholecystectomy, the fundoplication is a familiar laparoscopic procedure and one of the most common operations in pediatric minimally invasive general surgery. It also has a modest level of minimally invasive complexity because of the suturing requirements making it even more preferable than the cholecystectomy for learning. The procedures are usually performed in a nonurgent manner and the size of the patients can vary considerably making the fundoplication a great opportunity to see how the size of the patient impacts the port placement decisions. The fundoplication has also been a benchmark procedure in standard laparoscopic surgery and often used to assess one's skills and establish a learning curve. Therefore, it makes sense to utilize this procedure to train robotic surgeons. We have also learned that the selection of port sites in the robotic version has some subtle differences from laparoscopic surgery which highlight the differences between the two technologies. Understanding these differences is vital in the robotic learning curve process and will help the surgeon take these learned lessons to more complex cases. The importance of starting with familiar laparoscopic procedures long before proceeding to more challenging cases cannot be overstated.

The 360° Nissen is the most common fundoplication and performed through an abdominal approach [5]. Other partial wrap fundoplications such as the Toupet and Thal are somewhat less common. The choice of the fundoplication type is surgeon preference but all have been shown to be effective [6]. The learning curve for the laparoscopic approach has been estimated somewhere between 25 and 30 cases [7]. We have found that the robotic learning curve is much shorter when compared to laparoscopy, perhaps as short as five cases [8].

When selecting your port locations, remember that robotic surgery is all about the angles of the arms in relation to each other and not necessarily the distance between them. The ultimate goal for proper port placement is proper angles and not so much the distance. These angles are important to maintain so as to avoid robotic arm collisions. The angle between the camera and the left and right arms should be about 45° each which creates an angle of about 90° between the left and right working arms (Fig. 16.5). Port locations for a small child are shown in Fig. 16.5. Notice the

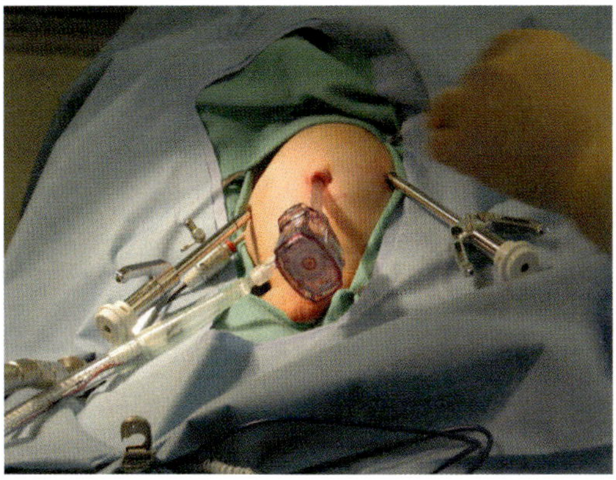

Fig. 16.5 Port locations for a small child

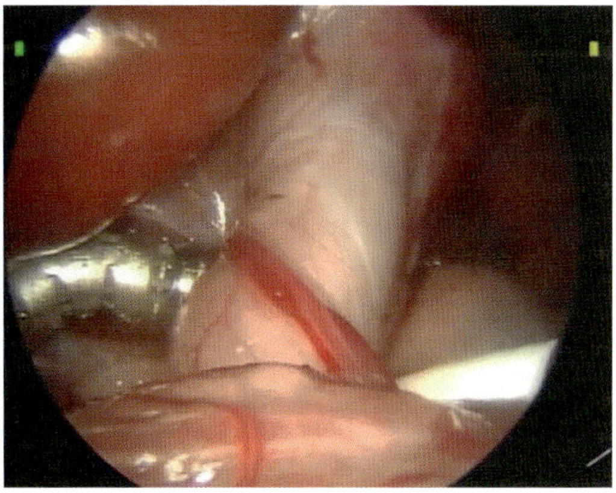

Fig. 16.6 Esophageal bougie, retracted during the retroesophageal dissection

more lateral placement of the left and right working arms.

The robot cart is positioned directly over the patient's head. We use the 8 mm camera and the 5 mm instruments. Dissection begins by exposing the hiatus and taking down the short gastric vessels as necessary. Regardless of using the laparoscopic or robotic approach, we minimize these two steps. We prefer a minimal hiatal dissection due to the risk of a slipped fundoplication and find that overdissection does very little to improve the case visually. We also minimize the number of short gastrics taken whenever possible. A common complication in fundoplication is a gastric perforation, likely caused by injury to the greater curve of the stomach while taking short gastrics. We take only a small amount of short gastrics at the most superior aspect of the greater curve and then proceed with attempting the wrap. If the fundus is not mobile enough, it is easy to go back and take a little more. Once this is accomplished, the posterior dissection is begun. A bougie placed at the beginning of the case is retracted by the anesthesiologist temporarily while we begin the retroesophageal dissection (Fig. 16.6). An adequate window is constructed taking care not to damage the vagus nerve (Fig. 16.7). The 5 mm Maryland is used for most of this dissection and also used to grasp the fundus when we eventually pass it retroesophageally (Fig. 16.8). Once we have an adequate window, the hiatus is assessed. Reapproximating of the crura is done with nonabsorbable suture as

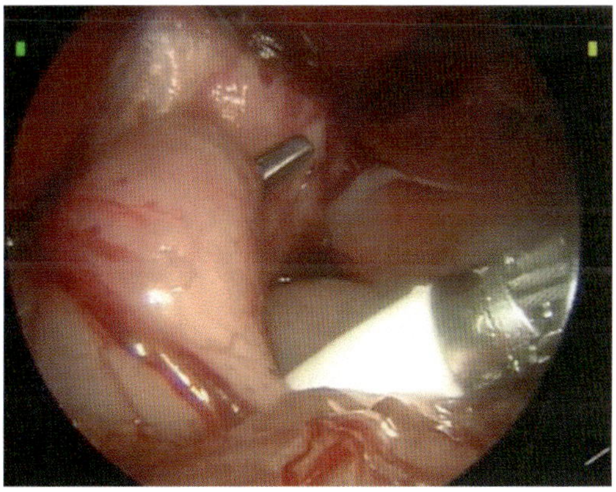

Fig. 16.7 Retroesophageal window

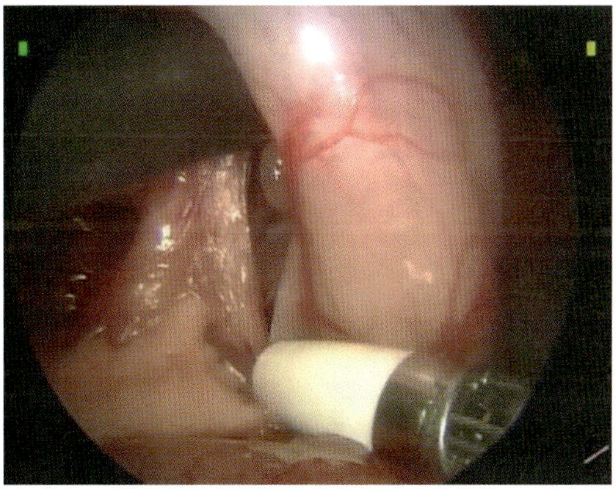

Fig. 16.8 Maryland retroesophageal passage

necessary but is not performed if the crura is already well approximated. Large hiatal defects may require a patch. There are many commercially available patches but a nonabsorbable mesh-based patch seems to work best. Once the hiatus has been addressed, the wrap is constructed. Grasp the mobilized fundus through the retroesophageal window and bring it posteriorly to begin the creation of the wrap (Fig. 16.9). The wrap is constructed with nonabsorbable simple interrupted sutures and generally should be at least 3 cm in length (Fig. 16.10). Suturing the completed wrap to the underside of the diaphragm is optional.

A gastrostomy tube is commonly required in fundoplication patients. Once we finish the fundoplication, we routinely undock the robot and proceed with the g-tube using handheld laparoscopic instruments through the already present 5 mm ports. The camera is held by the bedside assistant.

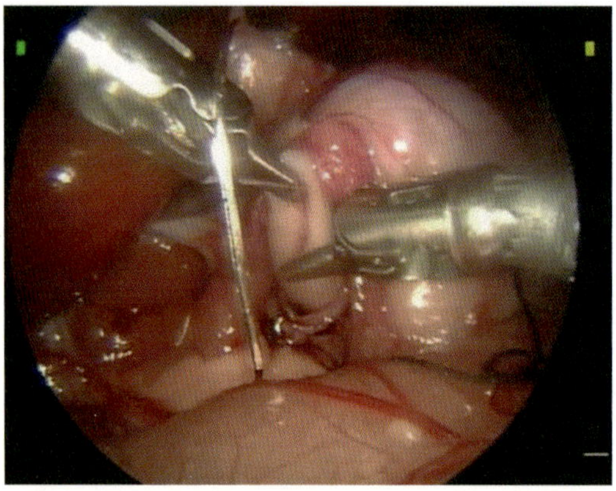

Fig. 16.9 Fundus mobilization through the retroesophageal window

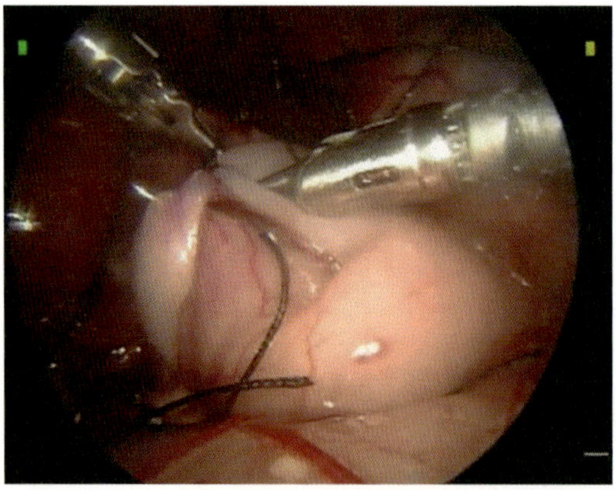

Fig. 16.10 Wrap construction with nonabsorbable simple interrupted sutures

16.7 Discussion

The variety of general intra-abdominal procedures which have been accomplished in children robotically is extensive (Table 16.1). This is largely due to the wide range of pediatric congenital anomalies and acquired diseases that exist in the general population. A review of the literature suggests that a fundoplication is probably the most commonly performed robotic procedure [8–11]. Some papers suggest that this procedure is not cost effective since it can be done laparoscopically with similar results [11]. Fundoplications performed laparoscopically have historically taken the pediatric surgeon at least 25 cases before proficiency can be expected [7, 12]. Robotically performed fundoplications may have a learning curve of less than five cases [8]. Using the fundoplication as the introductory robotic teaching case is further enhanced by the relative frequency of fundoplications with the opportunity for repetitive experience in a relatively short period of time. It can also be advantageous either for redo fundoplications or when a gastrostomy tube is already present. In nearly 15 years of using the robot, we have never needed to take down a preexisting gastrostomy tube in any robotic fundoplication and have always been able to articulate around the stomach when already attached to the anterior abdominal wall. Other papers have since been published with similar experiences [13]. This can be problematic for the pediatric laparoscopist using standard rigid laparoscopic instruments and the gastrostomy sight is often taken down at the beginning of the case only to be required for placement once again at the end of the case. The articulating robotic instruments make it quite easy to steer around this distraction.

Results comparing robotic versus laparoscopic surgery in children are lacking. Freidmacher and

Till reviewed 20 papers on five common robotic pediatric procedures but had difficulty drawing outcome conclusions since there were no level 1 or 2 studies [14]. However, they did report that fundoplication robotically had shorter hospital length of stay but an added expense. Mahida drew similar conclusions [15]. Alqhantai reported on a large series of patients with multiple diagnoses and robotic procedures including 39 fundoplication but had one esophageal perforation [16].

The biggest criticism of robotic surgery remains the cost and increased expense of the robot [11, 14]. Although the cost of the procedures was higher in the robotic group, Albassam's comparative analysis between laparoscopic and robotic fundoplication failed to show any differences in resolution of symptoms, length of stay, or complications leading them to the conclusion that robotic surgery had no benefit in the fundoplication for children [11]. And while we see benefit by using the robot in the fundoplication for learning purposes, it will ultimately be difficult to prove its merit unless the expense is reduced.

In conclusion, the fundoplication is an excellent learning procedure for the eager robotic surgeon. The great advantage of the robot will ultimately lie in more complicated procedures requiring high precision and fine suturing capabilities. Pediatric robotic surgeons need to learn how to walk before they can run. Learning robotics with the fundoplication is a key step in the progression towards more complex operations.

References

1. Meehan JJ. Robotic surgery in small children: is there room for this? J Laparoendosc Adv Surg Tech A. 2009;19(5):707–12.
2. Meehan JJ, Sandler A. Robotic repair of a Bochdalek congenital diaphragmatic hernia in a small neonate: robotic advantages and limitations. J Pediatr Surg. 2007;42(10):1757–60.
3. Meehan JJ, Francis P, Sandler A. Robotic repair of duodenal atresia. J Pediatr Surg. 2007;42(7):E31–3.
4. Meehan JJ, Phearman L, Sandler A. Robotic pulmonary resections in children: series report and introduction of a new robotic instrument. J Laparoendosc Adv Surg Tech. 2008;18(2):293–5.
5. Abdullah F, Salazar JH, Gause CD, Gadepalli S, Biester TW, Azarow KS, Brandt ML, Chung DH, Lund DP, Rescorla FJ, Waldhausen JH, Tracy TF, Fallat ME, Klein MD, Lewis FR, Hirschl RB. Understanding the operative experience of the practicing pediatric surgeon: implications for training and maintaining competency. JAMA Surg. 2016; doi:10.1001/jamasurg.2016.0261.
6. C E, Montupet P, van Der Zee D, Settimi A, Paye-Jaouen A, Centonze A, Bax NK. Long-term outcome of laparoscopic Nissen, Toupet, and Thal antireflux procedures for neurologically normalchildren with gastroesophageal reflux disease. Surg Endosc. 2006;20(6):855–8.
7. Meehan JJ, Georgeson KE. The learning curve associated with laparoscopic antireflux surgery in infants and children. J Pediatr Surg. 1997;32(3):426–9.
8. Meehan JJ, Meehan TD, Sandler A. Robotic fundoplication in children: resident teaching and a single institutional review of our first 50 patients. J Pediatr Surg. 2007;42(12):2022–5.
9. Lehnert M, Richter B, Beyer PA, Heller K. A prospective study comparing operative time in conventional laparoscopic and robotically assisted Thal semifundoplication in children. J Pediatr Surg. 2006;41(8): 1392–6.
10. Meehan JJ, Sandler A. Pediatric robotic surgery: a single-institutional review of the first 100 consecutive cases. Surg Endosc. 2008;22(1):177–82.
11. Albassam AA, Mallick MS, Gado A, Shoukry M. Nissen fundoplication, robotic-assisted versus laparoscopic procedure: a comparative study in children. Eur J Pediatr Surg. 2009;19(5):316–9.
12. Rothenberg SS. Experience with 220 consecutive laparoscopic Nissen fundoplications in infants and children. J Pediatr Surg. 1998;33(2):274–8.
13. Margaron FC, Oiticica C, Lanning DA. Robotic-assisted laparoscopic Nissen fundoplication with gastrostomy preservation in neurologically impaired children. J Laparoendosc Adv Surg Tech A. 2010;20(5):489–92. doi:10.1089/lap.2009.0367.
14. Friedmacher F, Till H. Robotic-assisted procedures in pediatric surgery: a critical appraisal of the current best evidence in comparison to conventional minimally invasive surgery. J Laparoendosc Adv Surg Tech A. 2015;25(11):936–43.
15. Mahida JB, Cooper JN, Herz D, Diefenbach KA, Deans KJ, Minneci PC, McLeod DJ. Utilization and costs associated with robotic surgery in children. J Surg Res. 2015;199(1):169–76. doi:10.1016/j.jss.2015.04.087.
16. Alqahtani A, Albassam A, Zamakhshary M, Shoukri M, Altokhais T, Aljazairi A, Alzahim A, Mallik M, Alshehri A. Robot-assisted pediatric surgery: how far can we go? World J Surg. 2010;34(5):975–8. doi:10.1007/s00268-010-0431-6.

Colectomy

17

Giuseppe Spinoglio, Paolo Bellora,
and Manuela Monni

Pediatric colectomy (PC) is currently mainly performed, urgent or elective, for IBD [1], malformation with poor functional patterns, or congenital diseases as Hirschsprung's agangliosis: however PC can also be performed for colonic malignancies, even in childhood. Colorectal adenocarcinoma is a rare pediatric tumor, 1% of all pediatric malignances, with an incidence of about 1 per million; other pediatric colonic non-adenocarcinoma malignancies are classified as mucinous adenocarcinoma, carcinoids, lymphomas, and carcinoma developed on familiar adenomatous polyposis (FAP). As for adults, also PC can be complicated by postoperative fistulas, strictures, bowel obstruction, perforation, or bleeding: only few studies about pediatric robotic surgery are available [2, 3]: but minimally invasive surgery, including robotic approaches, can be performed also in pediatric patients, according to the improved functional outcomes obtained in urological robotic surgery [4, 5].

G. Spinoglio (✉)
Hepatobiliary-Pancreatic and Digestive Program,
IEO Istituto Europeo di Oncologia, Milan, Italy
e-mail: giuseppe.spinoglio90@gmail.com

P. Bellora • M. Monni
Clinica Chirurgica - General Surgery Department,
"Maggiore della Carita" Hospital, Corso Mazzini 18,
Novara, 28100 Italy
e-mail: paolobellora@me.com;
monni.manuela@gmail.com

17.1 Right Colonic Surgery

17.1.1 Introduction

Right colonic surgery with intracorporeal anastomosis can be performed laparoscopically, even if the instrumental stricness causes many technical challenges: following the improvements reported in adults, robotic colonic approach is developing also for pediatric patients, by the two available robotic systems: da Vinci Si® and da Vinci Xi® that can support pediatric sized instruments.

Even if the main indications for colonic pediatric surgery are related to benign disease, and don't require extended resections and lymphectomies with central vascular ligature as for malignancies, the robotic approach can be proposed to perform limited resections, with peripheric vessel transection, in order to offer the child the same benefits in terms of fast recovering, lower postoperative pain, and quick recovery to everyday activities.

We describe a full robotic procedure.

17.1.2 Patient Positioning

The first step is narcosis and subsequent placement of nasogastric probe and urinary catheter.

The patient is placed on the operative table in supine position, the arms are placed along the body, and the legs are closed. After port placement, the patient is settled in a 5–10°

G. Mattioli, P. Petralia (eds.), *Pediatric Robotic Surgery*, DOI 10.1007/978-3-319-41863-6_17

Trendelenburg position with a left tilt of 5–10°. This placement allows the small bowel to move aside under gravity and expose the right and transverse mesocolon. The head plate is tilted down (10–15°) to avoid facial soft-tissue injury from the robotic arm movement.

17.1.3 Trocar Placement

The distance of each trocar from the others depends on the size of the patient that can vary during pediatric age. The superior mesenteric axis (SMA) is considered the "target" organ.

17.1.3.1 da Vinci Si® System, Trocars Are Placed as Follows (Fig. 17.1)

The camera port is placed in the midpoint of the left spinoumbilical line: from the left iliac fossa, the complete visualization of the abdominal right quadrants and the course of SMA is feasible.

- R1 is placed laterally to the left midclavicular line and below the costal margin.
- R2 is placed on the midline above the symphysis pubis.

The R1 and R2 trocars are used for dissection.

- R3 is located just below the xiphoid process.

The assistant port is positioned between the camera port and R1 in the left flank: its role is to allow suction/irrigation, clipping, stapling, and additional retraction.

The anatomical umbilicus is considered to be the midpoint between the xiphoid process and the pubis.

17.1.3.2 da Vinci Xi® System, Trocars Are Placed as Follows (Fig. 17.2)

All ports are placed on a straight vertical line parallel on the left of the middle line:

- The camera port (P2) is placed, on this line, below the transversal umbilical line.
- Port 1 is placed along the vertical line distant below P2.
- Ports 3 (P3) and Port 4 (P4) are placed above to Port 2, away from each other.

Airseal® trocar is triangulated on P2 and P3, usually on transversal umbilical line: it allows the assistant to perform suctioning, stapling, or retractioning. P4 is generally used for retraction while P3 supports monopolar device as scissors, and P1 the bipolar instruments.

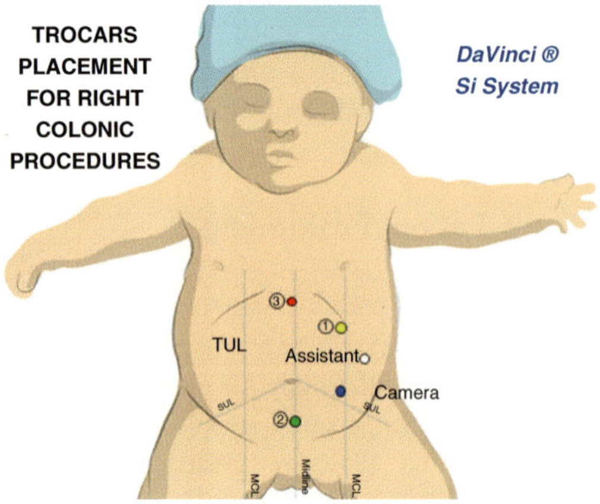

Fig. 17.1 Trocar placement for right colonic procedures

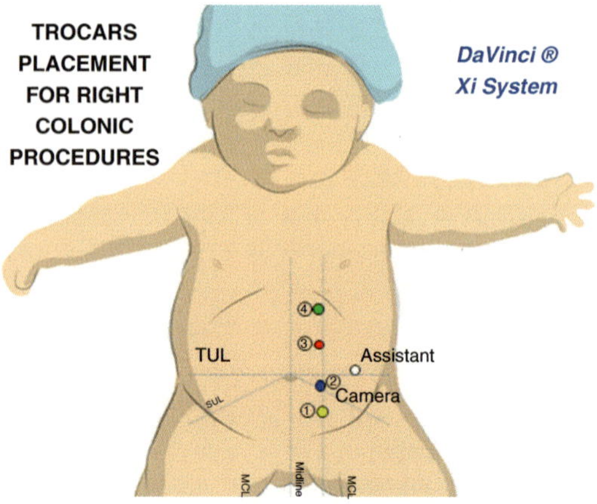

Fig. 17.2 Trocar placement for right colonic procedures

17.1.4 Robot Positioning and Docking

The surgical cart is located at the patient's right hemithorax level with a 45° angle; the vision cart is on the right side of the surgical cart; and the robot arms are docked to the trocars. The first assistant stands on the patient's left side.

17.1.5 Procedure Description

17.1.5.1 Device Placement

A 30° down endoscope is used for both systems. The device placement is as follows:

For **da Vinci Si® system:**

R1: monopolar curved scissors or cautery hook
R2: bipolar fenestrated forceps
R3: Cadiere forceps
R4: camera arm

For **da Vinci Xi® system:**

P1: bipolar fenestrated forceps
P2: camera arm
P3: monopolar curved scissors or cautery hook
P4: prograsp forceps

17.1.5.2 Mesocolic Exposure and Traction on the Superior Mesenteric Axis

The first mandatory step is to achieve the ileocolic vessels through the exposure of the right and transverse mesocolon: bipolar fenestrated forceps, Cadiere device, or prograsp forceps are used to keep the superior mesenteric axis in traction while the monopolar cautery hook/scissors are used for dissection.

17.1.5.3 Vessel Management and Bowel Transection

Segmental resections with peripheral vessel ligature are performed with lateral-to-medial approach while a medial-to-lateral approach with the central vessel ligature is chosen for extended resections, as hemicolectomies with complete mesocolon excision (CME) for cancer.

The trocar layout allows better arm movement avoiding external collisions without any difficulties in the far lateral and superior extension or the blind spots.

A gentle traction on the transverse mesocolon is performed with the grasp, and the ileocolic vessels are identified and lifted up; the peritoneum is then opened just below their prominence along the left anterior side.

After the ileocolic vessel dissection, their ligature can be performed on different levels, near versus far from their root, depending on the disease to treat.

We use clip applier (Hem-o-lok®, Weck) through the assistant port.

For limited resection, after the peripheral ileocolic vessel ligature, we proceed with the gentle dissection of the mesentery until the site chosen for the ileal transection that is performed with a linear stapler.

In a similar way, the mesocolon is divided until the colonic margin adequate for the resection.

Another linear stapler is used for colonic transection.

In case of malignancies it is mandatory to perform an oncologically adequate transection, associated to extended lymphectomy with central vascular ligature, as the CME technique described for adult patient [6].

Both ileal and colonics stumps are evaluated for perfusion with indocyanine green ICG-NIR fluorescence imaging system and sectioned in a well-perfused site. After the complete coloparietal detachment, the specimen is inserted in an Endobag, introduced through the assistant port, and then it is placed in the right upper quadrant.

17.1.5.4 Intracorporeal Anastomosis and Specimen Extraction

The colon and the ileum, either the two colonic stumps, are approximated to choose the correct enterotomy sites, then the monopolar curved scissors are used to perform enterotomies on the antimesenteric border of the ileum and the free taenia of the colon, and then the monopolar device is replaced by a needle driver.

A linear stapler is introduced through the assistant port to perform an isoperistaltic side-to-side anastomosis and the enterotomies are closed with a robotically hand-sewn double-layer running suture (using absorbable monofilament barbed knotless sutures; V-Loc™, Covidien). A continuous suture is sewn to mesenteric defect to prevent internal hernias. The specimen is then extracted into a plastic bag through a mini-suprapubic incision. The intracorporeal anastomosis limited chance for bowel and anastomotic twisting.

17.1.5.5 Wall Closure and Abdominal Reevaluation

After specimen removal and mini-laparotomy closure, the PNP is reestablished for a final robotic check of the operative field. Usually no drains are needed. No drain is usually placed. Left in place. The trocars are removed under direct vision and the port sites are closed with absorbable sutures at the fascial level.

17.1.6 Conclusions

Robotic colonic resections are safe and feasible and short-term postoperative outcomes are comparable to those of conventional laparoscopic surgery: indeed a lower conversion rate is noticed for robotic (0–4%) compared to laparoscopic colonic resections (16–25%) in adult patients.

17.2 Left Colonic Surgery

17.2.1 Introduction

Robotic surgical approach reduces the surgical invasiveness and improves the adequacy especially for cancer: the devices also help to overcome the poor ergonomics of laparoscopic instruments, making narrow fields as pelvis easy to be reached.

In children, left colonic surgery has its indications include severe left colonic or sigmoidal IBD, resistant to pharmacological therapies to drugs located in left colon or involving sigmoid, FAP, aganglіosis, and, more rarely primitive neoplasms.

17.2.2 Procedure Overview

Robotic left colonic management is not a hard technical challenge for surgeons compared to other procedures as rectal anterior resection: its advantages are more evident for splenic flexure mobilization, pelvic dissection, and intracorporeal sutures and anastomosis, in which the robotic technology overcomes the difficulties related to laparoscopic device strictness. These improvements are more favorable for pediatric surgery, where the smallness of surgical fields makes the laparoscopic approach more harder.

17.2.3 Patient Positioning and Docking

The supine position with arms alongside the trunk and legs abducted is the most performed: to expose the operative field from the ileal loops, we place the operative bed in a slight Trendelenburg position and a right tilt. The pneumoperitoneum (PNP) is induced through Veress needle placed in the left hypochondrium.

17.2.4 Trocar Placement

The sigmoid colon is considered the "target" organ for left colonic procedures.

17.2.4.1 da Vinci Si® System, Trocars Are Placed as Follows (Fig. 17.3)

- The camera port is placed right of the midline along an ideal line passing through the left anterosuperior iliac spine and right hypochondrium.
- R1 is placed in the right iliac fossa.
- R2 is placed in the left iliac fossa.
- R3 is located in right hypochondrium.

17.2.4.2 da Vinci Xi® System, Trocars Are Placed as Follows (Fig. 17.4)

P1 is placed on the middle line at a median distance of 4 cm from P2.

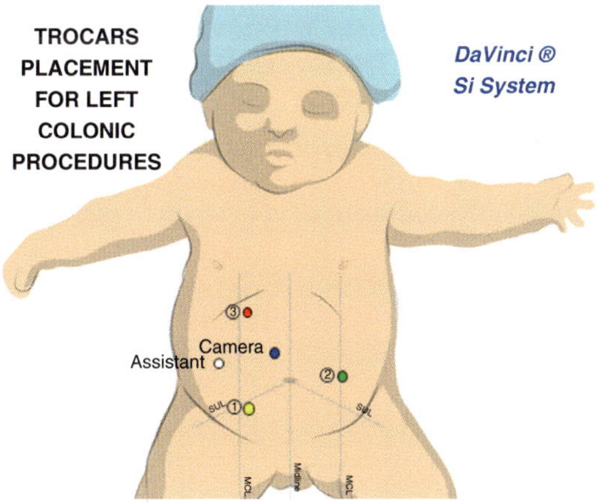

Fig. 17.3 Trocar placement for left colonic procedures

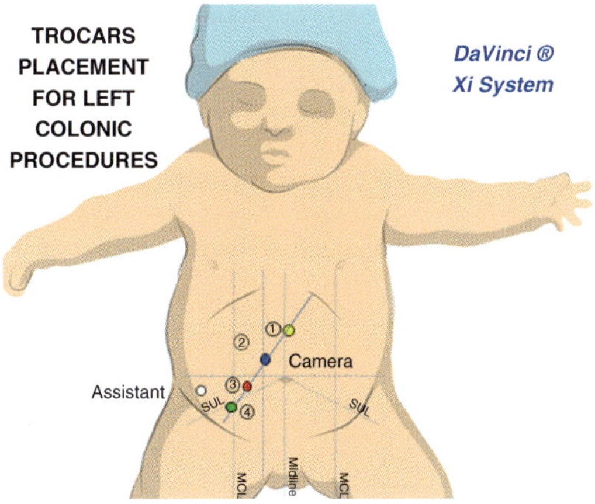

Fig. 17.4 Trocar placement for left colonic procedures

P2: camera port placed above and on the right of the umbilicus.

P3 and P4 are placed on a line drawn between P1 and P2, at a median distance of 4 cm from each other.

This is the starting placement: however, with da Vinci Xi® it is possible to switch the camera from P2 to P3 during the various phases of the procedure. Endoscope in P3 is useful for vessel ligation and pelvic dissection, while camera in P2 is adequate for splenic flexure mobilization. Airseal® port is triangulated on P3 and P4, on the right side.

17.2.5 Robot Positioning and Docking

The robotic cart approaches the operative table from the left side of the patient; the assistant takes place on the right side.

17.2.6 Procedure Description

17.2.6.1 Device Placement

A 30° down endoscope is used for both systems. The device placement is as follows:

For **da Vinci Si® system:**

R1: robotic monopolar hook/scissors
R2: robotic grasper
R3: bipolar grasper
R4: camera arm

For **da Vinci Xi® system:**

P1: bipolar forceps
P2: camera port
P3: monopolar scissors
P4: prograsp forceps

17.3 Splenic Flexure Resection

17.3.1 Procedure Overview

Splenic flexure (SF) resection is a challenging procedure in minimally invasive surgery, both for anatomical and technical aspects: SF is mainly close to splenocolic ligament and sustentaculum lienis, therefore carefull dissective maneuvers should be done to avoid any trauma or bleeding of the spleen. SF can be sometimes defined as "high" or "bulky," as it is difficult to reach by available laparoscopic devices. The main challenges during SF resection are the detection and dissection of the supply vessels, the left colic artery, originating from the IMA, and the middle colic artery, originating from SMA. For malignancies it is mandatory to associate an adequate lymphectomy including the dissection around the middle colic vein.

The resection requires a reconstructive step with an intracorporeal colo-colonic anastomosis: the robotic technology, with endowristed devices, provides a stable three-dimensional vision of the anatomy, a fine vascular dissection, and an easy fashioning of the intracorporeal anastomosis.

17.3.2 Splenic Flexure Mobilization

The procedure starts with the detection of the inferior mesenteric vein (IMV) at the angle of Treitz and inferior mesenteric artery (IMA) and the dissection of the left colonic vein (LCV) and artery (LCA).

According to disease behavior and position, IMV can be preserved by sectioning the LCV alone.

Left colic vessels are clipped by the assistant or by the clip applier and sectioned by the robotic scissors. After the complete SF mobilization, the descending colon is mobilized up to the sigmoid loop to avoid any tension of the anastomosis.

17.3.3 Left Branch of the Middle Colic Vessel Dissection

The robotic grasper retracts the distal transverse colon to expose the transverse mesocolon and facilitates vascular dissection. The transverse colon is pulled upward providing tension on the root of the transverse colon. After the detection of the root of the middle colic vessels, for segmental resections, it is not mandatory to perform their ligature at their root, while it could be transected the left branch alone, in order to preserve the common origin and the right branch, many important, according to spare most vessels as possible in a young body with progressive growing. The precise dissection of the left branch of the MCV is performed by the robotic scissors or hook. The vessels are clipped by the robotic clip applier and sectioned by the robotic scissors. Differently from cancer, for benign diseases, lymphectomy is not required.

17.3.4 Transverse and Descending Colon Transection and Anastomosis

After SF mobilization and vessel dissection have been performed, the transverse colon and the left colon are transected by the assistant trocar with a linear stapler. The use of both laparoscopic and robotic instruments allows an increased freedom of movement and an easy transection of both the descending and transverse colon. After transection a robotic stitch is placed to sew together the colonic stumps; the wristed robotic needle holder facilitates the intraoperative movements as in open surgery. The robotic bipolar gasper holds the descending colon stump while a colotomy is performed at the level of the tenia, with the robotic monopolar hook or scissors.

While the transverse colonic stump is held by assistant grasper, a second incision is performed at the level of the tenia of the transverse colon stump with the robotic monopolar hook, so the laparoscopic linear stapler is introduced by the assistant through the trocar in the right flank and the surgeon at the console facilitates the introduction of the two branches of the stapler inside the colonic stumps with the robotic grasper. A colo-colic side-to-side mechanical anastomosis is then performed: the adequate stump perfusion can be evaluated by the use of ICG fluorescence and near-infrared image, to reduce the risk of an ischemic anastomotic damage. The colotomies are closed by two running sutures starting from the opposite angles: the first running suture is performed from the inferior angle upward so the tails of upper and inferior suture are tied together. After completing the first layer, the second suture is sewn from the upper angle downward, so the two suture tails are tied together. Then a suprapubic mini-laparotomy is performed to extract the specimen inside an endo-bag.

17.4 Left Colectomy and Sigmoidectomy

It is mandatory to explore the abdominal cavity with robotic camera or with a standard laparoscope to complete the macroscopic evaluation of disease extension: when some adhesions are detected, they can be removed before starting colonic mobilization and respective procedures.

17.4.1 Splenic Flexure Mobilization

The inferior mesenteric vein (IMV) is detected at the inferior border of the pancreas and its saliency is discovered after the incision of the peritoneum below IMV by the robotic monopolar hook or scissor: this maneuver exposes the avascular plane between the two folds of the Toldt's fascia, so it can be proceeded with the medial-to-lateral dissection along the avascular plane.

While for malignancies we have to dissect the whole mesocolon until the end of the pancreatic tail, for benign lesions, it is adequate to dissect the mesocolon until the disease development ends, to obtain surgical stumps on healthy tissue.

The lateral mobilization of the descending colon is performed by the dissection of the parietocolic ligament using the monopolar hook but not mandatory until the splenic flexure: the extension of the lateral mobilization depends on the length of the specimen to remove and the length of the stump to pull down to fashion the anastomosis.

17.4.2 Inferior Mesenteric Artery Dissection

The dissected IMV is pulled upward to expose the inferior mesenteric artery (IMA), and then the space between the IMA and the aorta is exposed: at this level the para-aortic nerves lie over the preaortic plane and the superior hypogastric plexus can be detected: for segmental resections we don't need to dissect the IMA until the aortic plane, so by performing a lower ligature of the IMA, we are able to spare safely the nervous structures. The wristed ergonomics of monopolar hook or scissors facilitates the dissection of the IMA surrounded by the lymphatic tissue, so an adequate lymphadenectomy can be performed in case of malignancies: the isolated IMA is clipped by the assistant and then sectioned by the robotic scissors.

17.4.3 Distal Colonic Transection and Anastomosis

The colonic distal transection lays a few centimeters below the distal disease margin, on healthy tissue, so it can be sited on distal descending colon, in sigmoid colon, or in the rectum.

The colonic resection is performed by the assistant with a linear stapler, and then the anastomosis is fashioned according to the Knight and Griffen technique. A mini-Pfannestiel incision is performed to extract the descending colon that is transected proximally. The anvil of a circular stapler is inserted into the colon stump and sutured by using a manual purse string. The colon is repositioned, then the laparotomy is sewn the transanal end-to-end mechanical colorectal anastomosis is fashioned by laparoscopic assistance.

17.5 Transverse Colectomy

It's an unusual procedure related to pediatric age: it has main indication due to FAP or agangliosis or when a total colectomy is required.

17.5.1 Patient Positioning and Docking

The required position is the anti-Trendelenburg with the arms along the trunk and the legs abducted with a slight tilt to the right, in order to roll off the small bowel from the operative field. A 12 mmHg PNP is induced with the insertion of the Veress needle in the left hypochondrium.

17.5.2 Trocar Placement

The camera targeting for transverse colectomy is focused on the middle transverse colon, near the field of middle colonic vessels.

17.5.2.1 da Vinci Si® System, Trocars Are Placed as Follows (Fig. 17.5)

- The camera port.
- R1 is placed in the left hypochondrium.
- R2 is placed in the right hypochondrium.
- R3 is located in the right flank.

The assistant trocar is placed in the left flank while the robotic cart approaches the operative table from the patient's head.

17.5.2.2 da Vinci Xi® System, Trocars are Placed as Follows (Fig. 17.6)

P1 is placed on the same line on the right of P2.

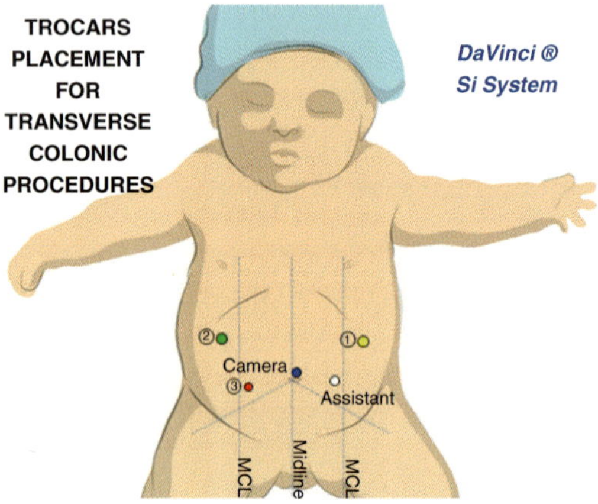

Fig. 17.5 Trocar placement for transverse colonic procedures

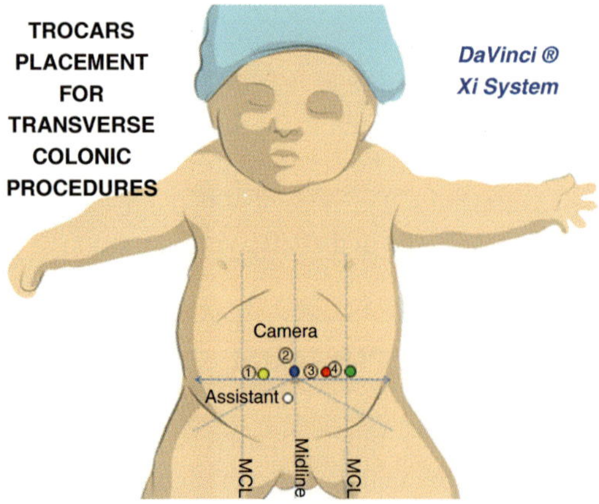

Fig. 17.6 Trocar placement for transverse colonic procedures

P2: camera port placed near the umbilicus.
P3 and P4 are placed at the same distance each from the other on the left of P2.

Airseal® port is placed under the transumbilical line, in a triangle shape with P1 and P2.

17.5.3 Procedure Description

17.5.3.1 Device Placement

A 30° down endoscope is used for both systems. The device placement is as follows:

For **da Vinci Si® system:**

R1: robotic monopolar hook/scissors
R2: robotic grasper
R3: bipolar grasper
R4: camera arm

For **da Vinci Xi® system:**

P1: bipolar grasper
P2: camera arm
P3: robotic monopolar hook/scissors
P4: robotic grasper

17.5.4 Dissection of the Middle Colic Vessels

The transverse colonic exposition is necessary to discover the proper site and extension of disease: it is performed by the pulling up of the greater omentum by assistant's grasper. The transverse colon is then placed up to enhance the main trunk of the MC that is circumferentially dissected, then clipped by the robotic clip applier, and then sectioned by the robotic or assistant's scissors.

Dissection of the transverse mesocolon follows a medial-to-lateral pathway: the robotic grasper provides a stable tension on the transverse colon and mesocolon; the robotic bipolar device pulls up the mesocolon while the robotic monopolar tool performs a dissection of the transverse mesocolon from the posterior peritoneal layer toward the right colic flexure. Transverse mesocolon dissection is achieved providing a V-shape that is pulled down.

17.5.5 Mobilization of the Left and Right Colic Flexures and of the Transverse Colon

The medial retraction of the proximal descending colon and of the SF is provided by the bipolar grasper while the robotic monopolar device sections the parietocolic ligament to the left colic flexure, the phrenocolic, the splenocolic ligament, and the sustentaculum lienis. The transverse colon is pulled down with a grasper by the assistant, while the robotic bipolar forceps lifts up the proximal side of the gastrocolic ligament. The ligament is then dissected below the gastroepiploic vessels by the robotic monopolar device, up to the right flexure. The right colon is then retracted medially by the assistant's grasper and by the robotic grasper, allowing the dissection of the right parietocolic ligament, performed by the robotic monopolar hook: total mobilization of both the right and left colic flexures and of the transverse colon is completed with a robotic single docking approach.

17.5.6 Transverse Colon Transection and Anastomosis

The assistant transects the transverse colon with a laparoscopic linear stapler on both left and right sides: so both stumps are joined by graspers and then opened at distal site by robotic scissors, in order to perform an intracorporeal colo-colonic end-to-end anastomosis with a double-running suture.

The robotic grasper holds the right colon and the assistant holds the left colon: the wristed robotic needle holders facilities intracorporeal manual end-to-end anastomosis fashioning, as well as the 3D view provided by the robotic system.

17.6 Discussion and Conclusions

Weber reported the first robot-assisted colectomy in 2002; since then, many results of robotic colorectal surgery in adults have been reported, about its feasibility and its satisfactory functional and oncological outcomes; however, only few studies on robotic colorectal surgery in childhood have been reported so far.

Robotic devices offer many advantages due to their wristed technology that make even narrow abdominal fields reachable, and the 3D stable vision that allows an improved vision for detection and dissection of vessels and the ICG fluorescence that allows the real-time evaluation of surgical stump perfusion.

Pediatric surgery is expected to benefit from the robotic technology (RT), because of the gentle and precise movements in small fields that are allowed by RT that are of main importance expecially in small anatomic structures as children abdomen: sized pediatric robotic instruments as 5 mm ports are available, and 0 and 30° cameras too. For adolescents the same trocars as for adults can be used.

Minimally invasive trocars reduce also the risk of postoperative herniation due to the weakness of abdominal wall.

References

1. Page AE, Sashittal SG, Chatzizacharias NA, et al. The role of laparoscopic surgery in the management of children and adolescents with inflammatory bowel disease. Medicine. 2015;94(21):e874.
2. Mahida JB, Cooper JN, Herz D, Diefenbach KA, et al. Utilization and costs associated with robotic surgery in children. J Surg Res. 2015;199:169–76.
3. Cundy TP, Shetty K, Clark J, Chang TP, et al. The first decade of robotic surgery in children. J Pediatr Surg. 2013;48:858–65.
4. Finkelstein JB, Levy AC, Silva MV, Murray L, Delaney C, Casale P. How to decide which infant can have robotic surgery? Just do the math. J Pediatr Urol. 2015;11:170.e1–4.
5. Cundy TP, Marcus HJ, Hughes-Hallett A, Sanjeev Khurana S, Darzi A. Robotic surgery in children: adopt now, await, or dismiss? Pediatr Surg Int. 2015;31:1119–25.
6. Spinoglio G. Robotic Surgery: Current Applications and New Trends. Springer Verlag. 2015.

18 Robotic Assisted Proctectomy and Ileal J-Pouch Anorectal Anastomosis

Luca Pio and Girolamo Mattioli

18.1 Background

The reconstructive surgery plays a fundamental role in the quality of life of children with complicated ulcerative colitis (UC), and in recent years pediatric minimally invasive surgery is becoming a surgical standard (UC) [1–5].

Currently the main type of surgical reconstruction involves the use of a reservoir from an ileal pouch [6], with or without endorectal pull through (ERPT) and mucosectomy.

The original technique provided an open approach that has been translated to the minimally invasive surgery (MIS) during the years [7].

The cardinal principle of proctectomy is to leave the minor amount of rectal tissue guaranteeing sphincter preservation and fecal continence.

Proctectomy may cause fertility complications because of the proximity to the seminal vesicles in male and the vagina in female patients. Dissection in deep pelvis is largely considered at risk for the poor vision and limited space to operate with possibility of nerve, vascular, and urogenital injury.

In adult da Vinci robotic surgery (RS) has the main application for the deep pelvis site for prostate cancer treatment and gained popularity for the better nervous tissue visualization and the faster learning curve when compared to conventional minimally invasive laparoscopic surgery [8–10].

Based on promising results of the current application of RS in pediatric surgery and the recognized role in deep pelvis, this type of surgical approach may be used in reconstructive surgical step of patients with rectal disorders.

We describe for the first time the technical aspects of restorative proctectomy and ileal J-pouch anorectal anastomosis with robotic approach.

18.2 Technique

A 3-cm J-pouch ileal reservoir with vascular supply control was created using the stoma incision (Fig. 18.1). The head of the circular stapler is inserted and stabilized, then the J-pouch is replaced in abdomen, and a multichannel-access flexible SILS® Port (Covidien plc, Cherrywood Business Park, Loughlinstown Co. Dublin, Ireland) is placed in the ileostomy site and used for two 5 mm service instruments (for needle insertion and for suction) and one 8 mm da Vinci robotic port.

L. Pio (✉) • G. Mattioli
Pediatric Surgery Unit, Istituto Giannina Gaslini, Largo G. Gaslini 5, Genoa 16147, Italy

DINOGMI, University of Genoa, Genoa, Italy
e-mail: lucakeats@hotmail.it

G. Mattioli, P. Petralia (eds.), *Pediatric Robotic Surgery*, DOI 10.1007/978-3-319-41863-6_18

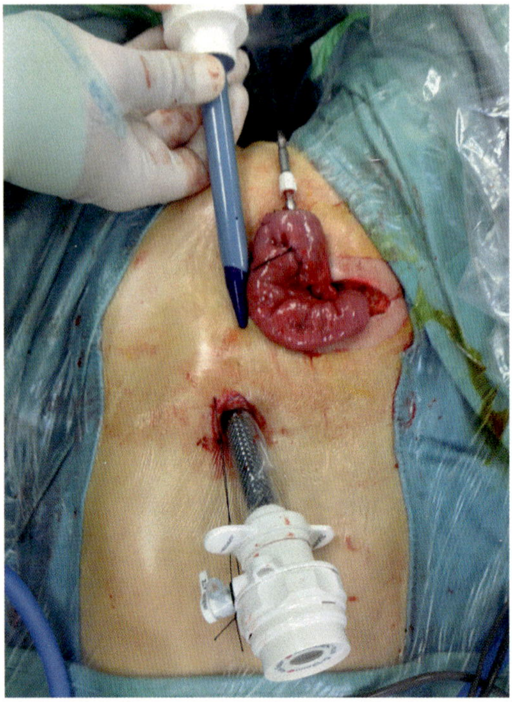

Fig. 18.1 J-Pouch creation using single-port incision

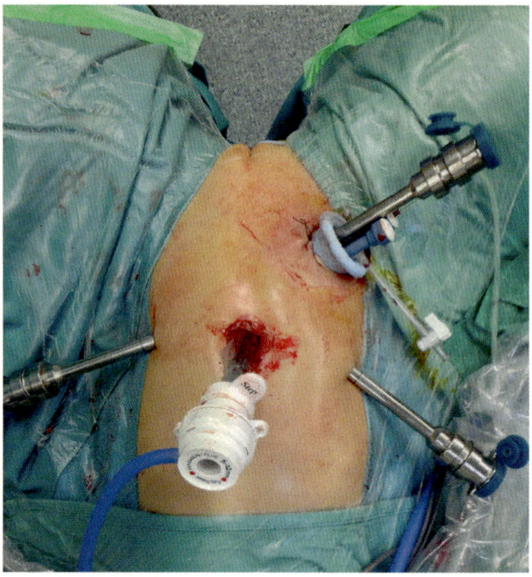

Fig. 18.2 Robotic trocars setting

After the SILS® insertion a 12 mm port and three operative 8 mm ports are, respectively, placed in the umbilical, left paraumbilical, and right subcostal space (Fig. 18.2).

A 12 mm Hg CO_2 pneumoperitoneum is created and robotic docking is completed with utilization of four arms: one for the camera, two for operative instruments, and one for bladder/uterus retraction, which avoid the need of the assistant, who is involved only for introduction of the suture and anal manipulation through the anus.

First step of robotic time was the identification of the rectal stump, the ureters, and the vagina (Fig. 18.3). Proctectomy is performed using the monopolar hook, close to the rectum or inside the muscular rectal wall (ERPT), to preserve innervation and integrity of pelvic organs. The hook allows tissue traction and despite its fulguration action the rectal planes are well identified and easily dissected without bleeding. Mesorectal vessels are well identified too, as well as vaginal wall, and coagulated close to the rectum.

Dissection has gone up to the levator ani muscle and residual rectum stump is resected with a flexible linear stapler. The rectal stump is removed at the end of procedure through the previous stoma incision.

The circular stapler is used for the side-to-end anastomosis through the anus. Before connection of the head of the stapler previously placed in the J-pouch, a careful control avoiding any J-pouch torsion is performed which can compromise the vascular supply of the anastomosis and cause very important complication as pouchitis or anastomotic dehiscence (Fig. 18.4).

Reinforcement sutures in the deep pelvis are easily performed.

At the end of the procedure a terminal ileostomy is created in the preexisting SILS incision site in order to protect the J-pouch anal anastomosis.

Neither drainage nor nasogastric tube are necessary.

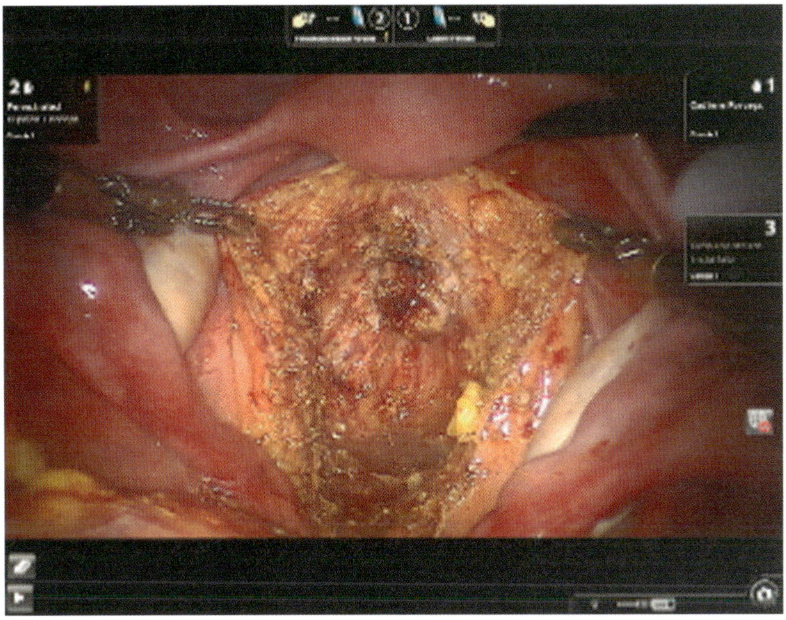

Fig. 18.3 Identification of the rectal stump, the ureters, and the vagina

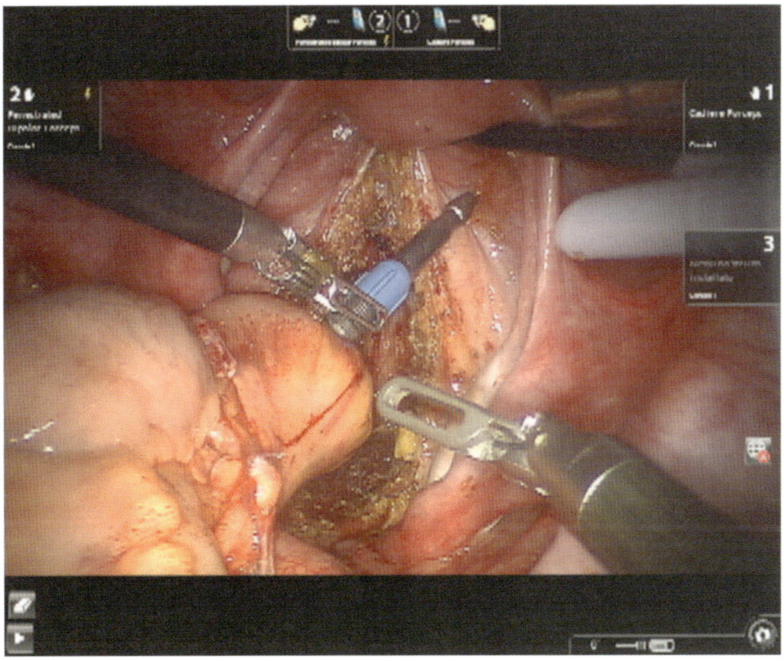

Fig. 18.4 Preparation of ilal-J-pouch anorectal anastomosis

18.3 Discussion

In recent years MIS gained a more recognized role for the treatment of pediatric UC [11] and the development of new technologies helped surgeons to reduce surgical invasiveness until the application of RS for the treatment of children disease.

Reconstructive surgery represents the more delicate process of the different surgical phases for UC treatment, and it is characterized by a series of potential complications that may irreversibly compromise the quality of life of children in their adult development as vaginal fistula, seminal vesicle damage, bladder fistula, J-pouch anastomotic leak, J-pouch torsion, pouchitis, and denervation of pelvic floor with risk of neurogenic bladder and fecal incontinence.

All these complications must be considered when pediatric surgeon performs residual proctectomy to leave the lesser intestinal tissue to avoid the risk of cancer.

It is well known that RS overcome several potential complications of deep pelvis conventional MIS in adult populations and some technical disadvantages as the lack of tactile feedback are compensated by 3-D visualization giving the possibility to play an important role also for the minimally invasive approach of rectal cancer and for radical prostatectomy [9, 10, 12, 13].

da Vinci® system gives the surgeons a better control of the entire phases of the second surgical step for UC: it allows a better manipulation of the intra-abdominal J-pouch in the anastomotic time, thanks to its major degrees of freedom compared to conventional MIS; proctectomy has several advantages in terms of anatomic 3-D visualization of rectum, bladder neck, prostatic, and vaginal plane during dissection; J-pouch anorectal anastomosis is better controlled, with the possibility to easily perform reinforced hand sutures.

The main limitation of RS is related to the higher cost for procedure compared to traditional MIS, but if robotic approach allows a better surgical control of all the delicate phases of reconstructive UC treatment, we can speculate that it avoids frequency of postoperative sequelae traducing with cost of surgical reinterventions and hospitalization, and of utmost importance, it can reduce the risk of complications.

A safety deep pelvis approach is appealing in pediatric surgery and could be applied to other pediatric diseases for the ERPT procedures as anorectal malformations or Hirschsprung's disease, thanks to the progressive miniaturization of robotic instruments. Considering this aspect, restorative proctectomy may be the initial procedure to introduce robotic assisted laparoscopic pull-through in children.

These considerations are possible only if pediatric diseases are centralized in selected centers that can offer a da Vinci robotic system. Centralization is a cornerstone to reduce the relevant costs of RS for the pediatric community.

Obviously, larger series is necessary to confirm the functional outcomes in patients treated with robotic reconstructive surgery for UC.

Conclusion

Pediatric da Vinci® robotic assisted laparoscopic restorative proctectomy and ileal J-pouch anal anastomosis offer advantages in terms of tissue visualization and a better working space; thanks to the robotic arms with more degrees of freedom, it is feasible, easy, and safe; provides good functional outcomes; and must be offered to all children.

References

1. Larson DW, Cima RR, Dozois EJ, Davies M, Piotrowicz K, Barnes SA, Wolff B, Pemberton J. Safety, feasibility, and short-term outcomes of laparoscopic ileal-pouch-anal anastomosis: a single institutional case-matched experience. Ann Surg. 2006;243(5):667–70.
2. Simon T, Orangio G, Ambroze W, Schertzer M, Armstrong D. Laparoscopic-assisted bowel resection in pediatric/adolescent inflammatory bowel disease: laparoscopic bowel resection in children. Dis Colon Rectum. 2003;46(10):1325–31.
3. Linden BC, Bairdain S, Zurakowski D, Shamberger RC, Lillehei CW. Comparison of laparoscopic-assisted and open total proctocolectomy and ileal pouch anal anastomosis in children and adolescents. J Pediatr Surg. 2013;48(7):1546–50.

4. Diamond IR, Gerstle JT, Kim PC, Langer JC. Outcomes after laparoscopic surgery in children with inflammatory bowel disease. Surg Endosc. 2010;24(11):2796–802.
5. Flores P, Bailez MM, Cuenca E, Fraire C. Comparative analysis between laparoscopic (UCL) and open (UCO) technique for the treatment of ulcerative colitis in pediatric patients. Pediatr Surg Int. 2010;26(9):907–11.
6. Griffen FD, Knight CD Sr, Whitaker JM, Knight CD Jr. The double stapling technique for low anterior resection. Results, modifications, and observations. Ann Surg. 1990;211(6):745–51.
7. Mattioli G, Guida E, Pini-Prato A, Avanzini S, Rossi V, Barabino A, Coran AG, Jasonni V. Technical considerations in children undergoing laparoscopic ileal-J-pouch anorectal anastomosis for ulcerative colitis. Pediatr Surg Int. 2012;28(4):351–6.
8. Haglind E, Carlsson S, Stranne J, Wallerstedt A, Wilderäng U, Thorsteinsdottir T, Damber JE, Bjartell A, Hugosson J, Wiklund P, Steineck G. LAPPRO steering committee. Urinary incontinence and erectile dysfunction after robotic versus open radical prostatectomy: a prospective, controlled, nonrandomised trial. Eur Urol. 2015;68(2):216–25.
9. Asimakopoulos AD, Miano R, Di Lorenzo N, Spera E, Vespasiani G, Mugnier C. Laparoscopic versus robot-assisted bilateral nerve-sparing radical prostatectomy: comparison of pentafecta rates for a single surgeon. Surg Endosc. 2013;27(11):4297–304.
10. Ploussard G, de la Taille A, Moulin M, Vordos D, Hoznek A, Abbou CC, Salomon L. Comparisons of the perioperative, functional, and oncologic outcomes after robot-assisted versus pure extraperitoneal laparoscopic radical prostatectomy. Eur Urol. 2014;65(3):610–9.
11. Mattioli G, Barabino A, Aloi M, Arrigo S, Caldaro T, Carlucci M, Cucchiara S, De Angelis P, Di Leo G, Illiceto MT, Impellizzeri P, Leonelli L, Lisi G, Lombardi G, Martelossi S, Martinelli M, Miele E, Randazzo A, Romano C, Romeo C, Romeo E, Selvaggi F, Valenti S, Dall'Oglio L. Paediatric ulcerative colitis surgery: Italian survey. J Crohns Colitis. 2015;9(7):558–64.
12. Midura EF, Hanseman DJ, Hoehn RS, Davis BR, Abbott DE, Shah SA, Paquette IM. The effect of surgical approach on short-term oncologic outcomes in rectal cancersurgery. Surgery. 2015;158(2):453–9.
13. Tam MS, Kaoutzanis C, Mullard AJ, Regenbogen SE, Franz MG, Hendren S, Krapohl G, Vandewarker JF, Lampman RM, Cleary RK. A population-based study comparing laparoscopic and robotic outcomes in colorectal surgery. Surg Endosc. 2016;30:455–63.

Part 4

Oncology Surgery and Thoracic Surgery

Principles of Minimally Invasive Surgery Applied to Oncology Patients

19

Girolamo Mattioli, Luca Pio, Stefano Avanzini, Claudio Granata, Thomas Blanc, and Sabine Sarnacki

19.1 Introduction

Surgical resection is one of the cornerstones of multimodal treatment strategies for many paediatric solid tumours. Overall cure rates for childhood cancers are nowadays approaching 80%. Efforts are therefore directed towards decreasing sequels and improving quality of life. In the surgical field, the use of MIS may be one way to do it. In 1995 Holcomb et al. reported on a first series of children with thoracic and abdominal cancer undergoing biopsy thanks to MIS [1] and many authors confirmed then the feasibility and accuracy of MIS for diagnostic purposes in paediatric oncological patients [1–3]. The use of MIS for resection of children solid cancers developed however more slowly for essentially three reasons: (1) the indications are few as most of children cancers are embryonic tumours with a huge size at diagnosis that let few space in the thorax or abdomen to work, even after size reduction by neoadjuvant chemotherapy; (2) paediatric oncologists were reluctant for such an approach for a long time, fearing incomplete resection and most of all peritoneal dissemination with higher rate recurrence as it was described in adults [4, 5]; (3) paediatric surgeons involved historically in children cancer were not those that were the pioneers of MIS and it took some time to merge both expertise.

A relevant number of paediatric surgeons now perform demanding laparoscopic, thoracoscopic, or robotic oncological procedures [4–22]. By now however, most of the retrospective analyses simply underline the feasibility and the advantages of this approach [23] and there is clearly a lack of worldwide-accepted guidelines [24, 25] and of randomized prospective clinical trials. Although MIS does carry some risks such as CO_2 embolism, increased abdominal pressure decreasing lung compliance, and increased cardiac overload [26], a minimally invasive approach offers on the other hand many proved advantages. Besides the well-recognized cosmetic advantage of MIS, by reducing parietal injury, it also decreases the need of narcotic analgesics and time to complete post-operative mobilization and

G. Mattioli • S. Avanzini (✉)
Pediatric Surgery Department, Giannina Gaslini Research Institute, Genoa, Italy
e-mail: stefanoavanzini@gaslini.org

L. Pio
Department of Neurosciences, Rehabilitation, Ophthalmology, Genetics, Maternal and Child Health (DINOGMI), University of Genoa, Genoa, Italy

Pediatric Surgery Department, Giannina Gaslini Research Institute, Genoa, Italy

C. Granata
Pediatric Radiology Unit, Giannina Gaslini Research Institute, Genoa, Italy

T. Blanc • S. Sarnacki
Pediatric Surgery and Urology Department, AP-HP, Hopital Necker Enfants Malades, Université Paris Descartes, Sorbonne Paris Cité, Paris, France

G. Mattioli, P. Petralia (eds.), *Pediatric Robotic Surgery*, DOI 10.1007/978-3-319-41863-6_19

oral feeding. In addition, this approach ensures less bowel adhesion formation [27] and less risk of wound infections and incisional hernias [14]. Altogether these advantages should allow earlier post-operative recovery and thus reduce time for adjuvant therapy [5, 7, 9, 16, 28, 29]. Finally, the development of MIS in paediatric oncology showed that the wide range of technical and ergonomic enhancements displayed by robotic surgical technology [16, 22] offers a better access and view of some anatomical regions and allows then an optimized dissection and resection of the tumour. The use of MIS in paediatric oncology is thus now a part of the tools offered to cure children from cancer and should be discussed when appropriate, provided the surgery follows the same basic oncologic than those applied to open surgery [13].

The extrapolation of data and results from the literature dealing with MIS in oncological adult patients is not applicable to children as tumour origin, biology, treatment, and prognosis are completely different.

19.2 Case Selection and Indications

In absence of official guidelines, the indication for minimally invasive diagnostic biopsy or ablative surgery is generally considered and approved by an interdisciplinary panel, including paediatric oncologists, surgeons, radiologists, radiotherapists, and pathologists. The expertise of the surgical team not only with MIS but also with open procedures being acquired, some indications and contraindications are currently well recognized and consisted the basis for the patient-specific discussion confirming or discouraging MIS [6].

The main obvious contraindications for MIS in paediatric oncology are huge and fragile tumour carrying a high risk of tumour spillage, extensive previous surgery resulting in dense intra-abdominal or thoracic adhesions, and severe respiratory impairment [24–32]. Tumour spillage results indeed in intensified chemotherapy regimens and radiotherapy in these children with a high risk of recurrence impairing their prognosis.

19.3 Abdominal Tumours

19.3.1 Technical Notes

From the technical point of view, four different approaches may be considered [16]: prone retroperitoneoscopic, lateral retroperitoneoscopic, anterior laparoscopic, and lateral laparoscopic, mostly depending on the localization and the size of the tumour.

In 2010 the International Pediatric Endosurgery Group (IPEG) issued guidelines for laparoscopic adrenalectomy confirming the feasibility of the technique and recommending both laparoscopic and retroperitoneoscopic approaches, with the choice being dictated by the surgeon's experience and preference [33–35]. Similarly, Wilms tumour has been approached both laparoscopically and retroperitoneoscopically [15, 36]. The limits of the retroperitoneal approach lie in the absence of ability to explore the abdominal cavity and to perform lymph node sampling or dissection easily. Laparoscopic approach is generally preferred because of a larger working space and more familiar anatomic landmarks, which are crucial to the surgeon.

The antibiotic prophylaxis is the same than the one used for open procedure and is usually administered intra-operatively and during the first 24 hours post-operatively. After induction of general anaesthesia, the patient is positioned in a prone or in a 60°–90° lateral decubitus (for midline or lateral localization of the tumour respectively), elevated on a soft roll, to guarantee the best exposure. Understanding the "geometry" of laparoscopy, choosing the optimal trocar position, and using trans-abdominal stay sutures are all strategic key factors allowing for a better tumour exposure thus significantly reducing the number of additional trocars to handle the tumour, suturing, and knotting [16]. A 10 mm umbilical camera with 30° should be privileged for a better anatomical magnification. Nearly all authors work with three or four trocars. Exploration of the renal pedicle can be improved with a trans-abdominal traction suture around the ureter. Stay sutures on the back wall of the stomach and duodenum lead to an excellent exposure of the pancreas head for pancreatic tumours.

Sutures, mono- or bipolar electro-coagulation, harmonic scalpel, and/or vessel sealing devices may be alternatively and complementarily used to ensure an optimal haemostasis. Monofilament polydioxanone sutures are generally indicated for large vessel securement. Metallic clips or Hemoloc may quickly fix small bleeding vessels, although they carry a significant risk of dislocation when touching or mobilizing the stump during further dissection. Intra-abdominal pressure may be temporarily increased up to 12 mmHg to provide a larger working space and/or to manage bleeding [16].

Whenever recommended, lymph node sampling should precede tumour excision, as tissues may retract following tumour ablation and limit lymph nodes exposure. Once completely dissected, tumours are most commonly removed from the abdomen in an endoscopic bag by enlarging the umbilical port site or through a supra-pubic incision [16]. This step of the procedure should be considered as important as the dissection steps in order to avoid bag rupture and tumour spillage, whatever the nature of the tumour.

19.3.2 Neuroblastoma and Adrenal Tumours

Neuroblastomas (NBs) are the most common extracranial solid tumours in children. They mostly arise from the abdomen (adrenal gland 48%, extra-adrenal retroperitoneum 25%), less frequently from the chest (16%), and rarely from the pelvis (3%) or the neck (3%). They are known to derive from the sympathetic nervous system originating from neural crests cells (NCCs), and thus may theoretically arise from any migratory pathways. These tumours are associated with remarkable biological heterogeneity and outcome. Some NBs may undergo spontaneous regression and some are cured by surgery alone or after chemo-reduction, while others have an extremely aggressive behaviour with metastases and recurrences despite intensive treatments. In patients affected by NB MIS may be indicated in the following circumstances:

19.3.2.1 Tumour Biopsy

Procurement of tumour tissue is mandatory to assign the patient to the appropriate treatment group. Although percutaneous biopsy is usually sufficient for tumour tissue analysis, a minimally invasive approach is the optimal way to obtain a huge amount of tissue when required. It allows histopathological investigation with a nearly 100% diagnostic accuracy and biological and genetic analysis which are key elements of the risk stratification [12, 14] for further multimodality treatment [37]. MIS is particularly interesting in case of recurrence when a large amount of tissue is now needed for potential targeted therapies screening.

19.3.2.2 Tumour Resection

The introduction of Image-Defined Risk Factors (IDRF) in the clinical practice has brought more objective criteria to define the surgical risk of tumour removal [38, 39]. In the absence of IDRF, regardless of the size of the tumour, MIS has been established as a safe alternative to open ablative surgery [35, 39–42] essentially in adrenal tumours and thoracic neuroblastoma arising from the paravertebral parasympathetic chain.

Regarding adrenal tumours, Kelleher et al. demonstrated that MIS in adrenal neuroblastoma can be performed with comparable recurrence and mortality rates in low, intermediate, and high risk patients [41]. Interestingly, the first reports on NB treated by MIS included a high percentage of infants diagnosed postnatally or even antenatally with an adrenal tumour that would not have been operated today with the current European low and intermediate risk neuroblastoma protocol (LINES). Regarding the high rate of tumour spontaneous regression and/or maturation in this population, an expectant observation is currently recommended, provided that the patient has no life-threatening symptoms and that the tumour is of favourable biology and not increasing in size. When persisting after 12 months with no IDRFs, these adrenal tumours are good candidates for surgical resection with MIS. In contrast, when IDRFs are persisting after this wait and see strategy, the question of surgery in tumour with good biology is still debated whatever the surgical approach, open or MIS [43].

The presence of IDRFs in most of the other locations of NBs developing in the abdomen [38] explained that MIS has been poorly reported for extra-adrenal NBs [21, 39].

In the thorax, NBs arising from the paravertebral parasympathetic chain appeared as the best indication for MIS. The spare of the osteomuscular thoracic wall is not only less painful post-operatively but also decrease the risk of scoliosis that may be the result of a thoracotomy. This is particularly interesting in mature neurogenic tumours as ganglioneuroblastoma and ganglioneuroma, not only in the thorax but also in the abdomen or the pelvis as the benefit of surgery for those tumours is still debated [40, 41].

Adrenocortical tumours are rare tumours, representing 0.2% of all paediatric malignancies, i.e. 0.1–0.4 out of one million [44]. Complete excision is the treatment of choice, as they usually do not respond to chemo- or radiotherapy. The risk of spillage is considerably high due to the friability of the tumour's capsule [34] and impairs notably the prognosis of these very aggressive tumours. Biopsy is thus formally contraindicated and although surgery may appear not difficult when the tumour is small and localized to the adrenal gland, laparoscopic resection should be discouraged when clinical presentation and imaging favour this diagnosis [45, 46].

Pheochromocytoma is a rare catecholamine-secreting tumour in children, benign in approximately 90% of cases. Regarding the possible cardiac impact of the associated hypertension, a pre-operative preparation of the patient is usually mandatory. Surgical resection is the main treatment. The advantage of MIS on open procedure is well recognized, as it allows less manipulation of the lesion, less delivery of catecholamines during the procedure, and thus less tensional instability. Although only case reports are documented [47, 48], MIS is an accepted procedure for pheochromocytoma, especially when bilateral [44].

19.3.3 Renal Tumours

Wilms tumour or nephroblastoma is the most common malignant renal tumour of childhood, representing 90% of all malignant renal tumours. Complete surgical resection, without spillage, associated with a sufficient lymph node sampling is the main goal of surgical treatment and strongly predicts final outcome [49, 50]. Intra-operative tumour spillage influences the multimodality treatment intensity as it upgrades the local staging to stage III and requires thus post-operative irradiation of the whole abdominal cavity, worsening the overall prognosis. Therefore, the standard surgical approach is open total nephrectomy without microscopic residue or spillage. Limited working space, risk of tumour rupture, and difficulties in correct lymph node sampling are factors that explain that MIS may greatly affect the safety of the procedure especially in large tumours [15, 51–54]. Varlet et al. concluded that only lesion that is not extending beyond the midline may be a potential candidate for MIS, whereas the presence of inferior vena cava or renal thrombosis, adhesions to other organs, and initial tumour rupture would strongly contraindicate such an approach [15]. Beyond these criteria that should be respected, the possibility of conversion during the procedure should be always present in the surgeon's mind in order not to take any oncological risk. Moreover, whenever a small Wilms tumour would be considered for minimally invasive tumour nephrectomy, this approach often competes against open nephron sparing surgery (NSS). This later option should be discussed and preferred if possible, as it has the advantage to preserve renal function [21]. Anecdotal reports have described the use of laparoscopic [55] or retroperitoneoscopic approach to perform NSS [56]. They reported tumour dissemination confirming that MIS is contraindicated in NSS for Wilms [56].

Renal Cell Carcinoma accounts for 2–6% of paediatric renal malignancies. Complete radical resection together with extended lymph nodes dissection is the cornerstone of treatment. This is a contraindication of MIS.

19.3.4 Germ Cell Tumours—Ovarian

Germ cell tumours in children and adolescents most commonly originate from the ovaries, including benign conditions (mature teratoma, cystic tumours) as well as malignant tumours

(Granulosa-theca cell tumours, germ cell tumours, immature teratoma, gonadoblastoma, dysgerminoma). Laparoscopy has been widely used for ovarian-sparing procedures in documented benign tumours [57–59]. Preservation of healthy ovarian tissue is crucial to minimize the risk of long-term ovarian failure and infertility [60, 61]. However, in cases of malignant ovarian tumours, laparoscopy is not recommended because of the risk of peroperative rupture or spillage [57, 59, 62]. If it happens, the treatment is radically changed, as adjuvant chemotherapy is mandatory while surgery alone would have been sufficient in case of appropriate surgical resection. If laparoscopy is useful for an appropriate staging, especially because the inspection of the peritoneum and omentum is not possible by a sus-pubic incision [58, 63], the preferred approach for any malignant ovarian lesion should be a sus-pubic incision that allows protection of the operative field and a safe ovariectomy or salpingo-ovariectomy. As the malignant or benign nature of these ovarian lesions are not always easy to determine (malignant non-secreting tumours), some teams preferred to approach any ovarian lesion by a sus-pubic approach, even for an ovarian-sparing surgery.

Patients requiring pelvic radiation may benefit from laparoscopic ovarian transposition to preserve fertility. Ovaries may be shifted laterally, contralaterally, or in line with the iliac crest, according to the radiation field. Good function with normal pregnancies has been described, without the need for the ovaries to be relocated following radiotherapy [64]. Similarly, ovarian tissue cryopreservation has been described as a valid option to preserve fertility and laparoscopy is certainly the best approach to do it [62, 65].

19.3.5 Pancreatic Tumours

Tumours of the pancreas are rare in children and cover different pathologies of benign (serous or mucinous cystadenoma), malignant (pancreatoblastoma, carcinoma), and borderline type (solid pseudopapillary tumour or Frantz tumour, endocrine tumours) [66, 67]. Pancreatoblastoma are mainly seen in young children under 10 years of age and Frantz tumour in older ones. Complete tumour excision in the absence of rupture is of utmost importance in the treatment of those malignancies and decisive for the outcome. Biopsies should be avoided as tumour recurrence has been reported after intra-operative cell spillage. While the impact of tumour rupture is still debated in Frantz tumours, incomplete resection clearly increases the risk of recurrence. Concerns with MIS for pancreatic tumours in children are mainly directed towards the requested experience in all advanced surgical techniques of pancreatic surgery including the Whipple procedure. However, spleen-preserving distal pancreatectomy and central pancreatectomy with pancreaticogastrostomy for pseudopapillary tumours have been described [16, 68–70].

19.3.6 Liver Tumours

Liver tumours in childhood (hepatoblastoma and hepatocellular carcinoma) are rare tumours. Complete tumour resection is the key factor for survival. Most of the studies dealing with the role of MIS in liver tumours report on resection of benign lesions such as focal nodular hyperplasia, hamartoma, hemangioma, or dysontogenetic cysts [71, 72]. Minimally invasive resection for malignant tumours is more rarely reported and should certainly be developed with highly trained surgeons, like adult liver surgeons [16].

19.3.7 Lymph Nodes Sampling

Paratesticular rhabdomyosarcomas or germinal cell tumours of the testis may metastasize to the retroperitoneal lymph nodes. MIS staging sampling performed by retroperitoneoscopy [36] or laparoscopy [73, 74] has been described.

19.4 Thoracic Tumours and Lung Metastasis

19.4.1 Technical Notes

Thoracic oncological MIS procedures should follow analogous principles described for abdominal tumours, with specific peculiarity related to thoracoscopy. Anesthesiological setting plays a relevant role in this scenario. Single lung ventilation is generally recommended. In small children and infants this can be relevantly hampered because of airway and/or lung compression, increased intra-thoracic pressure, and intra-operative carbon dioxide uptake [8, 17–19, 75]. Whenever possible a 10 mm camera should be positioned along the axillary line. Trocars in the lower intercostal spaces should be positioned under direct vision to avoid diaphragmatic and liver/spleen damage. A retrieval bag and eventually a mini-thoracotomy help in removal of the resected specimen from the thoracic cavity [20, 28, 76]. Fragmentation of the tumour is discouraged because of the risk of rupture of the retrieval bag and subsequent pleural spillage. Moreover, histopathological detection of tumour architecture may be compromised by fragmentation.

19.4.2 Neurogenic Tumours

Besides the high interest of MIS in resection of neurogenic tumours in the thorax (see above) [16, 19, 20, 28], thoracoscopy could be proposed for the biopsy of any thoracic lesion discovered during the staging of any cancer.

19.4.3 Germ Cell Tumours

Germ cell tumours of the thorax are rare, usually located in the mediastinum (anterior or medium) and infiltrating lesions. Complete surgical resection is mandatory and MIS is not a good option to achieve this goal [77].

19.4.4 Lung Metastases

The rate of MIS resection of lung metastases mostly from Wilms tumour as well as from osteogenic sarcoma has been strongly increased especially following the introduction of localization techniques by interventional radiologists (the most common being coils, coil wires, colour dye, or radionuclide as well as minimally invasive thoracoscopic ultrasound) to overcome the lack of tactile abilities and the inability to visualize intra-parenchymal lesions [78–85]. However, as the surgical outcome in these patients highly depends on tumour biology and associated treatments, MIS for lung metastases should be performed in targeted patients with respect to protocol guidelines [18, 86–89] and contraindicated in some malignancies as in case of metastasectomy for synovial sarcoma [90].

19.4.5 Ewing's Sarcoma

Minimally invasive surgery for Ewing sarcoma is rarely reported for mediastinal location [91] and when originated in the chest wall [92].

19.4.6 Nonsolid Tumours

Hodgkin and non-Hodgkin lymphoma represent 6–7% of all paediatric malignancies, generally originating from the anterior mediastinal lymph nodes, causing relevant tracheal compression with a high risk of intra-operative anesthesiological complications [1, 2, 8, 93]. The essential role of surgery is focused on a representative tumour biopsy for diagnostic workup and risk stratification if no peripheral accessible lymph nodes are available for biopsy.

19.5 Supportive Care

Although MIS was largely described for supportive care in paediatric oncology, robotic surgery has not yet developed.

Supportive care procedures include gastrostomy for enteral feeding, ovarian transposition to preserve fertility for girls with pelvic cancer that requiring irradiation [64], and ovarian cryopreservation to preserve fertility for prepubertal girls who underwent gonadotoxic treatments for malignant tumours [94].

Another supportive care treatment was described by Irtan, describing bowel protection for irradiation treatment using sigmoid as an hammock [95].

19.6 Outcome and Discussion

The potential of MIS in paediatric oncology has been mostly derived from small retrospective series of patients who underwent biopsy or resection of limited disease. The fear of tumour spillage, previously reported in adult cancers, was a brake for its development but neuroblastoma offered a field of investigation as fragmentation of these lesions is unavoidable in many cases in open surgery and does not seem to impair prognosis. The advantages of MIS in many aspects of the supportive care requested by cancer patients (gastrostomy, fertility preservation techniques) also contributed to the introduction of this approach in the landscape of paediatric oncology. The spectrum of malignancies included now is larger including liver, pancreatic, and germ cell tumours but the series are small in number and difficult to analyse. The recent introduction of nephroblastoma as a potential indication, with strict criteria of inclusion, of MIS is certainly reflecting the favourable experience generally acquired with minimally invasive approaches in paediatric oncology [1, 2, 5, 7, 9–12]. A meta-analysis of randomized trials and controlled clinical trials conducted to ascertain the differences in outcome between MIS and open approach with respect to the overall and event-free survival could not retrieve any eligible study [23]. In 2002 an attempt to build such a study failed due to lack of patient recruitment, lack of surgical expertise with MIS procedures within surgical teams, and preconceived surgeon bias towards MIS or open surgery [24]. Since then, however, the feasibility and accuracy of minimally invasive approach for diagnostic and therapeutic purposes in paediatric oncological patients have been widely reported [6, 16, 21, 22]. Appropriate patient selection, detailed evaluation of surgical risk factors, and conformity to oncological principles have led to nearly 100% of diagnostic accuracy [6] and more than 90% of completeness of resection [20, 39, 40, 64], regardless of the size of the mass [35, 41, 44], with conversion rates ranging from less than 5% in thoracoscopic procedures to 10–20% in laparoscopic operations, both improving over time [5, 6, 16, 26, 41, 96, 97]. Conversion is mainly required in case of poor visibility and/or complications. These percentages are slightly higher than those reported in patients with non-malignant conditions [98]. Surgical complication rates for abdominal tumour surgery in general are reported to be as high as 30% [99]. Although biased by patient selection, no statistically significant difference has emerged in complication (ranging from 10 to 30%) or relapse rate in the examined series [16].

Fuchs has recently pointed out the following specific challenges in MIS of paediatric solid tumours: (1) Small working space in large tumours; (2) Risk of tumour spillage; (3) Tactile restriction; (4) Retrieval of large tumours; (5) Management of tumours with vascular encasement; (6) Learning curve. These principles should be kept in mind especially if the minimally invasive surgeon is not routinely committed to oncological surgery. Limited tactile feedback, limited visualization of the borders between tumour and unaffected tissue, or intraoperative detection of radiologically unexpected vessel infiltration should prompt the surgeon to convert to open approach, thus limiting the possibility of leaving residual tumour or damaging healthy organs with subsequent worse outcome [16, 100, 101].

Little is known about the impact of MIS and carbon dioxide pneumoperitoneum on tumour growth or biology [102–104]. However, after being used for a relevant time with respective follow-up, clinical experiences did not highlight relevant differences in outcome compared to open surgical procedures [16]. Similarly, other authors found no evidence of recurrence or port-site metastasis after resection of adrenal neuroblastoma and various other tumours [2, 7, 30, 96].

Future directions are being already explored in the paediatric field and include 3D minimally invasive surgery, single incision surgery, navigation, and robotic surgery. 3D MIS offers advantages in visualization and spatial orientation [105]. The single incision MIS, providing excellent cosmetic result, seems to have good indications in tumour biopsies [106, 107]. The endoscopic navigation, fluorescent imaging, and other localization techniques do improve the identification of tumours or metastases [108, 109].

19.7 Robotic Surgery

As happened to traditional MIS, also the idea of applying robotic surgery (RS) to paediatric oncological patients was subsequent to the progressive acceptance of the same in adult cancer. Cumby et al. [22] recently reviewed the available series reported in the literature concerning robot-assisted solid tumour resection procedures in children identifying at least 40 eligible procedures [110–129]. With a maximum diameter ranging from 1 to 11 cm, two thirds of tumours were located in the abdomen/pelvis, whereas the remaining involved the thoracic and cervical compartments. Of note, less than 15% of children were younger than teenage years at the time of surgery. Overall conversion rate was 12.5%, mainly due to anatomical difficulties and/or to guarantee an appropriate management of intra-operative complications (10%).

Clear and demonstrated advantages of RS over conventional MIS include restoration of organic faculties enjoyed by open surgery, such as three-dimensional vision and highly redundant manual dexterity [22]. These technical advancements allow a finer tumour manipulation and dissection, greatly facilitate intra-corporeal suturing, and, lastly, offer obvious ergonomic benefits for the surgeon, which might be able to undertake cases that would not be approachable with conventional MIS [110–114, 118, 119, 122, 124–127, 129]. Moreover, Nakib et al. demonstrated that lower pneumoperitoneum insufflation pressures may be required compared to conventional laparoscopy if using the distal instrument shaft to mechanically elevate the abdominal wall directly over the operative site [126].

On the other hand, the lack of haptic feedback is frequently cited as a primary technical disadvantage [110, 111, 114, 119], although maybe partially compensated by 3D magnified vision and surgeon's experience [114, 119, 126]. Learning curve for paediatric surgeons may be speeded up by a teamwork together with a more experienced adult robot-assisted surgical oncologist acting as a proctor [110, 118]. Another limiting factor for younger patients is the unavailability of appropriately sized paediatric instrumentation, causing frequent robot arm conflicts due to extremely narrow distance between port-site [110]. Lastly, RS is currently expensive and savings from reduced length of hospital stay with current low case volume in the paediatric field do not seem to compensate the costs [118, 130–132].

19.8 Robotic Adrenalectomy for Neuroblastoma

Surgical treatment of localized cancer is nowadays shifting the world widely from open to MIS approach with evidence-based benefits in terms of hospitalization and possibility to promptly resume chemotherapy and/or radiotherapy. Oncological criteria and risk factors should be clearly evaluated when planning surgery [133] as these may contraindicate a MIS approach.

Preoperative CT scan or MR imaging is mandatory in order to carefully evaluate risk factors. Vascular or organ involvement/encasement should be pointed out and therefore lead the surgeon to choose the safest procedure to carry out.

Encasement of major vascular structures is the most troublesome feature as the so-called Image-Defined Risk Factors (IDRFs) [134]. Recent studies by Mattioli and Irtan showed that vascular encasement did represent a contraindication to complete MIS resection, whereas open surgery seemed to be the approach of choice [35, 39].

Regarding Robotic Surgery (RS) of neuroblastoma few studies were reported in literature.

In the recent review of Meehan and Cundy in the last 10 years were reported less than ten neuroblastoma resected with robotic approach, without data regarding IDRFs or tumour margins and long-term follow-up [22, 135].

19.8.1 Technique

A good preparation of the patient, a reliable central venous line, and intra-operative stability are mandatory to avoid serious sequelae in case of complications. For the transperitoneal approach of perinephric area in children the patient usually lies in a supine or lateral decubitus [136]. Strategic ports positioning is of utmost importance. 8.5 mm scope, two (10 or 5 mm) operative ports for the surgeon, and at least a third operative access managed by the assistant are absolutely necessary for an optimal tissue exposition and manipulation.

Exposition of the mass is usually gained by gentle dissection of the peritoneal bowel attachments towards the posterior peritoneal space. As in open surgery, the chance to remove a tumour highly depends on a correct vascular display and vascular security [137]. Vascular dissection is usually commenced in the disease-free tissues surrounding the tumour. Major abdominal tumours are progressively exposed by blunt dissection to define the proximal and distal vascular supply to the mass.

Once the vascular supply to the mass is identified, the Bipolar Maryland forceps® is usually employed in order to avoid thermal injuries to contiguous structures.

In case of bleeding, it can be controlled by employing a grasping instrument to secure the vessel and consequently apply a stay suture, using bipolar forceps or Valleylab® LigaSure™ vessel sealing system introduced by the assistant in the third operative port.

In such an event, we would not recommend the use of metal clips, as it may result extremely difficult to manipulate tissue or to perform further tissue dissection once a clip has been positioned because of the risk of slippage and electricity conduction.

Monopolar coagulation applied to scissors or hook dissection is generally not employed, in order to reduce the risk of bleeding and to increase the possibility to correctly identify tissue limits. Coagulation devices are of little use in case of biopsies, unless a single vessel is clearly identified. Therefore, a stay suture is usually prepared in order to control parenchymal bleeding. However, before applying any suture, a few minutes pad compression with a gauze or pad is performed on the site of bleeding.

Whenever resection is preoperatively planned, a progressive dissection in a disease-free plane is carried on. Once all the vascular supplies are identified and properly divided, the mass is gently placed in a plastic endo-bag and consequently retrieved through one of the ports or, if necessary, through an accessory mini-umbilical laparotomy.

It is well known that robotic surgery allows better visualization of the tissues, reveals more anatomical details thanks to image magnification and 3D visualization, and can guarantee effective bleeding control with multiple devices (endoclips, bipolar forceps). Combined with the fact that many children affected by cancer are likely to undergo multiple surgical procedures, as MIS, RS theoretically allows for minimal inflammation, fewer adhesions, decreased pain, and quicker resumption to normal activities, facilitating subsequent initiation of chemotherapy and delayed surgery or further surgical procedures.

On the other hand, limitations of RS include the inability to palpate tissue to identify deep or central lesions.

In conclusion, as far as oncological criteria are respected in terms of SRFs and risk of tumour spreading, RS can represent the mean to obtain an accurate complete resection.

Further prospective studies are needed to confirm equivalent oncological outcomes in patients treated with a robotic approach.

RS provided a better visualization and more precision than conventional laparoscopy; then in future the limit represented by the presence of IDRFs can be exceeded.

Conclusions

MIS, regardless of the different techniques—thoracoscopy, laparoscopy, retroperitoneoscopy, robot-assisted—is increasingly being used as a surgical approach in children with cancer and will certainly have a definitive place in the future in this field. Unfortunately, although case control studies have shown its non-inferiority to open approach, neither randomized clinical trials nor worldwide-accepted guidelines to date have clearly demonstrated its routine applicability. The decision whether to use MIS or not is therefore generally demanded for an interdisciplinary panel and a meticulous patient selection. The clinical variety among these patients, among different pathological entities, and among different stages of the same entity is probably precluding short-term comparative studies. Efforts from the various surgical panels should be addressed to formulating guidelines for MIS in paediatric solid tumours within specific protocols. An expertise in MIS and surgical oncology is essential for operating surgeons and treating centres to guarantee acceptable treatment outcomes. RS—with its already-mentioned advantages in terms of restoration of organic functions enjoyed by open surgery compared to conventional MIS—has been cautiously introduced in the field of paediatric oncological surgery, showing good versatility for thoracic and abdominal tumour surgery and complications as well as conversion rates in line with data from open and conventional MIS literature [22]. It seems therefore reasonable, in the absence of relevant contraindications and/or worse outcome reported for treated patient, to encourage further experiences with RS, progressively adopting and configuring technical achievements from adult to paediatric oncological surgery.

References

1. Holcomb GW 3rd, Tomita SS, Haase GM, et al. Minimally invasive surgery in children with cancer. Cancer. 1995;76:121–8.
2. Spurbeck WW, Davidoff AM, Lobe TE, Rao BN, Schropp KP, Shochat SJ. Minimally invasive surgery in pediatric cancer patients. Ann Surg Oncol. 2004;11:340–3.
3. Sailhammer E, Jackson CC, Vogel AM, et al. Minimally invasive surgery for pediatric solid neoplasms. Am Surg. 2003;69:566–8.
4. Holcomb GW 3rd. Minimally invasive surgery for solid tumors. Semin Surg Oncol. 1999;16:184–92.
5. Warmann S, Fuchs J, Jesch NK, Schrappe M, Ure BM. A prospective study of minimally invasive techniques in pediatric surgical oncology: preliminary report. Med Pediatr Oncol. 2003;40:155–7.
6. Metzelder ML, Kuebler JF, Shimotakahara A, Glueer S, Grigull L, Ure BM. Role of diagnostic and ablative minimally invasive surgery for pediatric malignancies. Cancer. 2007;109(11):2343–8.
7. Iwanaka T, Arai M, Kawashima H, et al. Endosurgical procedures for pediatric solid tumors. Pediatr Surg Int. 2004;20:39–42.
8. Smith TJ, Rothenberg SS, Brooks M, et al. Thoracoscopic surgery in childhood cancer. J Pediatr Hematol Oncol. 2002;24:429–35.
9. Saenz NC, Conlon KC, Aronson DC, LaQuaglia MP. The application of minimal access procedures in infants, children, and young adults with pediatric malignancies. J Laparoendosc Adv Surg Tech A. 1997;7:289–94.
10. Sandoval C, Strom K, Stringel G. Laparoscopy in the management of pediatric intraabdominal tumors. J Soc Laparoendosc Surg. 2004;8:115–8.
11. Silecchia G, Silecchia G, Fantini A, et al. Management of abdominal lymphoproliferative diseases in the era of laparoscopy. Am J Surg. 1999;177:325–30.
12. Waldhausen JH, Tapper D, Sawin RS. Minimally invasive surgery and clinical decision-making for pediatric malignancy. Surg Endosc. 2000;14:250–3.
13. Cecchetto G, Riccipetitoni G, Inserra A, et al. Minimally invasive surgery in paediatric oncology: proposal of recommendations. Pediatr Med Chir. 2010;32(5):197–201.
14. Malkan AD, Loh AH, Sandoval JA. Minimally invasive surgery in the management of abdominal tumors in children. J Pediatr Surg. 2014;49(7):1171–6.
15. Varlet F, Petit T, Leclair MD, et al. Laparoscopic treatment of renal cancer in children: a multicentric study and review of oncologic and surgical complications. J Pediatr Urol. 2014;10(3):500–5.
16. Fuchs J. The role of minimally invasive surgery in pediatric solid tumors. Pediatr Surg Int. 2015;31(3):213–28. doi:10.1007/s00383-015-3660-9.
17. Malkan AD, Loh AH, Fernandez-Pineda I, Sandoval JA. The role of thoracoscopic surgery in pediatric oncology. J Laparoendosc Adv Surg Tech A. 2014;24(11):819–26.
18. Guye E, Lardy H, Piolat C, et al. Thoracoscopy and solid tumors in children: a multicenter study. J Laparoendosc Adv Surg Tech A. 2007;17(6):825–9.
19. Petty JK, Bensard DD, Partrick DA, Hendrickson RJ, Albano EA, Karrer FM. Resection of neurogenic

tumors in children: is thoracoscopy superior to thoracotomy? J Am Coll Surg. 2006;203(5):699–703.
20. Fraga JC, Rothenberg S, Kiely E, Pierro A. Video-assisted thoracic surgery resection for pediatric mediastinal neurogenic tumors. J Pediatr Surg. 2012;47(7):1349–53.
21. Peycelon M, Audry G, Irtan S. Minimally invasive surgery in childhood cancer: a challenging future. Eur J Pediatr Surg. 2014;24:443–9.
22. Cundy TP, Marcus HJ, Clark J, Hughes-Hallett A, Mayer EK, Najmaldin AS, Yang GZ, Darzi A. Robot-assisted minimally invasive surgery for pediatric solid tumors: a systematic review of feasibility and current status. Eur J Pediatr Surg. 2014;24:127–35.
23. van Dalen EC, de Lijster MS, Leijssen LGJ, Michiels EMC, Kremer LCM, Caron HN, Aronson DC. Minimally invasive surgery versus open surgery for the treatment of solid abdominal and thoracic neoplasms in children (review). Cochrane Database Syst Rev. 2015;1:CD008403.
24. Ehrlich PF, Newman KD, Haase GM, Lobe TE, Wiener ES, Holcomb GW. Lessons learned from a failed multi-institutional randomized controlled study. J Pediatr Surg. 2002;37(3):431–6.
25. Shamberger RC. Cooperative group trials in pediatric oncology: the surgeon's role. J Pediatr Surg. 2013;48(1):1–13.
26. Cribbs RK, Wulkan ML, Heiss KF, Gow KW. Minimally invasive surgery and childhood cancer. Surg Oncol. 2007;16(3):221–8.
27. Barmparas G, Branco BC, Schnüriger B, Lam L, Inaba K, Demetriades D. The incidence and risk factors of post-laparotomy adhesive small bowel obstruction. J Gastrointest Surg. 2010;14(10):1619–28.
28. Malek MM, Mollen KP, Kane TD, Shah SR, Irwin C. Thoracic neuroblastoma: a retrospective review of our institutional experience with comparison of the thoracoscopic and open approaches to resection. J Pediatr Surg. 2010;45(8):1622–6.
29. Kim T, Kim DY, Cho MJ, Kim SC, Seo JJ, Kim IK. Use of laparoscopic surgical resection for pediatric malignant solid tumors: a case series. Surg Endosc. 2011;25(5):1484–8.
30. Metzelder M, Ure B. Port-site metastasis after laparoscopic biopsy of a posttransplant Burkitt lymphoma in a child. Eur J Pediatr Surg. 2009;19(2):126–7.
31. Hayes-Jordan AA, Daw NC, Furman WL, Hoffer FA, Shochat SJ. Tumor recurrence at thoracostomy tube insertion sites: a report of two pediatric cases. J Pediatr Surg. 2004;39(10):1565–7.
32. Bhatnagar S, Sarin YK. Scope and limitations of minimal invasive surgery in practice of pediatric surgical oncology. Indian J Med Paediatr Oncol. 2010;31(4):137–42.
33. International Pediatric Endosurgery Group. IPEG guidelines for the surgical treatment of adrenal masses in children. J Laparoendosc Adv Surg Tech A. 2010;20(2):vii–x. doi:10.1089/lap.2010.9999.
34. Heloury Y, Muthucumaru M, Panabokke G, Cheng W, Kimber C, Leclair MD. Minimally invasive adrenalectomy in children. J Pediatr Surg. 2012;47(2):415–21.
35. Mattioli G, Avanzini S, Pini Prato A, Pio L, Granata C, Garaventa A, Conte M, Manzitti C, Montobbio G, Buffa P. Laparoscopic resection of adrenal neuroblastoma without image-defined risk factors: a prospective study on 21 consecutive pediatric patients. Pediatr Surg Int. 2014;30(4):387–94.
36. Theilen TM, Paran TS, Rutigliano D, Wexler L, Sonoda Y, LaQuaglia MP. Experience with retroperitoneoscopy in pediatric surgical oncology. Surg Endosc. 2011;25(8):2748–55.
37. Cohn SL, Pearson AD, London WB, Monclair T, Ambros PF, Brodeur GM, Faldum A, Hero B, Iehara T, Machin D, Mosseri V, Simon T, Garaventa A, Castel V, Matthay KK, INRG Task Force. The International Neuroblastoma risk group (INRG) classification system: an INRG Task Force report. J Clin Oncol. 2009;27(2):289–97.
38. Monclair T, Brodeur GM, Ambros PF, et al. The International Neuroblastoma risk group (INRG) staging system: an INRG Task Force report. J Clin Oncol. 2009;27(2):298–303.
39. Irtan S, Brisse HJ, Minard-Colin V, Schleiermacher G, Canale S, Sarnacki S. Minimally invasive surgery of neuroblastic tumors in children: indications depend on anatomical location and image-defined risk factors. Pediatr Blood Cancer. 2015;62(2):257–61.
40. Iwanaka T, Kawashima H, Uchida H. The laparoscopic approach of neuroblastoma. Semin Pediatr Surg. 2007;16(4):259–65.
41. Kelleher CM, Smithson L, Nguyen LL, et al. Clinical outcomes in children with adrenal neuroblastoma undergoing open versus laparoscopic adrenalectomy. J Pediatr Surg. 2013;48(8):1727–32.
42. Lopes RI, Denes FT, Bissoli J, Mendonca BB, Srougi M. Laparoscopic adrenalectomy in children. J Pediatr Urol. 2012;8(4):379–85.
43. Nuchtern JG, London WB, Barnewolt CE, et al. A prospective study of expectant observation as primary therapy for neuroblastoma in young infants: a Children's oncology group study. Ann Surg. 2012;256(4):573–80.
44. Cheng SP, Saunders BD, Gauger PG, Doherty GM. Laparoscopic partial adrenalectomy for bilateral pheochromocytomas. Ann Surg Oncol. 2008;15(9):2506–8.
45. Hubertus J, Boxberger N, Redlich A, von Schweinitz D, Vorwerk P. Surgical aspects in the treatment of adrenocortical carcinomas in children: data of the GPOH-MET 97 trial. Klin Padiatr. 2012;224(3):143–7.
46. Miller BS, Ammori JB, Gauger PG, Broome JT, Hammer GD, Doherty GM. Laparoscopic resection is inappropriate in patients with known or suspected adrenocortical carcinoma. World J Surg. 2010;34(6):1380–5.
47. Soheilipour F, Pazouki A, Ghorbanpour S, Tamannaie Z. Laparoscopic adrenalectomy for pheochromocytoma in a child. APSP J Case Rep. 2013;4(1):2.
48. Al-Shanafey S, Habib Z. Feasibility and safety of laparoscopic adrenalectomy in children: special emphasis on neoplastic lesions. J Laparoendosc Adv Surg Tech A. 2008;18(2):306–9.

49. Fuchs J, Kienecker K, Furtwangler R, et al. Surgical aspects in the treatment of patients with unilateral wilms tumor: a report from the SIOP 93-01/German Society of Pediatric Oncology and Hematology. Ann Surg. 2009;249(4):666–71.
50. Godzinski J, van Tinteren H, de Kracker J, et al. Nephroblastoma: does the decrease in tumor volume under preoperative chemotherapy predict the lymph nodes status at surgery? Pediatr Blood Cancer. 2011;57(7):1266–9.
51. Duarte RJ, Denes FT, Cristofani LM, Srougi M. Laparoscopic nephrectomy for Wilms' tumor. Expert Rev Anticancer Ther. 2009;9(6):753–61.
52. Varlet F, Stephan JL, Guye E, Allary R, Berger C, Lopez M. Laparoscopic radical nephrectomy for unilateral renal cancer in children. Surg Laparosc Endosc Percutan Tech. 2009;19(2):148–52.
53. Duarte RJ, Dénes FT, Cristofani LM, Odone-Filho V, Srougi M. Further experience with laparoscopic nephrectomy for Wilms' tumour after chemotherapy. BJU Int. 2006;98(1):155–9.
54. Ko EY, Ritchey ML. Current management of Wilms' tumor in children. J Pediatr Urol. 2009;5(1):56–65.
55. Chui CH, Lee AC. Peritoneal metastases after laparoscopic nephron-sparing surgery for localized Wilms tumor. J Pediatr Surg. 2011;46(3):e19–21.
56. Piche N, Barrieras D. Minimally invasive nephron-sparing surgery for unilateral Wilms tumor. J Pediatr Surg. 2012;47(7):E1–4.
57. Grabowski A, Korlacki W, Pasierbek M. Laparoscopy in elective and emergency management of ovarian pathology in children and adolescents. Wideochir Inne Tech Malo Inwazyjne. 2014;9(2):164–9.
58. Rescorla FJ. Pediatric germ cell tumors. Semin Pediatr Surg. 2012;21(1):51–60.
59. Mayer JP, Bettolli M, Kolberg-Schwerdt A, et al. Laparoscopic approach to ovarian mass in children and adolescents: already a standard in therapy. J Laparoendosc Adv Surg Tech A. 2009;19(Suppl 1):S111–5.
60. Pontarelli EM, Emami C, Nguyen NX, Torres M, Anselmo DM. Single-incision laparoscopic resection of ovarian masses in children: a preliminary report. Pediatr Surg Int. 2013;29(7):715–8.
61. Chabaud-Williamson M, Netchine I, Fasola S, et al. Ovarian-sparing surgery for ovarian teratoma in children. Pediatr Blood Cancer. 2011;57(3):429–34.
62. Sarnacki S. Ovarian tissue cryopreservation in children with cancer. Lancet Oncol. 2014;15(10): 1049–50.
63. Ehrlich PF, Teitelbaum DH, Hirschl RB, Rescorla F. Excision of large cystic ovarian tumors: combining minimal invasive surgery techniques and cancer surgery—the best of both worlds. J Pediatr Surg. 2007;42(5):890–3.
64. Irtan S, Orbach D, Helfre S, Sarnacki S. Ovarian transposition in prepubescent and adolescent girls with cancer. Lancet Oncol. 2013;14(13):e601–8.
65. Babayev SN, Arslan E, Kogan S, Moy F, Oktay K. Evaluation of ovarian and testicular tissue cryopreservation in children undergoing gonadotoxic therapies. J Assist Reprod Genet. 2013;30(1):3–9.
66. Dall'igna P, Cecchetto G, Bisogno G, et al. Pancreatic tumors in children and adolescents: the Italian TREP project experience. Pediatr Blood Cancer. 2010;54(5):675–80.
67. Ellerkamp V, Warmann SW, Vorwerk P, Leuschner I, Fuchs J. Exocrine pancreatic tumors in childhood in Germany. Pediatr Blood Cancer. 2011;58(3):366–71.
68. Fais PO, Carricaburu E, Sarnacki S, et al. Is laparoscopic management suitable for solid pseudo-papillary tumors of the pancreas? Pediatr Surg Int. 2009;25(7):617–21.
69. Sokolov YY, Stonogin SV, Donskoy DV, Povarnin OY, Vilesov AV. Laparoscopic pancreatic resections for solid pseudopapillary tumor in children. Eur J Pediatr Surg. 2009;19(6):399–401.
70. Uchida H, Goto C, Kishimoto H, et al. Laparoscopic spleen-preserving distal pancreatectomy for solid pseudopapillary tumor with conservation of splenic vessels in a child. J Pediatr Surg. 2010;45(7):1525–9.
71. Dutta S, Nehra D, Woo R, Cohen I. Laparoscopic resection of a benign liver tumor in a child. J Pediatr Surg. 2007;42(6):1141–5.
72. Yeung CK, Chowdhary SK, Chan KW, Lee KH, Till H. Atypical laparoscopic resection of a liver tumor in a 4-year-old girl. J Laparoendosc Adv Surg Tech A. 2006;16(3):325–7.
73. Abhijith SM, Nerli RB, Weiss D, Srinivasan A. Laparoscopic retroperitoneal lymph node dissection for paratesticular rhabdomyosarcoma in older children/adolescents. Indian J Surg Oncol. 2013;4(4):341–4.
74. Tomaszewski JJ, Sweeney DD, Kavoussi LR, Ost MC. Laparoscopic retroperitoneal lymph node dissection for high-risk pediatric patients with paratesticular rhabdomyosarcoma. J Endourol. 2010;24(1):31–4.
75. Bishay M, Giacomello L, Retrosi G, et al. Hypercapnia and acidosis during open and thoracoscopic repair of congenital diaphragmatic hernia and esophageal atresia: results of a pilot randomized controlled trial. Ann Surg. 2013;258(6): 895–900.
76. Lawal TA, Gosemann JH, Kuebler JF, Gluer S, Ure BM. Thoracoscopy versus thoracotomy improves midterm musculoskeletal status and cosmesis in infants and children. Ann Thorac Surg. 2009;87(1):224–8.
77. Schneider DT, Calaminus G, Reinhard H, et al. Primary mediastinal germ cell tumors in children and adolescents: results of the German cooperative protocols MAKEI 83/86, 89, and 96. J Clin Oncol. 2000;18(4):832–9.
78. Fuchs J, Seitz G, Ellerkamp V, et al. Analysis of sternotomy as treatment option for the resection of bilateral pulmonary metastases in pediatric solid tumors. Surg Oncol. 2008;17(4):323–30.
79. Kayton ML, Huvos AG, Casher J, et al. Computed tomographic scan of the chest underestimates the

number of metastatic lesions in osteosarcoma. J Pediatr Surg. 2006;41(1):200–6.
80. Burdine J, Joyce LD, Plunkett MB, Inampudi S, Kaye MG, Dunn DH. Feasibility and value of video-assisted thoracoscopic surgery wedge excision of small pulmonary nodules in patients with malignancy. Chest. 2002;122(4):1467–70.
81. Gow KW, Saad DF, Koontz C, Wulkan ML. Minimally invasive thoracoscopic ultrasound for localization of pulmonary nodules in children. J Pediatr Surg. 2008;43(12):2315–22.
82. Martin AE, Chen JY, Muratore CS, Mayo-Smith WW, Luks FI. Dual localization technique for thoracoscopic resection of lung lesions in children. J Laparoendosc Adv Surg Tech A. 2009;19(Suppl 1):S161–4.
83. Parida L, Fernandez-Pineda I, Uffman J, Davidoff AM, Gold R, Rao BN. Thoracoscopic resection of computed tomography-localized lung nodules in children. J Pediatr Surg. 2013;48(4):750–6.
84. Fuchs J, Seitz G, Handgretinger R, Schafer J, Warmann SW. Surgical treatment of lung metastases in patients with embryonal pediatric solid tumors: an update. Semin Pediatr Surg. 2012;21(1):79–87.
85. Castagnetti M, Delarue A, Gentet JC. Optimizing the surgical management of lung nodules in children with osteosarcoma: thoracoscopy for biopsies, thoracotomy for resections. Surg Endosc. 2004;18(11):1668–71.
86. Warmann SW, Furtwangler R, Blumenstock G, et al. Tumor biology influences the prognosis of nephroblastoma patients with primary pulmonary metastases: results from SIOP 93-01/GPOH and SIOP 2001/GPOH. Ann Surg. 2011;254(1):155–62.
87. Tronc F, Conter C, Marec-Berard P, et al. Prognostic factors and long-term results of pulmonary metastasectomy for pediatric histologies. Eur J Cardiothorac Surg. 2008;34(6):1240–6.
88. Metzelder ML, Schober T, Grigull L, et al. The role of laparoscopic techniques in children with suspected post-transplantation lymphoproliferative disorders. J Laparoendosc Adv Surg Tech A. 2011;21(8):767–70.
89. Shamberger RC, Holzman RS, Griscom NT, Tarbell NJ, Weinstein HJ. CT quantitation of tracheal cross-sectional area as a guide to the surgical and anesthetic management of children with anterior mediastinal masses. J Pediatr Surg. 1991;26(2):138–42.
90. Ang KL, Tan C, Hsin M, Goldstraw P. Intrapleural tumor dissemination after video-assisted thoracoscopic surgery metastasectomy. Ann Thorac Surg. 2003;75(5):1643–5.
91. Koizumi K, Haraguchi S, Mikami I, et al. Video-assisted thoracic surgery for Ewing's sarcoma of the mediastinum in a 3-year-old girl. Ann Thorac Cardiovasc Surg. 2005;11(2):117–20.
92. Gera PK, La Hei E, Cummins G, Harvey J. Thoracoscopy in chest wall Ewing's sarcoma. J Laparoendosc Adv Surg Tech A. 2006;16(5):509–12.
93. Chan KW, Lee KH, Tam YH, Yeung CK. Minimal invasive surgery in pediatric solid tumors. J Laparoendosc Adv Surg Tech A. 2007;17(6):817–20.
94. Sarnacki S. Ovarian tissue cryopreservation in children with cancer. Lancet Oncol. 2014;15(10):1049–50.
95. S I, Mascard E, Bolle S, Brugières L, Sarnacki S. The small bowel in its hammock: how to avoid irradiation thanks to the sigmoid. J Laparoendosc Adv Surg Tech A. 2015;25(1):77–80.
96. De Lagausie P, Berrebi D, Michon J, et al. Laparoscopic adrenal surgery for neuroblastomas in children. J Urol. 2003;170:932–5.
97. Leclair MD, de Lagausie P, Becmeur F, et al. Laparoscopic resection of abdominal neuroblastoma. Ann Surg Oncol. 2008;15(1):117–24.
98. St Peter SD, Valusek PA, Hill S, et al. Laparoscopic adrenalectomy in children: a multicenter experience. J Laparoendosc Adv Surg Tech A. 2011;21(7):647–9.
99. Ure BM, Bax NM, Zee v d. Laparoscopy in infants and children: a prospective study on feasibility and the impact on routine surgery. J Pediatr Surg. 2000;35:1170–3.
100. Günther P, Tröger J, Holland-Cunz S, et al. Surgical complications in abdominal tumor surgery in children. Experiences at a single oncological center. Eur J Pediatr Surg. 2009;19(5):297–303.
101. Cotton CA, Peterson S, Norkool PA, et al. Early and late mortality after diagnosis of wilms tumor. J Clin Oncol. 2009;27(8):1304–9.
102. Schmidt AI, Reismann M, Kubler JF, et al. Exposure to carbon dioxide and helium reduces in vitro proliferation of pediatric tumor cells. Pediatr Surg Int. 2006;22:72–7.
103. Metzelder M, Kuebler J, Shimotakahara A, Vieten G, von Wasielewski R, Ure BM. CO(2) pneumoperitoneum increases systemic but not local tumor spread after intraperitoneal murine neuroblastoma spillage in mice. Surg Endosc. 2008;22(12):2648–53.
104. Reismann M, Wehrmann F, Schukfeh N, Kuebler JF, Ure B, Gluer S. Carbon dioxide, hypoxia and low pH lead to overexpression of c-myc and HMGB-1 oncogenes in neuroblastoma cells. Eur J Pediatr Surg. 2009;19(4):224–7.
105. Zdichavsky M, Schmidt A, Luithle T, Manncke S, Fuchs J. Three-dimensional laparoscopy and thoracoscopy in children and adults: a prospective clinical trial. Minim Invasive Ther Allied Technol. 2015;27:1–7.
106. Lacher M, Kuebler JF, Yannam GR, et al. Single-incision pediatric endosurgery for ovarian pathology. J Laparoendosc Adv Surg Tech A. 2013;23(3):291–6.
107. Luithle T, Szavay P, Fuchs J. Single-incision laparoscopic nephroureterectomy in children of all age groups. J Pediatr Surg. 2013;48(5):1142–6.
108. Till H, Bergmann F, Metzger R, et al. Videoscopic fluorescence diagnosis of peritoneal and thoracic metastases from human hepatoblastoma in nude rats. Surg Endosc. 2005;19(11):1483–6.

109. Till H, Metzger R, Bergmann F, et al. Tumor model for laparoscopy in pediatric oncology: subperitoneal inoculation of human hepatoblastoma cells in nude rats. Eur J Pediatr Surg. 2006;16(4):231–4.
110. Urla C, Armeanu-Ebinger S, Fuchs J, Seitz G. Successful in vivo tumor visualization using fluorescence laparoscopy in a mouse model of disseminated alveolar rhabdomyosarcoma. Surg Endosc. 2015;29(5):1105–14.
111. Anderberg M, Backman T, Annerstedt M. Robot-assisted radical cystoprostatectomy in a small child with rhabdomyosarcoma: a case report. J Robot Surg. 2008;2:101–3.
112. Meehan JJ, Sandler A. Pediatric robotic surgery: a single-institutional review of the first 100 consecutive cases. Surg Endosc. 2008;22(1):177–82.
113. Meehan JJ, Sandler AD. Robotic resection of mediastinal masses in children. J Laparoendosc Adv Surg Tech A. 2008;18(1):114–9.
114. Akar ME, Leezer KH, Yalcinkaya TM. Robot-assisted laparoscopic management of a case with juvenile cystic adenomyoma. Fertil Steril. 2010;94(3):e55–6. author reply e57
115. Backes FJ, Seamon LG, Fowler JM. Robotic radical hysterectomy and pelvic lymphadenectomy for uterine rhabdomyosarcoma. J Robot Surg. 2008;2:197–200.
116. Camps JI. The use of robotics in pediatric surgery: my initial experience. Pediatr Surg Int. 2011;27(9):991–6.
117. Choy B, Gordetsky J, Varghese M, Lloyd GL, Wu G, Miyamoto H. Mixed epithelial and stromal tumor of the kidney in a 14-year-old boy. Urol Int. 2012;88(2):247–8.
118. Cost NG, Geller JI, WR DF Jr, Wagner LM, Noh PH. A robotic-assisted laparoscopic approach for pediatric renal cell carcinoma allows for both nephron-sparing surgery and extended lymph node dissection. J Pediatr Surg. 2012;47(10):1946–50.
119. Cost NG, DaJusta DG, Granberg CF, et al. Robot-assisted laparoscopic retroperitoneal lymph node dissection in an adolescent population. J Endourol. 2012;26(6):635–40.
120. DeUgarte DA, Teitelbaum D, Hirschl RB, Geiger JD. Robotic extirpation of complex massive esophageal leiomyoma. J Laparoendosc Adv Surg Tech A. 2008;18(2):286–9.
121. Dumitrascu T, Stanciulea O, Herlea V, Tomulescu V, Ionescu M. Central pancreatectomy for pancreatoblastoma in a 16-year-old girl. J Pediatr Surg. 2011;46(8):e17–21.
122. Gutt CN, Markus B, Kim ZG, Meininger D, Brinkmann L, Heller K. Early experiences of robotic surgery in children. Surg Endosc. 2002;16(7):1083–6.
123. Hassan M, Smith JM. Robotic assisted excision of a left ventricular myxoma. Interact Cardiovasc Thorac Surg. 2012;14(1):113–4.
124. Hsu SD, HS W, Kuo CL, Lee YT. Robotic-assisted laparoscopic resection of ectopic pancreas in the posterior wall of gastric high body: case report and review of the literature. World J Gastroenterol. 2005;11(48):7694–6.
125. Lee J, Kang SW, Jung JJ, et al. Multicenter study of robotic thyroidectomy: short-term postoperative outcomes and surgeon ergonomic considerations. Ann Surg Oncol. 2011;18(9):2538–47.
126. Lee KE, Koo H, Kim SJ, et al. Outcomes of 109 patients with papillary thyroid carcinoma who underwent robotic total thyroidectomy with central node dissection via the bilateral axillo-breast approach. Surgery. 2010;148(6):1207–13.
127. Nakib G, Calcaterra V, Scorletti F, et al. Robotic assisted surgery in pediatric gynecology: promising innovation in mini invasive surgical procedures. J Pediatr Adolesc Gynecol. 2013;26(1):e5–7.
128. Rogers CG, Blatt AM, Miles GE, Linehan WM, Pinto PA. Concurrent robotic partial adrenalectomy and extra-adrenal pheochromocytoma resection in a pediatric patient with von Hippel-Lindau disease. J Endourol. 2008;22(7):1501–3.
129. Park BJ, Flores RM, Rusch VW. Robotic assistance for video-assisted thoracic surgical lobectomy: technique and initial results. J Thorac Cardiovasc Surg. 2006;131(1):54–9.
130. St Julien J, Ball D, Schulick R. Robot-assisted cortical-sparing adrenalectomy in a patient with von Hippel-Lindau disease and bilateral pheochromocytomas separated by 9 years. J Laparoendosc Adv Surg Tech A. 2006;16(5):473–7.
131. Anderberg M, Kockum CC, Arnbjornsson E. Paediatric robotic surgery in clinical practice: a cost analysis. Eur J Pediatr Surg. 2009;19(5): 311–5.
132. Rowe CK, Pierce MW, Tecci KC, et al. A comparative direct cost analysis of pediatric urologic robot-assisted laparoscopic surgery versus open surgery: could robot-assisted surgery be less expensive? J Endourol. 2012;26(7):871–7.
133. Cecchetto G, Mosseri V, De Bernardi B, et al. Surgical risk factors in primary surgery for localized neuroblastoma: the LNESG1 study of the European International Society of Pediatric Oncology Neuroblastoma Group. J Clin Oncol. 2005;23(33):8483–9.
134. Monclair T, Brodeur GM, Ambros PF, et al. The International Neuroblastoma risk group (INRG) staging system: an INRG Task Force report. J Clin Oncol. 2009;27(2):298–303.
135. Meehan JJ. Robotic surgery for pediatric tumors. Cancer J. 2013;19(2):183–8.
136. Mattioli G, Avanzini S, Pio L, et al. Transperitoneal laparoscopic approach to the Perinephric area in children: technical report and lessons learned. J Laparoendosc Adv Surg Tech A. 2015;25(10):841–6.
137. Kiely E. Technique for excision of abdominal and pelvic neuroblastomas. Ann R Coll Surg Engl. 2007;89(4):342–8.

Pediatric Thoracic Robotic Surgery 20

John Meehan

The da Vinci surgical robot excels in many procedures inside the chest when compared to more traditional thoracoscopic procedures. The robotic articulations are particularly useful for navigating around difficult rigid anatomy such as mediastinal masses thereby. Areas that are difficult to reach with nonarticulating thoracoscopic instruments such as the foramen of Bochdalek are also more easily approached with the articulating arms of the robot. We anticipate that robotic surgery will eventually prove to be superior to the thoracoscopic approach but the current instrument selections and diameter are limiting our progress. However, we believe that robotic surgery will eventually prevail as technology improves.

20.1 Mediastinal Mass

There are several types of mediastinal masses in children. Masses are classified according to their location followed by characteristics. The type of mass includes both benign and malignant tumors as well as congenital anomalies. Identifying the location and radiographic characteristics of the mass will often lead to the most likely diagnosis. Congenital anomalies with cystic characteristics include bronchogenic cyst, lymphangioma, and esophageal duplication. Bronchogenic cysts are often located at the carina but occasionally found in other locations. Thoracic enteric duplications may be found along the esophagus. Patients may present with dysphagia, odynophagia, or reflux. Resection is usually straightforward for small enteric duplications but can become more complex if the duplication is long. In some cases, removal may require an esophageal segmentectomy. Primary closure of small defects is preferred but segmentectomy would require an end-to-end anastomosis. Rarely, a reversed gastric tube may be required in long segments which would need a combined abdominal and thoracic approach. Most esophageal duplications are resected via a thoracoscopic approach while a few carefully selected low lesions may be accessible from the abdomen.

Lymphangiomas are particularly challenging postoperatively due to their high propensity to leak chyle. Surgical treatment of thoracic lymphangiomas has been replaced by sclerotherapy for macrocystic lesions whenever possible. Newer modalities such as rapamycin are also being trialed and all treatment options should be discussed using a multidisciplinary approach [1]. Problematic lymphangiomas not amenable to sclerotherapy could be resected but all nonoperative avenues should be sought first.

As stated previously, mediastinal location and radiographic features often predict the cell line of a mediastinal mass. Classification begins with the determination of either an anterior or a

J. Meehan
Division of Pediatric Surgery, Seattle Children's Hospital, Seattle, WA 98105, USA
e-mail: john.meehan@seattlechildrens.org

G. Mattioli, P. Petralia (eds.), *Pediatric Robotic Surgery*, DOI 10.1007/978-3-319-41863-6_20

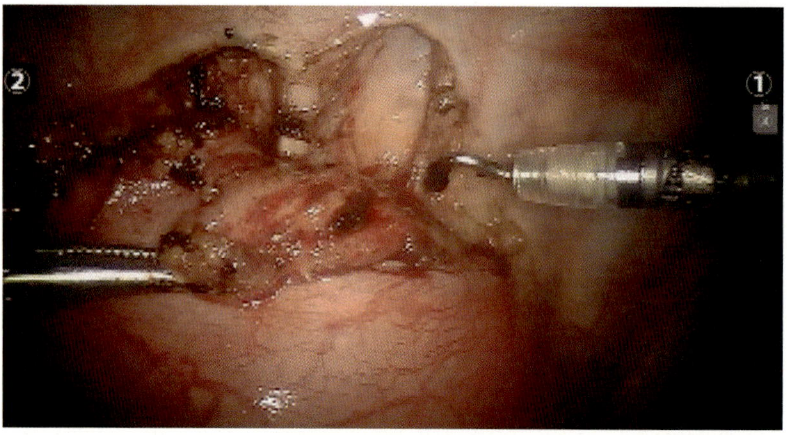

Fig. 20.1 Resection of a ganglioneuroma

posterior mass. The differential diagnosis for the posterior mass includes ganglioneuroma, ganglioneuroblastoma, and neuroblastoma which all arise from the sympathetic chain. If surgery is required, MIS had replaced open surgery for many of these masses but the location can be challenging for the nonarticulating instruments. The robot is our preferred method for resection. Some may cross the diaphragm which then requires a combined abdominal and thoracic approach. Alternatively, the diaphragm could be opened and then reapproximated following the resection.

Ganglioneuromas are slow-growing benign tumors (Fig. 20.1). Primary resection had been the only therapy required for these tumors although recent debate questions whether or not these even need resection. Location, size, and perceived difficulty may influence the decision on whether or not to proceed with resection. Neuroblastomas are malignant and can be quite large on initial presentation. Although small lesions may be amenable to a primary resection on initial presentation, biopsy followed by chemotherapy is almost always the best option, particularly for large lesions. Depending on tumor biology, resection remains the mainstay of therapy after adequate chemotherapy. Recent unpublished trends within the Children's Oncology Group (COG) suggest that subsequent resection may not always be required for low-grade or intermediate-grade lesions. The current recommendation on intermediate grade is a 50% or more resection based on tumor volume while low-grade lesions may be observed. We caution the reader that this is an ongoing investigation and details are still emerging. Finally, ganglioneuroblastomas carry an intermediate classification due to their occasional propensity to recur locally but require primary resection only.

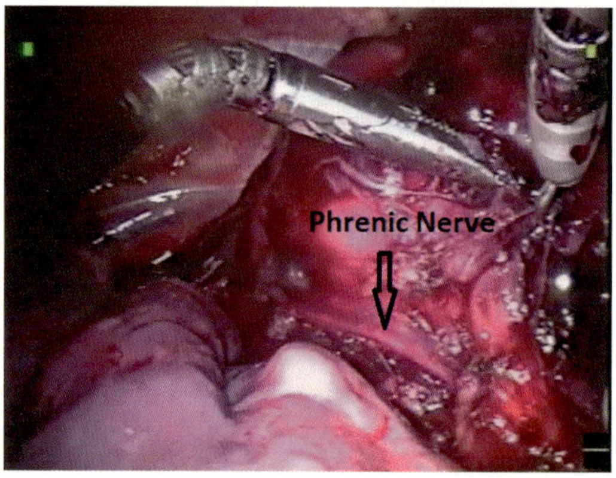

Fig. 20.2 A large germ cell tumor adherent to the pericardium. Note the proximity of the phrenic nerve (*arrow*)

Anterior mediastinal tumors include teratomas, germ cell tumors, and thymomas. The potential for a teratoma to be malignant can be predicted if the alpha fetoprotein (AFP) and beta human chorionic gonadotropin levels (beta-HCG) are elevated. Surveillance serum measurements of AFP and beta-HCG following resection are helpful to monitor for recurrence of malignant teratomas [2]. If the serum levels are normal at presentation, the teratoma is usually a benign mature teratoma. Thymic tumors include thymomas and germ cell tumors. Germ cell tumors may also have increased beta-HCG and AFP and can grow to an enormous size (Fig. 20.2).

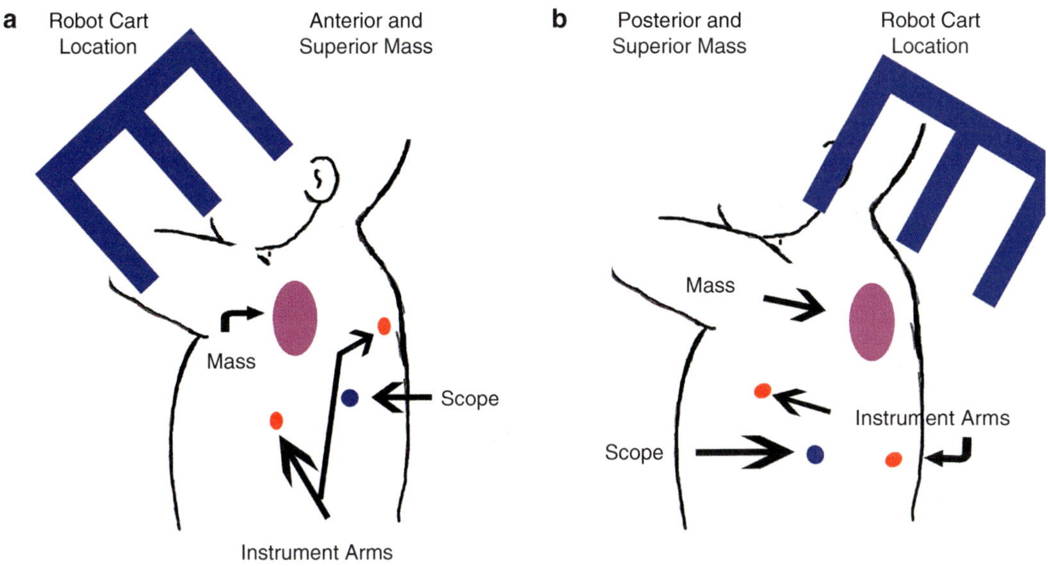

Fig. 20.3 Representative port locations and robot cart positioning for mediastinal masses; (**a**) anterior and superior mass, (**b**) posterior and superior mass

Robotic resection of a mediastinal mass begins with proper cart placement. The easiest way to remember how to plan robot cart placement is to place the cart in the general location of the mass. For example, if the mass is anterior and superior, the robot is placed anterior and superior to the patient. If the mass is posterior and inferior, the robot will be placed in a posterior and inferior location (Fig. 20.3). Port placement should take in the considerations we discussed in the introduction section on fundoplications, taking care to maintain the proper robot arm angles, and also paying close attention to port depth. Careful review of the anatomy is paramount to a safe resection. A mass that crosses the diaphragm may require a combined thoracic and abdominal approach. The real benefit of the robot is the articulations allowing the surgeon to reach intrathoracic locations that are challenging with standard thoracoscopic instrumentation. Resections robotically are subjectively much easier as the articulations allow the surgeon to navigate around the solid mass in a more precise fashion. We predict that robotic resection of all mediastinal masses will become the gold standard in the future due to the ease of the procedure, reduction in number of ports, and superior visualization.

20.2 Congenital Diaphragmatic Hernia: Bochdalek Hernia

The posterolateral Bochdalek CDH occurs due to the failure of the diaphragm to close properly in embryology. The defect is always posterior and lateral but the size of the defect can be quite variable. The resultant effect is compression of the ipsilateral lung during embryogenesis creating a number of physiological challenges. Besides the lack of oxygenation and ventilation due to a decrease in pulmonary tissue, the resultant pulmonary hypertension is often the most limiting factor in determining survivability. Pulmonary hypertension can develop within the first few hours of life resulting in significant cardiopulmonary compromise and rapid deterioration. Support often escalates rapidly to include high-frequency ventilation and nitric oxide. Extracorporeal membrane oxygenation (ECMO) may be a lifesaving bridge. Overall survival is 70.3–81.0% [3–5]. Timing of the surgical repair may need to be dictated by the patient's overall status. Some patients with either cardiopulmonary sensitivity or those with large defects requiring a patch may not be good candidates for the MIS approach. Stable patients with small- or medium-size defect could be considered for either thoracoscopic or robotic repairs.

The most posterolateral rim may have no diaphragm making it difficult to find adequate tissue to complete the repair. Adding to the challenge, this anatomic location is hard to reach with standard MIS instruments because of the difficult angles. Failure rates using standard thoracoscopic instrumentation have been alarmingly high in some series [6, 7]. The abdominal approach has the advantage that reaching the posterolateral aspect may be more technically feasible. However, these children have a small intra-abdominal compartment because of the lack of abdominal domain as the viscera developed inside the chest. Bringing the viscera back into the abdomen crowds the already small abdominal compartment reducing the available working space. For these reasons, most pediatric surgeons prefer the thoracic approach when using MIS.

Reports have demonstrated that robotic surgery is feasible for the Bochdalek CDH repair with low recurrence rates [8]. But not all steps of the Bochdalek CDH are ideal for the robot. Large sweeping movements, like the movements necessary to reduce the viscera, are not easily done with the robot. Therefore, we reduce the viscera with standard thoracoscopic 5 mm peanuts before docking the robot. Defects that are too large for a primary repair can be accomplished with patch closure. Patch material is brought in through a 5 mm trocar rolled up like a carpet. Once inside, it can be unrolled and sewn in place. In patients with a tight primary closure, patch material can be used as reinforcement sewing it directly over the repair.

The patient is placed in a lateral decubitus position. The robot cart is placed at the patient's feet, in a slight angle towards the patient's back

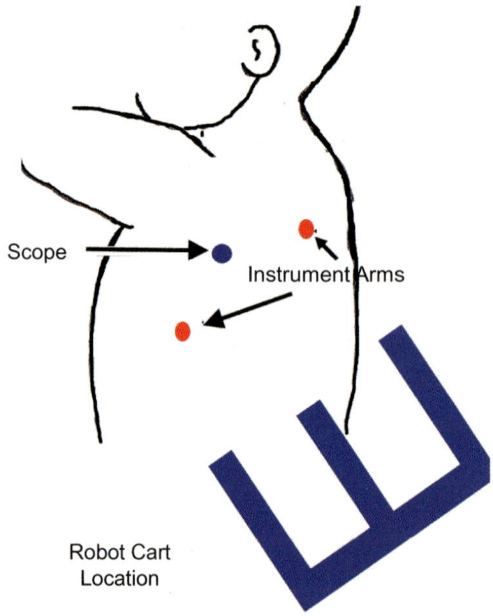

Fig. 20.4 Port placement for the neonatal Bochdalek CDH repair

(Fig. 20.4). For patient safety, it is important to place a protective solid barrier over the baby's head to prevent the robot arms from making inadvertent contact with the patient. We prefer a table-mounted laryngoscopy holder (Fig. 20.5).

Because the space in the chest of a neonate is so small, placement of the robotic ports must be carefully planned with a clear understanding of the arm movement limitations in the neonatal Bochdalek CDH. Withdrawing the port such that the remote center is just outside the chest gains critical robotic arm articulating length. The robotic ports are placed and the viscera is reduced with handheld laparoscopic peanuts and gentle traction (Fig. 20.6). After the viscera has been reduced, the robot is docked and robotic instruments are inserted. Begin by mobilizing the diaphragmatic edge of the defect as it fuses with the posterolateral chest wall with the hook cautery (Fig. 20.7). Once an adequate rim of tissue has been mobilized, primary closure can be attempted using nonabsorbable suture. We prefer to close the posterolateral aspect first and then proceed medially closing the defect using interrupted

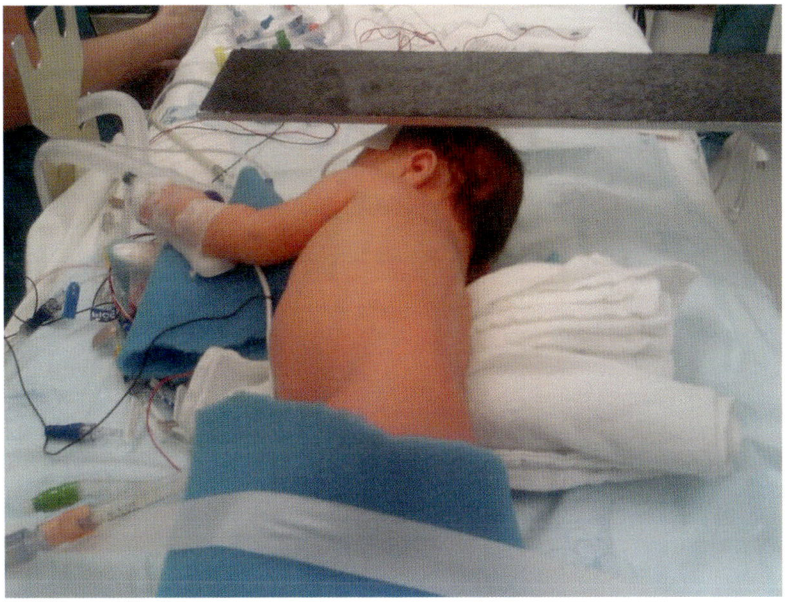

Fig. 20.5 A protective table-mounted barrier is positioned over the baby's head

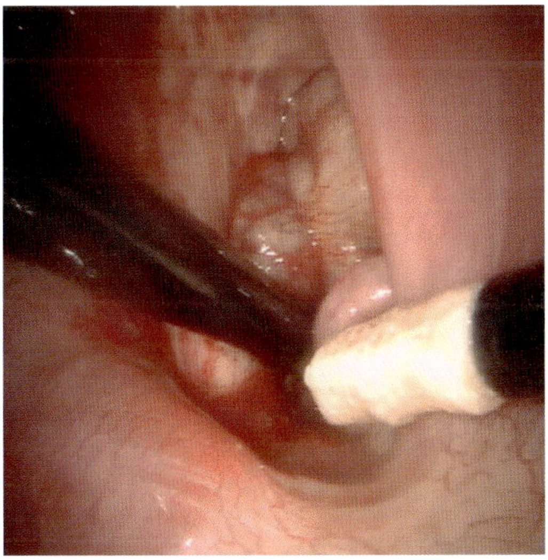

Fig. 20.6 Reduce the viscera with peanut dissectors in the neonatal CDH before the robot is docked. Using the robot for viscera reduction is not recommended

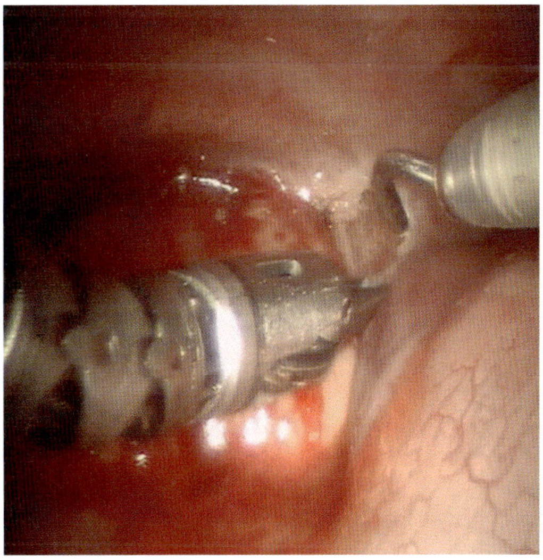

Fig. 20.7 Mobilizing lateral tissue to create a suitable rim for diaphragm repair

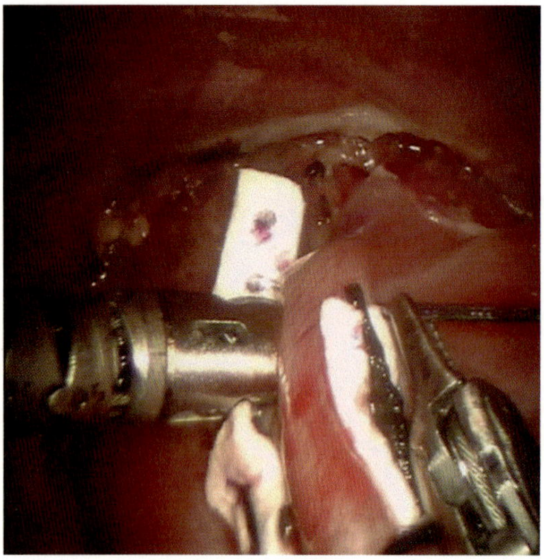

Fig. 20.8 Closure of the Bochdalek CDH using interrupted horizontal mattress sutures and pledgets

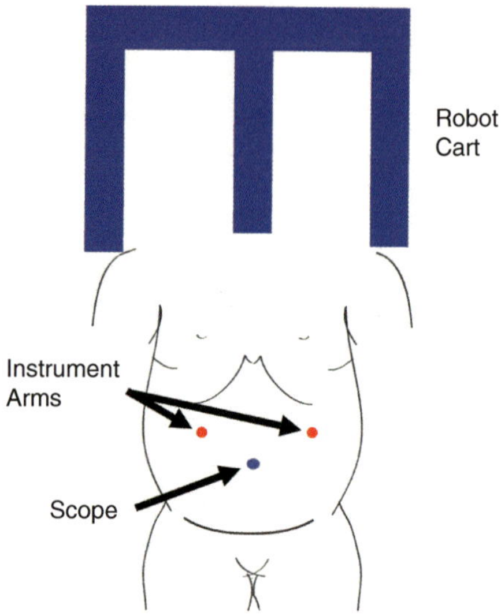

Fig. 20.9 Port placement for the Morgagni CDH repair

horizontal mattress sutures (Fig. 20.8). Pledgets help distribute the tension of the sutures on the diaphragm and may reduce tearing of the muscle. Patch closure, if necessary, is accomplished by suturing the lateral aspect first and proceeding medially. We do not leave a chest tube postoperatively.

20.3 Congenital Diaphragmatic Hernia: Morgagni Hernia

The Morgagni CDH is a fusion failure of the pleuroperitoneal surface of the diaphragm at the costo-sternal trigone. The defect is anterior and midline although it may be skewed slightly to the right. Repair is an abdominal procedure but we mention here for completeness. Unlike the Bochdalek CDH which often presents at birth with respiratory compromise, Morgagni CDH patients may go undiagnosed for many. Occasionally, the defect is found incidentally after a chest X-ray for unrelated issues. Most patients are asymptomatic although some will complain of mild substernal chest pain or indigestion. Rarely, a patient may present with a bowel obstruction from viscera trapped in the hernia. Because of its anterior location, the suturing angles needed to repair this defect using handheld laparoscopic instrumentation are challenging. The approach is from the abdomen and port placement is shown in Fig. 20.9. Typically, the camera port and two instrument ports are all that is required and there usually is no need for an accessory port. The visceral reduction is performed first (Fig. 20.10) followed by resection of the hernia sac if a sac is present. A rim of tissue on the anterior abdominal wall is mobilized with the hook cautery and repair is performed using

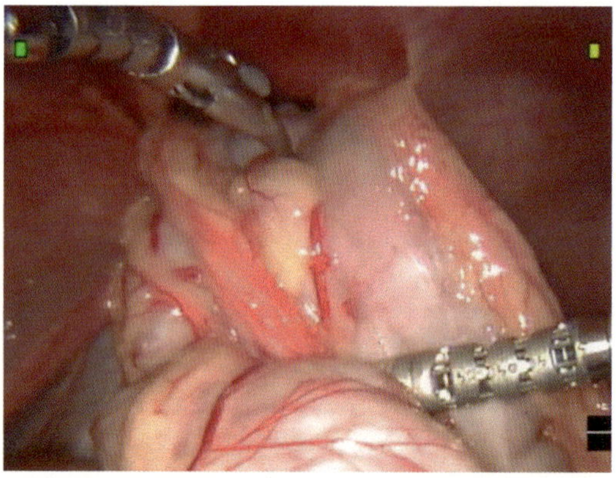

Fig. 20.10 Unlike the Bochdalek CDH, visceral reduction in the Morgagni CDH can be accomplished in the older patients with the robotic instruments

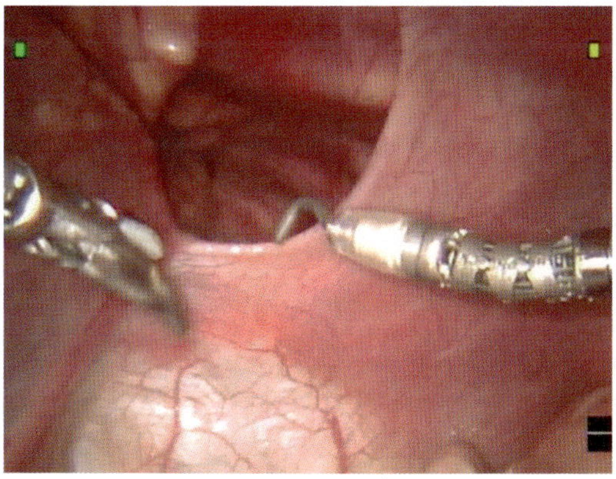

Fig. 20.11 The defect in some Morgagni hernia can be large. Mobilization of a rim of tissue on the anterior abdominal wall may facilitate closure

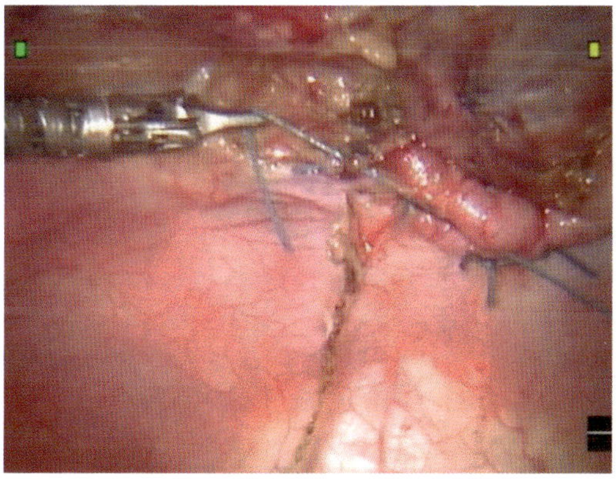

Fig. 20.12 Horizontal mattress sutures in the repair of the Morgagni CDH

pledgeted horizontal mattress sutures (Figs. 20.11 and 20.12). Primary repair is preferred although a patch closure may be required for larger defects.

20.4 Thymectomy

Myasthenia gravis (MG) is an autoimmune disorder where antibodies block muscle cells from receiving neurotransmitters from the nerve cell leading to weakness of the voluntary muscles. Patients present with fatigue, generalized weakness, facial paralysis, or breathing difficulties. The muscles around the eye may be affected early leading to the classic eye lid droop or double vision. The diagnosis is confirmed by nerve

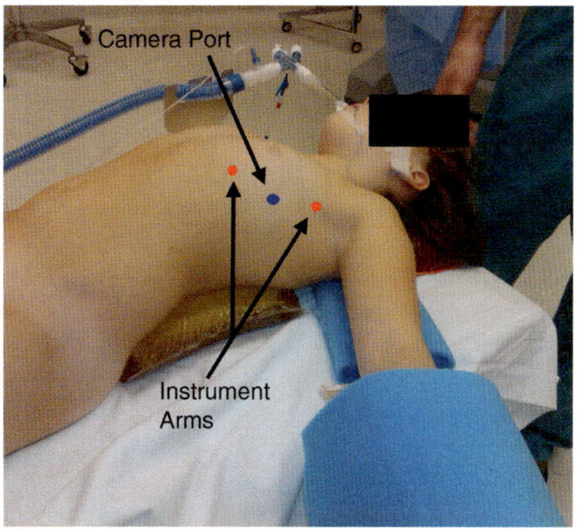

Fig. 20.13 Positioning and port placement for the robotic thymectomy. We prefer a left thoracic approach. The robot will come in over the patient's right shoulder

conduction studies and detection of acetylcholine receptor antibodies. Steroids are often prescribed to reduce the immune response while pyridostigmine is used to improve the communication between nerves and muscles. Exacerbations that lead to respiratory compromise may result in hospitalization. Thymectomy may alleviate symptoms in patients' refractory to medical management.

Thymectomy is ideally suited for the robotic approach. The thymus often extends beyond the mediastinum and up into the neck making the MIS approach with standard thoracoscopic instruments challenging. Preliminary studies comparing robotic thymectomy to alternative methods results are encouraging [9]. We perform this procedure exclusively using a left thoracic approach. A dual-lumen endotracheal tube will assist with lung isolation. The patient is placed in a supine position rolled slightly to the right with a small bump under the left scapula. The left arm is draped over the face and ports are placed as shown in Fig. 20.13. The entire procedure can be accomplished usually with only three ports utilizing a 30° scope. The scope is first placed in a downward orientation and the phrenic nerve is identified (Fig. 20.14). Resection is initiated using the hook electrocautery and progresses from the left chest into the right. A significant portion of the gland may extend up into the right neck (Fig. 20.15). These difficult areas are easily accessible from the left chest using the articulating robotic instruments. The camera may need to be switched to the 30° upward angle when dissecting in the neck. The thymus dissection will expose the innominate vein as the gland (Fig. 20.16). A complete resection is critical for the best chance for resolution of symptoms. A chest tube is usually not necessary. For precau-

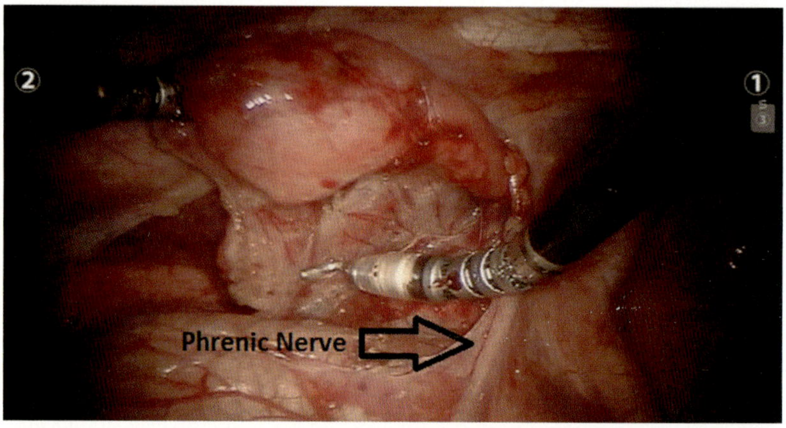

Fig. 20.14 Dissection in a robotic thymectomy. Note the phrenic nerve (*arrow*)

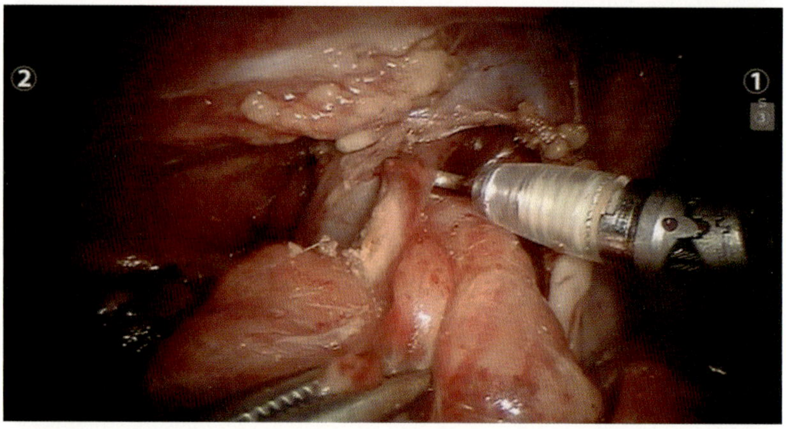

Fig. 20.15 The robotic articulating instruments facilitate dissecting the thymus from the superior mediastinum and the neck while approaching from the chest

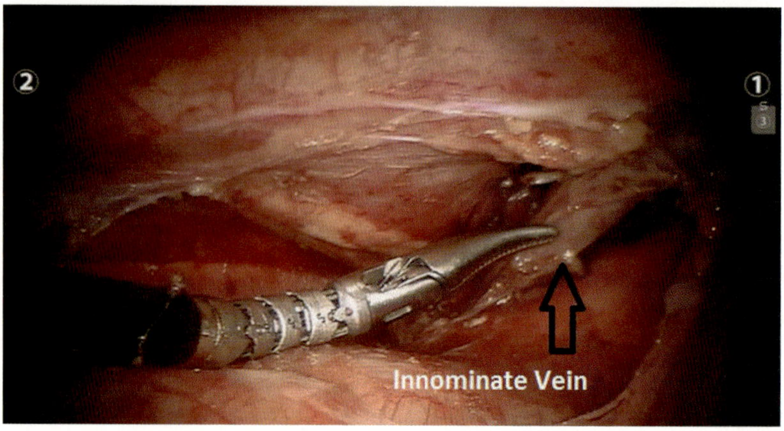

Fig. 20.16 Dissection of the thymus from around the innominate

tionary measures, we routinely admit all patients to the pediatric ICU because of their baseline weakness but have never had any postoperative respiratory issues and no one has required postoperative mechanical ventilation. Most patients are discharged in 24–48 h following surgery.

20.5 Esophageal Atresia with Tracheoesophageal Fistula

We commonly get asked about TEF repair and our brief experience with this treasured anomaly. Esophageal atresia with tracheoesophageal fistula (TEF) is one of the most fascinating anomalies encountered in pediatric surgery and absolute precision is required for the esophageal anastomosis in order to avoid leaks and structures. The first thoracoscopic TEF repair was reported in 1999 [10]. Several series have been reported but the procedure has not gained wide acceptance due to the technical challenges and less than optimal results. Initial stricture and leak rates for the thoracoscopic repair are relatively high [11]. Despite these shortcomings, MIS advantages include less pain, better cosmesis, and avoidance of the thoracotomy which may reduce the risk of scoliosis [12].

While we would like to see the robot eventually used for repair of the esophageal atresia and tracheoesophageal fistula, it will not likely become mainstream with the current robotic system simply because of the size of the instruments in relation to these newborns. The typical newborn with TEF is usually small and most weigh under 3 kg creating a significant size issue. Additionally, the robotic 8.5 mm scope may not fit between the ribs of some of these neonates. Finally, the amount of working space for the articulating robotic instruments is quite small. Simply put, this da Vinci robot is not the ideal device to be doing TEF repairs.

We did our first and only TEF repair in 2007 with a da Vinci standard system and used the two-dimensional 5 mm scope. Unfortunately, this scope is no longer supported. Moreover, the 5 mm 2-D scope was never adapted for the new Si system. It may be possible to perform the procedure with the 8.5 mm scope but the rib space will be very tight.

20.5.1 Pulmonary Resections

Lobectomies for pulmonary sequestration and congenital pulmonary adenomatoid formation (CPAM) are possible with the da Vinci robot and we first reported a small series nearly a decade ago. However, the key instrument for the MIS lobectomy is a thermal sealing device to seal the pulmonary parenchyma along the fissure. The da Vinci has a device called the tissue sealer which acts in a similar fashion but the company does not currently support or recommend its use in children for lobectomy. Until a thermal sealing alternative is cleared or pediatrics is available for robotics, we cannot support the use of the robot in pediatric pulmonary lobectomy.

References

1. Hammill AM, Wentzel M, Gupta A, Nelson S, Lucky A, Elluru R, Dasgupta R, Azizkhan RG, Adams DM. Sirolimus for the treatment of complicated vascular anomalies in children. Pediatr Blood Cancer. 2011;57(6):1018–24. doi:10.1002/pbc.23124.
2. Billmire DF, Grosfeld JL. Teratomas in childhood: analysis of 142 cases. J Pediatr Surg. 1986;21(6):548–51.
3. Ben-Ishay O, Johnson VM, Wilson JM, Buchmiller TL. Congenital diaphragmatic hernia associated with esophageal atresia: incidence, outcomes, and determinants of mortality. J Am Coll Surg. 2013;216(1):90–5.
4. Garriboli M, Duess JW, Ruttenstock E, Bishay M, Eaton S, De Coppi P, Puri P, Höllwarth ME, Pierro A. Trends in the treatment and outcome of congenital diaphragmatic hernia over the last decade. Pediatr Surg Int. 2012;28(12):1177–81.
5. Kimura O, Furukawa T, Higuchi K, Takeuchi Y, Fumino S, Aoi S, Tajiri T. Impact of our new protocol on the outcome of the neonates with congenital diaphragmatic hernia. Pediatr Surg Int. 2013;29:335–9.
6. Lansdale N, Alam S, Losty PD, Jesudason EC. Neonatal endosurgical congenital diaphragmatic hernia repair: a systematic review and meta-analysis. Ann Surg. 2010;252(1):20–6.
7. Arca MJ, Barnhart DC, Lelli JL Jr, Greenfeld J, Harmon CM, Hirschl RB, Teitelbaum DH. Early experience with minimally invasive repair of congenital

diaphragmatic hernias: results and lessons learned. J Pediatr Surg. 2003;38(11):1563–8. Review
8. Slater BJ, Meehan JJ. Robotic repair of congenital diaphragmatic anomalies. J Laparoendosc Adv Surg Tech A. 2009;19(s1):s123–7.
9. Hartwich J, Tyagi S, Margaron F, Oitcica C, Teasley J, Lanning D. Robot-assisted thoracoscopic thymectomy for treating myasthenia gravis in children. J Laparoendosc Adv Surg Tech A. 2012; 22(9):925–9.
10. Lobe TE, Rothenberg SS, Waldschmidt J, Stroeder L. Thoracoscopic repair of esophageal atresia in an infant. A surgical first. Pediatr Endosurg Innovative Tech. 1999;3:141–8.
11. Szavay PO, Zundel S, Blumenstock G, Kirschner HJ, Luithle T, Girisch M, Luenig H, Fuchs J. Perioperative outcome of patients with esophageal atresia and tracheo-esophageal fistula undergoing open versus thoracoscopic surgery. J Laparoendosc Adv Surg Tech A. 2011;21(5):439–43.
12. Sistonen SJ, Helenius I, Peltonen J, Sarna S, Rintala RJ, Pakarinen MP. Natural history of spinal anomalies and scoliosis associated with esophageal atresia. Pediatrics. 2009;124(6):e1198–204.

Printed by Printforce, the Netherlands